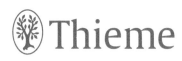

Video Atlas of Anterior Segment Repair and Reconstruction

Managing Challenges in Cornea, Glaucoma, and Lens Surgery

Amar Agarwal, MS, FRCS, FRCOphth
Chairman and Managing Director
Dr. Agarwal's Eye Hospital and Eye Research Centre
Chennai, Tamil Nadu, India

Priya Narang, MS
Director
Narang Eye Care and Laser Centre
Ahmedabad, Gujarat, India

732 illustrations

Thieme
New York • Stuttgart • Delhi • Rio de Janeiro

Library of Congress Cataloging-in-Publication Data
is available from the publisher.

Important note: Medicine is an ever-changing science undergoing continual development. Research and clinical experience are continually expanding our knowledge, in particular our knowledge of proper treatment and drug therapy. Insofar as this book mentions any dosage or application, readers may rest assured that the authors, editors, and publishers have made every effort to ensure that such references are in accordance with **the state of knowledge at the time of production of the book.**

Nevertheless, this does not involve, imply, or express any guarantee or responsibility on the part of the publishers in respect to any dosage instructions and forms of applications stated in the book. **Every user is requested to examine carefully** the manufacturers' leaflets accompanying each drug and to check, if necessary in consultation with a physician or specialist, whether the dosage schedules mentioned therein or the contraindications stated by the manufacturers differ from the statements made in the present book. Such examination is particularly important with drugs that are either rarely used or have been newly released on the market. Every dosage schedule or every form of application used is entirely at the user's own risk and responsibility. The authors and publishers request every user to report to the publishers any discrepancies or inaccuracies noticed. If errors in this work are found after publication, errata will be posted at www.thieme.com on the product description page.

Some of the product names, patents, and registered designs referred to in this book are in fact registered trademarks or proprietary names even though specific reference to this fact is not always made in the text. Therefore, the appearance of a name without designation as proprietary is not to be construed as a representation by the publisher that it is in the public domain.

©2020. Thieme. All rights reserved.

Thieme Medical Publishers New York
333 Seventh Avenue
New York, New York 10001 USA
+1 800 782 3488
customerservice@thieme.com

Thieme Publishers Stuttgart
Rüdigerstrasse 14, 70469 Stuttgart, Germany
+49 [0]711 8931 421, customerservice@thieme.de

Thieme Publishers Delhi
A-12, Second Floor, Sector-2, Noida-201301
Uttar Pradesh, India
+91 120 45 566 00, customerservice@thieme.in

Thieme Publishers Rio de Janeiro,
Thieme Publicações Ltda.
Edifício Rodolpho de Paoli, 25º andar
Av. Nilo Peçanha, 50 – Sala 2508,
Rio de Janeiro 20020-906 Brasil
+55 21 3172-2297

Cover design: Thieme Publishing Group
Typesetting by DiTech Process Solutions, India

Printed in USA by King Printing Company, Inc.   5 4 3 2 1

ISBN 978-1-68420-097-9

Also available as an e-book:
eISBN 978-1-68420-098-6

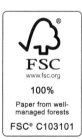

FSC
www.fsc.org
100%
Paper from well-managed forests
FSC® C103101

This book is dedicated to Dr. Kevin Miller who is a prolific surgeon, a wonderful human being, and a great friend.

Amar Agarwal and Priya Narang

Nothing in this world moves without Him. Writing this book was possible only because of His grace.

Amar Agarwal and Priya Narang

Contents

Dhivya Ashok Kumar, MD, FICO, FRCS, FAICO
Senior Consultant
Oculoplasty, Uvea, and Oncology Services
Dr. Agarwal's Group of Eye Hospitals and Eye
    Research Centre
Chennai, Tamil Nadu, India

Prafulla K. Maharana, MD
Assistant Professor
Department of Ophthalmology
Dr. Rajendra Prasad Centre for Ophthalmic Sciences
All India Institute of Medical Sciences
New Delhi, India

Ishani P. Majmudar
Medical Student
Honors Program in Medical Education
Northwestern University
Evanston, IL, USA

Parag A. Majmudar, MD
President and Chief Medical Officer
Chicago Cornea Consultants Ltd;
Associate Professor
Department of Ophthalmology
Rush University Medical Center
Chicago, IL, USA

Jodhbir S. Mehta, PhD, FRCOphth, FAMS, FRCS(Ed)
Head
Corneal and External Eye Disease Service;
Senior Consultant
Refractive Service
Singapore National Eye Centre;
Deputy Executive Director
Head
Tissue Engineering and Stem Cells Group
Singapore Eye Research Institute;
Deputy Vice Chair
Ophthalmology and Visual Sciences Academic Clinical
    Programme
SingHealth Duke-NUS Academic Medical Centre;
Professor
Duke-NUS Graduate Medical School;
Adjunct Professor
School of Material Science and Engineering
School of Mechanical and Aerospace Engineering
Nanyang Technological University;
Adjunct Professor
Department of Ophthalmology
Yong Loo Lin School of Medicine
National University of Singapore
Singapore, Singapore

Ritu Nagpal, MD
Research Officer
Department of Ophthalmology
Dr. Rajendra Prasad Centre for Ophthalmic Sciences
All India Institute of Medical Sciences
New Delhi, India

Priya Narang, MS
Director
Narang Eye Care and Laser Centre
Ahmedabad, Gujarat, India

Gregory S. H. Ogawa, MD
Partner
Eye Associates of New Mexico;
Assistant Clinical Professor
University of New Mexico School of Medicine
Albuquerque, NM, USA

Hon Shing Ong, FRCOphth, MSc, FRCS (Ed)
Associate Consultant
Corneal and External Diseases Department
Singapore National Eye Centre;
Stem Cells and Tissue Engineering Department
Singapore Eye Research Institute
Singapore, Singapore

Walter T. Parker, MD
Cornea, External Disease, Cataract, and Refractive Surgery
Alabama Ophthalmology Associates, P.C.
Birmingham, AL, USA

Pranita Sahay, MD
Senior Resident
Department of Ophthalmology
Dr. Rajendra Prasad Centre for Ophthalmic Sciences
All India Institute of Medical Sciences
New Delhi, India

Namrata Sharma, MD, DNB, MNAMS
Honorary General Secretary
All India Ophthalmological Society;
Professor
Cornea and Refractive Surgery Services
Dr. Rajendra Prasad Centre for Ophthalmic Sciences
All India Institute of Medical Sciences
New Delhi, India

Indu Singh, MS
Ophthalmic Consultant
Dr. Daljit Singh Eye Hospital
Amritsar, Punjab, India

Kiranjit Singh, MS
Ophthalmic Consultant
Dr. Daljit Singh Eye Hospital
Amritsar, Punjab, India

Ravijit Singh, MS
Ophthalmic Consultant
Dr. Daljit Singh Eye Hospital
Amritsar, Punjab, India

Michael E. Snyder, MD
Board of Clinical Directors
Cincinnati Eye Institute;
Chair
Clinical Research Steering Committee;
Associate Professor
Department of Ophthlamology
University of Cincinnati
Cincinnati, OH, USA

Sanjana Srivatsa, MS, FPRS
Fellow
Cornea and Refractive Services
Dr. Agarwal's Group of Eye Hospitals and Eye
    Research Centre
Chennai, Tamil Nadu, India

Claudia Perez Straziota, MD
Clinical Assistant Professor
Department of Ophthalmology
The Cleveland Clinic Cole Eye Institute
Cleveland, OH, USA

Sonal Tuli, MD
Professor and Chair
Department of Ophthalmology
University of Florida
Gainesville, FL, USA

Fasika A. Woreta, MD, MPH
Director
Eye Trauma Center;
Assistant Professor
Department of Ophthalmology
Residency Program Director
Wilmer Eye Institute
Johns Hopkins University School of Medicine
Baltimore, MD, USA

Shin Yamane, MD
Assistant Professor
Department of Ophthalmology
Yokohama City University Medical Center
Yokohama, Japan

Section I

Reconstructing the Cornea

1 Limbal Stem Cell Transplantation "Evolution and Techniques"

Ritu Nagpal, Prafulla K. Maharana, Pranita Sahay, Sreelakshmi P. Amar, Namrata Sharma

Summary

Stem cells are "pluripotent" cells which are capable of differentiating and proliferating into multiple lineages. Thus, they have an important role in reparative process. They are present in the cornea (limbus), conjunctiva, iris, ciliary body, trabecular meshwork, lens, retina, choroid, sclera, and the orbit. In some it has an established role as in limbal stem cell deficiency whereas in other further studies are still going on as in retinal diseases including age related macular degeneration, retinitis pigmentosa and Stargardt's disease, optic nerve disease, and glaucoma. Stem cells aims to provide a solution for diseases which have no cure at present and it will provide vision to such patients.

Keywords: Limbal stem cells, limbal stem cell deficiency, cultivated limbal epithelial transplantation, simple limbal epithelial transplantation

1.1 Introduction

Identification of limbal stem cells, their harvesting, expansion, and finally transplantation for the treatment of a wide variety of ocular surface pathologies has been a landmark innovation in the field of ophthalmology.

Limbal epithelial stem cells are basically a subpopulation of basal cells of the corneal epithelium with certain differences, as identified by nuclear labeling studies. Stem cells for the corneal epithelium have been seen to be preferentially located in a region called "limbus" and share common features with various types of other epithelial stem cells (palm, skin, hair, intestine) in terms of preferred location, pigment protection, and growth properties, all of which play an important role in maintaining their "stemness."[1] Stem cells located at all these sites exist as clusters in the basal region of their epithelium. Pigmentation and vascularity protect and nourish them and provide a specific microenvironment for their survival.[1] As evidenced by 3H-thymidine labeling, these cells are normally slow cyclers, but can be stimulated to proliferate in response to injury and various tumor promotors.[1] By a process of asymmetrical division, these cells give rise to a progeny of cells known as the transient amplifying cells (TAC). The TAC, unlike the stem cells, are capable of rapid division, but have limited potential to multiple. The TAC then finally divide to form a progeny of cells known as the terminally differentiated (TD) cells.[1] These properties of stem cells have been utilized by the researchers and clinicians, enabling them to culture these cells ex vivo and transplanting them to the affected site so that a small population of cells covers a much larger area of deficiency.

The corneal epithelium is a specialized structure with an exceptionally high regenerative capacity of basal cells and a turnover of 6 to 8 days. As per the Thoft's X, Y, Z hypothesis, the mass of corneal epithelium does not change under normal circumstances.[2] It is regulated by three separate, independent phenomena; the X component which is contributed by the proliferation of basal epithelial cells; the Y component, contributed by the centripetal movement of peripheral cells; and the Z component, representing epithelial cell loss from the surface. For normal homeostasis, the amount of cell loss must be balanced by the amount of cell formation; $X + Y = Z$.[2]

Limbus is a transition area between two different kinds of epithelial lineages; the conjunctiva and the corneal epithelium. It houses the stem cells for corneal epithelium located in specialized crypt-like structures known as the "palisades of Vogt."[3] These stem cells migrate centripetally and give rise to TAC, which reside in the basal layer of peripheral as well as the corneal epithelium. These cells become more mature as they migrate vertically into the suprabasal compartment of corneal epithelium to become TD cells.[4]

Limbal stem cell transplantation (LSCT) is currently the standard of care for treatment of eyes with limbal stem cell deficiency (LSCD). In eyes with unilateral involvement, the donor tissue is harvested from the unaffected fellow eye (autologous), while in patients with bilateral damage, the donor tissue is obtained from either a living related donor or from a cadaver (allogenic). The obvious advantage of using an autologous tissue over an allogenic tissue is the absence of immunological rejection, thereby avoiding the need for long-term systemic immunosuppression.[5,6] Harvesting of limbal tissue also carries a potential risk of induction of donor site complications such as conjunctivalization, perforation, filamentary keratitis, and scarring.[7,8,9,10,11,12,13,14,15,16] Various surgical techniques of LSCT have been evolved and modified from time and then to reduce these side effects and maximize the efficacy of procedure.

1.2 Evolution of Limbal Stem Cell Transplantation

Eduard Konrad Zirm, in 1905, performed the first full-thickness corneal transplant in a patient with bilateral severe lime burns.[17] The graft stayed clear for the initial postoperative period, but later on failed. The evolving patterns over a period of time have led to our current understanding that keratoplasty performed in eyes with ocular surface disease carries an extremely poor prognosis due to epithelial healing problems.

Maintenance of normal corneal epithelial homeostasis is an essential prerequisite for graft survival. Continuous renewal of epithelial cells is done by the stem cells, which as per our current understanding are located in the basal layer of limbal epithelium. The search for this location, however, began in late 1970s when conjunctiva was thought to be the source of renewal of corneal epithelium.

Shapiro et al, in their animal experiments, observed that following removal of the corneal epithelium, epithelial cells of conjunctival origin cover the exposed corneal surface followed by a morphologic transformation to normal-appearing corneal epithelium, about 4 to 5 weeks later.[18] This hypothesis was further supported by the observations that the conjunctival epithelium increases its mitotic rate in response to corneal epithelial injury.[19] Based on these findings, the concept of conjunctival transplantation[20] was proposed. For patients with bilateral ocular surface disease, keratoepithelioplasty[21] was considered as a modality of treatment. Both surgical techniques were based on the realization of the fact that either the peripheral cornea or conjunctiva is the source of corneal epithelial renewal.

This hypothesis was modified by the experiments of Lavker and Sun while they were working on epidermal stem cells.[22] The hypothesis that the epithelial stem cells are located in the limbal basal layer was finally given in 1986 by the findings of expression of 64K corneal keratin, which is a marker of advanced stage of corneal epithelial differentiation.[23] The 64K keratin was found to be expressed by all layers of corneal epithelium, while in the limbal epithelium, it was expressed only in the suprabasal layer suggesting that these cells are biochemically more primitive than the corneal basal cells. Conjunctival epithelium was found to be K3 negative suggesting that the conjunctiva and cornea are two distinct types of cell lineages.

Kenyon and Tseng,[24] who proposed the idea of limbal autografting, performed the first clinical translation of limbal location of epithelial stem cells in 1990, which was found to be much more effective than the conjunctival transplantation.[25] LSCT further went a revolutionary change when Pellegrini et al first reported the use of cultivated stem cells obtained from a 2 mm^2 limbal biopsy specimen.[26] This was a groundbreaking event as it reduced the size of limbal tissue to be harvested for transplantation. The technique was popularized as cultivated limbal epithelial transplantation (CLET). Sangwan et al further modified the technique from cultivating the stem cells in a laboratory to direct utilization of limbal biopsy for the expansion of stem cells.[27] This technique became popularly known as simple limbal epithelial transplantation (SLET).

1.3 Indications of Limbal Stem Cell Transplantation

LSCT is an established technique for ocular surface reconstruction in eyes with LSCD. This can occur either due to primary or secondary causes. The primary form is related to insufficient stromal microenvironment to support stem cell function. The causes include aniridia, congenital erythrokeratodermia, keratitis associated with multiple endocrine deficiencies, neurotrophic keratopathy, and chronic limbitis. The secondary causes are the more common form of insults and include various external factors which either acutely or chronically destroy the limbal stem cells. These include chemical or thermal injuries, ultraviolet and ionizing radiation, autoimmune disorders such as Stevens–Johnson syndrome, advanced ocular cicatricial pemphigoid, multiple surgeries, cryotherapy, chronic contact lens wear, and extensive/chronic microbial infections.[28,29,30,31]

1.4 Clinical Presentation and Diagnosis of Limbal Stem Cell Deficiency

Patients with LSCD present with complaints of reduced vision, photophobia, watering, blepharospasm, and recurrent episodes of pain due to epithelial breakdown. Slit lamp biomicroscopic findings at slit lamp examination may include a dull and irregular reflex of the corneal epithelium, absence of limbal palisades, presence of a thick fibrovascular pannus, and corneal scarring. Fluorescein staining shows abnormal pattern as the conjunctival epithelium is more permeable than the corneal epithelium.[32] The conjunctivalized corneal surface also shows a stippled late staining pattern as it is thinner and irregular compared to the adjacent normal corneal epithelium and therefore prone to recurrent erosions.[33,34] In eyes with partial stem cell deficiency, a demarcation line can be made out at the junction of corneal and conjunctival epithelium, where corneal epithelium can be seen extending into the conjunctivalized area via tiny "bud-like projections."[35,36]

The clinical diagnosis of LSCD is best confirmed by histologic findings of presence of goblet cell suggestive of conjunctival epithelium.[2,37] Immunohistochemically, the absence of keratin K3, which is a marker of corneal epithelial differentiation, suggests the presence of conjunctival epithelium.

1.5 Management of Limbal Stem Cell Deficiency

1.5.1 Preoperative Evaluation

A detailed preoperative evaluation is an important prerequisite before surgical planning in patients with LSCD. Severity of patient's symptoms, degree of conjunctivalization (total or partial), extent of symblepharon, amount of corneal scarring, and severity of corneal thinning should be noted prior to taking the patient for surgery. Anterior segment optical coherence tomography helps to assess the thickness of overlying fibrovascular pannus and the residual corneal stromal bed. Eyes with significant thinning of corneal stroma need additional lamellar or full-thickness keratoplasty along with stem cell transplantation (▶Video 1.1).

Asymptomatic patients with partial peripheral conjunctivalization of the corneal surface may not require any intervention. The corneal and conjunctival epithelial cell phenotypes have been known to coexist on the corneal surface without any significant extension of the conjunctivalized area or any transdifferentiation of conjunctival epithelium into cells of corneal phenotype.[33,34]

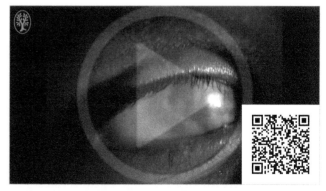

Video 1.1 Ocular surface disorders. https://www.thieme.de/de/q.htm?p=opn/tp/311890101/9781684200979_video_01_01&t=video

Patients with partial LSCD with involvement of visual axis and eyes with total LSCD need LSCT. The various surgical techniques for the transplantation of stem cells, their outcomes, complications, management, and modifications have been described as under, in the order of their evolution.

Conjunctival Transplantation

The technique involves transferring of conjunctival epithelial cells as a source of corneal epithelium. In eyes with unilateral ocular surface damage, conjunctival grafts are harvested from the uninjured fellow eye. Usually, four grafts are taken, one each from four quadrants, areas which are normally covered by the lids. Following removal of pannus tissue in the diseased eye, the grafts are transplanted with basal part anchored to the limbus using sutures while the apices are secured using a continuous suture, avoiding passage through corneal stroma. Conjunctival epithelial cells migrate from the grafts and cover the raw surface. The procedure helps by immediately halting the breakdown of ocular surface, thereby preventing further ulceration and scarring.[7]

Keratoepithelioplasty

This method was proposed as an alternative to conjunctivoplasty in patients with bilateral disease where healthy conjunctiva is not available. Keratoepithelioplatsy involves the use of donor lenticules consisting of corneal epithelium and with underlying stroma to serve as a carrier for corneal epithelium.[21] Four lenticules are placed equally around the corneoscleral limbus and sutured to the sclera with monofilament nylon sutures. The donor epithelium migrates centrally from the lenticules and covers the area of defect.

Conjunctival Limbal Autograft (CLAU) Transplantation

Limbal autografting procedure involves transfer of free limbal grafts from the uninjured donor eye to the recipient eye after pannus dissection. Two limbal grafts with adjacent conjunctiva are taken, each extending for about 4 clock hours circumferentially, measuring 3 × 10 mm. In a series of 26 patients reported by Kenyon and Tseng, epithelial outgrowths were seen to develop from the grafts within a period of 7 to 21 days in 22 eyes.[24] None of the eyes had infection, graft failure, or sloughing of the grafts. The success of procedure was attributed to the presence of limbal epithelium in the transplanted tissues.

The limbal donor eyes have been shown to be susceptible for developing LSCD.[36] Miri et al evaluated long-term changes at 50 donor sites, following limbal tissue harvesting for CLAU.[38] Limbal tissue of around 2 clock hours with 3 × 3 mm of adjacent conjunctiva was harvested both from superior as well as inferior quadrants. All donor sites showed re-epithelialization of the peripheral denuded limbus within 2 weeks. The re-epithelialized donor site was covered with conjunctival epithelium in 17 sites of 10 eyes and with corneal epithelium in 7 sites of 5 eyes. All cases had scarring at the donor site. Filamentary keratitis, negative staining with fluorescein, and subconjunctival hemorrhage were observed in the immediate postoperative period without any long-term consequences. None of the donor eye showed any signs of corneal epithelial instability or healing problems.

Most studies, wherein a total of 5 to 6 clock hours of limbus was removed, do not report long-term healing problems.[39,40,41,42] The use of amniotic membrane at the donor site has been suggested to reduce donor site complications in case larger amount of tissue is harvested.[43,44] The exact amount of donor limbus that can be safely removed is not known; however, it needs to be balanced against the proliferative potential of the limbal tissue.

Cultivated Limbal Epithelial Transplantation

CLET involves ex vivo cultivation of limbal epithelial stem cells rather than directly transplanting the limbal tissue. The technique has been shown to be as effective as direct limbal autografting with added advantages of requiring lesser amount of donor tissue and hence being a safer procedure for the donor eye.[3,24,26,45,46] The disadvantages include additional laboratory costs and theoretical risks associated with the use of xenobiotic materials for culture.[3,45,47] Ex vivo culture carries a risk of transfer of various infections both to the patient as well as to the laboratory personnel processing the tissue. For these reasons, consideration must be given to the screening of tissue donors and the risk of cross-contamination of cultures. All tissue donors should be screened for human immunodeficiency virus 1 and 2, human T-cell leukemia–lymphoma virus, hepatitis B and C, and syphilis. The techniques for the cultivation of stem cells can be broadly classified into two categories: explants and suspension culture technique.

The overall success rates of CLET, as reported in various studies, range between 50 and 100%.[1] The clinical outcomes based on the source of donor tissue (autologous or allogeneic), culture technique employed (explant or suspension), and the indication for surgery have been seen to be comparable.[3,45]

The surgical procedure is carried out in two phases: the first phase involves harvesting of limbal biopsy and in second phase, the cultivated stem cells are transplanted on the ocular surface.

Limbal Biopsy

Limbal biopsy is usually performed under peribulbar anesthesia. The conjunctiva is incised, starting 3 mm behind the limbus and dissection is carried out in the subconjunctival plane, taking care to avoid the underlying Tenon's capsule. The dissection is continued for about 1 mm into the clear cornea. Conjunctiva is then excised just behind the pigmented line (palisades of Vogt), and the dissected limbal tissue along with 1 mm of clear corneal tissue is excised. Both tissues are transported in tissue culture medium to the laboratory. Postoperatively, patients are prescribed topical antibiotics and corticosteroids in tapering doses.

In patients with bilateral ocular surface damage, limbal epithelial cells are obtained from cadaveric human corneas preserved under cold storage conditions in eye bank. The donor age should preferably be less than 40 years with less than 6-hour death enucleation time.

Suspension Culture Technique

Pellegrini et al first reported successful restoration of ocular surface using autologous corneal epithelial sheets generated by serial cultivation of limbal stem cells.[26] Epithelial cell cultures

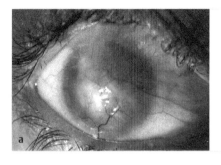
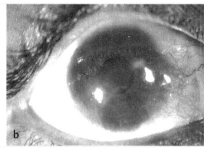

Fig. 1.4 Clinical photographs showing pre- (a) and postoperative appearance (b) of an eye with unilateral total LSCD. Patient underwent SLET and maintained a stable surface at 1-year follow-up. LSCD, limbal stem cell deficiency; SLET, simple limbal epithelial transplantation.

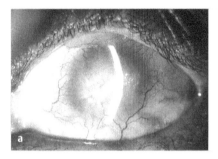
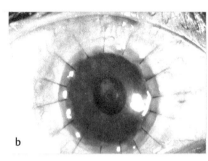

Fig. 1.5 Clinical photograph of the left eye (a) of a patient with total LSCD with central corneal scarring. (b) Postoperative photograph of the same eye showing a stable ocular surface following sequential limbal stem cell transplantation followed by deep anterior lamellar keratoplasty. LSCD, limbal stem cell deficiency.

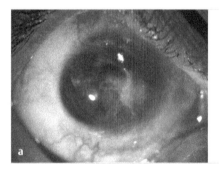
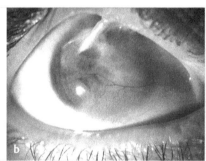

Fig. 1.6 Clinical photographs showing late postoperative complications in the form of recurrence of conjunctivalization (a) and focal symblepharon formation (b).

symblepharon at presentation, keratoplasty combined with SLET, and postoperative loss of explants.

Similar authors also studied the outcomes of SLET in eyes with prior failed CLET.[57] SLET was able to successfully restore a stable ocular surface in 80% eyes, at a mean follow-up of 2.3 years where CLET has previously failed once or twice. Overall, the technique was found to be more effective than repeat CLET across all age groups. None of the eye developed any donor site complication, even after undergoing multiple biopsies. Better outcomes with SLET were attributed to the transplantation of fresh unprocessed tissue without laboratory manipulation. Moreover, the size of the biopsy tissue, which is similar for both the surgical techniques in CLET, gets divided into two halves to be cultivated over two different culture plates, of which only one is used for transplantation while the other serves as a backup. Therefore, the effective number of limbal stem cells transplanted in SLET could be double than that of CLET.

Surgical Technique

A limbal-based peritomy is done after marking a 2 × 2 mm area over the superior limbus. The dissection is carried out in subconjunctival plane till the limbus, followed by a relatively shallow dissection extending for approximately 1 mm into the clear cornea. The limbal tissue was excised and placed in balanced salt solution.

The recipient bed is prepared before harvesting limbal biopsy. A 360° peritomy is done and performed followed by removal of vascular pannus. hAM graft is then secured over the ocular surface using fibrin glue with the edges well tucked underneath the surrounding conjunctiva. The limbal tissue is gently placed over the amniotic membrane using a nontraumatic forceps and divided into 8 to 10 pieces with the help of Vannas scissors. The tiny limbal explants are placed epithelial side up and distributed circumferentially in the midperipheral cornea avoiding visual axis. Fibrin glue is placed over the explants so as to adhere them well over the amniotic membrane. A soft bandage contact lens is placed and the eye is patched.[27]

Postoperatively topical antibiotics and corticosteroids are prescribed, which are gradually tapered. The bandage contact lens is removed once the epithelial defect heals.

Complications

Complications following SLET can occur either intraoperatively during pannus dissection and removal or in early or late postoperative period.

Intraoperative complications include corneal perforation while removal of fibrovascular pannus in eyes with extremely thinned and scarred cornea and damage to recti while removal of symblepharon. Early postoperative complications include loss of limbal explants due to displacement of bandage contact lens, occurrence of hemorrhage beneath the amniotic membrane, displacement of amniotic membrane, and sterile or infective keratitis causing corneal melting and perforation. Eyes receiving allogenic stem cell transplantation should be monitored for signs and symptoms of postoperative graft rejection. Delayed postoperative complications include recurrence of symblepharon formation and conjunctivalization of corneal surface.

Allogenic SLET

Allogenic SLET is a viable treatment option for the treatment of bilateral LSCD.[58] The limbal biopsy can be harvested either from living related donors or from cadaveric donors. Living donors are preferable for obtaining biopsy as the limbal cells obtained from cadavers have been shown to have a lower in vitro proliferative potential[59] and poorer in vivo corneal epithelialization rate.

Graft rejection is an important postoperative concern in these eyes due to the allogenic nature of the tissue and needs to be differentiated from recurrence of LSCD. It is important to the two entities as graft rejection promptly reverses with systemic immunosuppression, while the second entity requires repeat surgery. Failure of distinction between these entities can result in either a patient with acute allograft rejection receiving a second graft, which is bound to fail, or a patient with recurrence of LSCD being unnecessarily immunosuppressed.

Allograft rejection is usually suspected based on the acuteness of symptoms, presence of circumciliary congestion, engorged and tortuous perilimbal vessels with fine vascular ingrowths specifically directed towards the limbal grafts along with absence of generalized conjunctivalization, or large epithelial defects. These findings promptly reverse following administration of pulse intravenous and intensive topical steroids.[31,42,58]

Keratoplasty after SLET

Keratoplasty after Keratoplasty, either lamellar or full-thickness, has been performed with favorable outcomes once successful restoration of ocular surface is achieved following LSCT. Singh et al reported the outcomes of DALK following autologous SLET in 11 pediatric eyes (age < 16 years) with unilateral severe chemical injury.[60] Nine out of 11 eyes (81.82%) attained a stable ocular surface, while 2 eyes had failure of SLET requiring a repeat procedure. Gupta et al reported early results of PK following SLET in seven eyes with unilateral ocular surface burns.[61] The mean duration between SLET and PK was 9 months. SLET was successful in all seven eyes with six eyes maintaining a clear graft at a mean follow-up of 15 months.

Minor Ipsilateral Simple Limbal Epithelial Transplantation (mini-SLET)

mini-SLET is a novel technique, first described in 2015 for the management of eyes with pterygium, where conjunctival autograft cannot be performed. It involves the use of an AMG to cover the bare sclera area combined with a small autologous simple limbal epithelial transplant (mini-SLET) to provide stem cells at the limbal area.[62] The concept was based on the realization of the fact that pterygium involves localized LSCD or dysfunction.[63,64]

The surgical technique involves excision of pterygium along with underlying Tenon's capsule. The area of bare sclera measured is covered with AMG, measuring around 1 mm larger than the size of defect. The edges of the AMG are tucked under the margins of surrounding conjunctiva and fixed with fibrin glue. A 2 × 2 mm limbal biopsy is harvested from the ipsilateral eye, cut into 8 to 10 pieces using Vannas scissors and distributed along the conjunctival side of the limbus over the AMG. These limbal explants are glued, covered with a second small-sized amniotic membrane, which is applied as an overlaid graft. A soft bandage contact lens is then placed over the ocular surface. Topical antibiotics and corticosteroids are prescribed postoperatively.

Hernández-Bogantes et al performed mini-SLET in 10 eyes with pterygium with favorable results.[62] At 8 months follow-up, none of the patients had recurrence of fibrovascular growth. One patient developed pyogenic granuloma at the junction of amniotic membrane and conjunctiva, which resolved after stepping up of corticosteroids.

References

[1] Cotsarelis G, Cheng SZ, Dong G, Sun TT, Lavker RM. Existence of slow-cycling limbal epithelial basal cells that can be preferentially stimulated to proliferate: implications on epithelial stem cells. Cell 1989; 57(2):201–209

[2] Thoft RA, Friend J. The X, Y, Z hypothesis of corneal epithelial maintenance. Invest Ophthalmol Vis Sci 1983; 24(10):1442–1443

[3] Shortt AJ, Secker GA, Notara MD, et al. Transplantation of ex vivo cultured limbal epithelial stem cells: a review of techniques and clinical results. Surv Ophthalmol 2007; 52(5):483–502

[4] Taylor G, Lehrer MS, Jensen PJ, Sun TT, Lavker RM. Involvement of follicular stem cells in forming not only the follicle but also the epidermis. Cell 2000; 102(4):451–461

[5] Burman S, Sangwan V. Cultivated limbal stem cell transplantation for ocular surface reconstruction. Clin Ophthalmol 2008; 2(3):489–502

[6] Transplantation of ex vivo cultured limbal epithelial stem cells: a review of techniques and clinical results. PubMed—NCBI [online]. https://www.ncbi.nlm.nih.gov/pubmed/17719371. Accessed August 31, 2018

[7] Di Iorio E, Ferrari S, Fasolo A, Böhm E, Ponzin D, Barbaro V. Techniques for culture and assessment of limbal stem cell grafts. Ocul Surf 2010; 8(3):146–153

[8] Nakamura T, Inatomi T, Sotozono C, et al. Transplantation of autologous serum-derived cultivated corneal epithelial equivalents for the treatment of severe ocular surface disease. Ophthalmology 2006; 113(10):1765–1772

[9] Shimazaki J, Higa K, Morito F, et al. Factors influencing outcomes in cultivated limbal epithelial transplantation for chronic cicatricial ocular surface disorders. Am J Ophthalmol 2007; 143(6):945–953

[10] Di Girolamo N, Bosch M, Zamora K, Coroneo MT, Wakefield D, Watson SL. A contact lens-based technique for expansion and transplantation of autologous epithelial progenitors for ocular surface reconstruction. Transplantation 2009; 87(10):1571–1578

[11] Kolli S, Ahmad S, Lako M, Figueiredo F. Successful clinical implementation of corneal epithelial stem cell therapy for treatment of unilateral limbal stem cell deficiency. Stem Cells 2010; 28(3):597–610

[12] Gene expression profile of epithelial cells and mesenchymal cells derived from limbal explant culture [online]. https://www.ncbi.nlm.nih.gov/pmc/articles/PMC2903463/. Accessed August 31, 2018

[13] The use of human serum in supporting the in vitro and in vivo proliferation of human conjunctival epithelial cells. PubMed—NCBI [online]. https://www.ncbi.nlm.nih.gov/pubmed/15923513. Accessed August 31, 2018

[14] Mariappan I, Maddileti S, Savy S, et al. In vitro culture and expansion of human limbal epithelial cells. Nat Protoc 2010; 5(8):1470–1479

[15] Fatima A, Sangwan VS, Iftekhar G, et al. Technique of cultivating limbal derived corneal epithelium on human amniotic membrane for clinical transplantation. J Postgrad Med 2006; 52(4):257–261

[16] Sangwan VS, Vemuganti GK, Iftekhar G, Bansal AK, Rao GN. Use of autologous cultured limbal and conjunctival epithelium in a patient with severe bilateral ocular surface disease induced by acid injury: a case report of unique application. Cornea 2003; 22(5):478–481

[17] Zirm EK. Eine erfolgreiche totale Keratoplastik (A successful total keratoplasty). 1906. Refract Corneal Surg 1989; 5(4):258–261

[18] Shapiro MS, Friend J, Thoft RA. Corneal re-epithelialization from the conjunctiva. Invest Ophthalmol Vis Sci 1981; 21(1 Pt 1):135–142

[19] Danjo S, Friend J, Thoft RA. Conjunctival epithelium in healing of corneal epithelial wounds. Invest Ophthalmol Vis Sci 1987; 28(9):1445–1449

[20] Thoft RA. Conjunctival transplantation as an alternative to keratoplasty. Ophthalmology 1979; 86(6):1084–1092

[21] Thoft RA. Keratoepithelioplasty. Am J Ophthalmol 1984; 97(1):1–6

[22] Lavker RM, Sun TT. Epidermal stem cells. J Invest Dermatol 1983; 81(1, Suppl): 121s–127s

[23] Schermer A, Galvin S, Sun TT. Differentiation-related expression of a major 64K corneal keratin in vivo and in culture suggests limbal location of corneal epithelial stem cells. J Cell Biol 1986; 103(1):49–62

[24] Kenyon KR, Tseng SC. Limbal autograft transplantation for ocular surface disorders. Ophthalmology 1989; 96(5):709–722, discussion 722–723

[25] Tsai RJ, Sun TT, Tseng SC. Comparison of limbal and conjunctival autograft transplantation in corneal surface reconstruction in rabbits. Ophthalmology 1990; 97(4):446–455

[26] Pellegrini G, Traverso CE, Franzi aT, Zingirian M, Cancedda R, De Luca M. Long-term restoration of damaged corneal surfaces with autologous cultivated corneal epithelium. Lancet 1997; 349(9057):990–993

[27] Sangwan VS, Basu S, McNeil S, Balasubramanian D. Simple limbal epithelial transplantation (SLET): a novel surgical technique for the treatment of unilateral limbal stem cell deficiency. Br J Ophthalmol 2012; 96(7):931–934

[28] Holland EJ, Schwartz GS. Iatrogenic limbal stem cell deficiency. Trans Am Ophthalmol Soc 1997; 95:95–107, discussion 107–110

[29] Joseph A, Raj D, Shanmuganathan V, Powell RJ, Dua HS. Tacrolimus immunosuppression in high-risk corneal grafts. Br J Ophthalmol 2007; 91(1):51–55

[30] Sloper CM, Powell RJ, Dua HS. Tacrolimus (FK506) in the management of high-risk corneal and limbal grafts. Ophthalmology 2001; 108(10):1838–1844

[31] Tsai RJ, Tseng SC. Human allograft limbal transplantation for corneal surface reconstruction. Cornea 1994; 13(5):389–400

[32] Huang AJ, Tseng SC. Corneal epithelial wound healing in the absence of limbal epithelium. Invest Ophthalmol Vis Sci 1991; 32(1):96–105

[33] Coster DJ, Aggarwal RK, Williams KA. Surgical management of ocular surface disorders using conjunctival and stem cell allografts. Br J Ophthalmol 1995; 79(11):977–982

[34] Dua HS, Gomes JA, Singh A. Corneal epithelial wound healing. Br J Ophthalmol 1994; 78(5):401–408

[35] Dua HS, Forrester JV. The corneoscleral limbus in human corneal epithelial wound healing. Am J Ophthalmol 1990; 110(6):646–656

[36] Chen JJ, Tseng SC. Corneal epithelial wound healing in partial limbal deficiency. Invest Ophthalmol Vis Sci 1990; 31(7):1301–1314

[37] Tseng SC. Concept and application of limbal stem cells. Eye (Lond) 1989; 3(Pt 2): 141–157

[38] Miri A, Said DG, Dua HS. Donor site complications in autolimbal and living-related allolimbal transplantation. Ophthalmology 2011; 118(7):1265–1271

[39] Dua HS, Azuara-Blanco A. Autologous limbal transplantation in patients with unilateral corneal stem cell deficiency. Br J Ophthalmol 2000; 84(3):273–278

[40] Wylegała E, Tarnawska D, Wróblewska EM. [Limbal stem cell transplantation from HLA-compatible living donors. Long term observation] Klin Oczna 2003; 105(6):378–383

[41] Ivekovic R, Tedeschi-Reiner E, Novak-Laus K, Andrijevic-Derk B, Cima I, Mandic Z. Limbal graft and/or amniotic membrane transplantation in the treatment of ocular burns. Ophthalmologica 2005; 219(5):297–302

[42] Rao SK, Rajagopal R, Sitalakshmi G, Padmanabhan P. Limbal allografting from related live donors for corneal surface reconstruction. Ophthalmology 1999; 106(4):822–828

[43] Han ES, Wee WR, Lee JH, Kim MK. The long-term safety of donor eye for 180 degrees limbal transplantation. Graefes Arch Clin Exp Ophthalmol 2007; 245(5):745–748

[44] Meallet MA, Espana EM, Grueterich M, Ti S-E, Goto E, Tseng SCG. Amniotic membrane transplantation with conjunctival limbal autograft for total limbal stem cell deficiency. Ophthalmology 2003; 110(8):1585–1592

[45] Baylis O, Figueiredo F, Henein C, Lako M, Ahmad S. 13 years of cultured limbal epithelial cell therapy: a review of the outcomes. J Cell Biochem 2011; 112(4):993–1002

[46] Tan DT, Ficker LA, Buckley RJ. Limbal transplantation. Ophthalmology 1996; 103(1):29–36

[47] Schwab IR, Johnson NT, Harkin DG. Inherent risks associated with manufacture of bioengineered ocular surface tissue. Arch Ophthalmol 1960 2006; 124(12):1734–1740

[48] Sangwan VS, Basu S, Vemuganti GK, et al. Clinical outcomes of xeno-free autologous cultivated limbal epithelial transplantation: a 10-year study. Br J Ophthalmol 2011; 95(11):1525–1529

[49] Shortt AJ, Secker GA, Rajan MS, et al. Ex vivo expansion and transplantation of limbal epithelial stem cells. Ophthalmology 2008; 115(11):1989–1997

[50] Inatomi T, Nakamura T, Koizumi N, Sotozono C, Yokoi N, Kinoshita S. Midterm results on ocular surface reconstruction using cultivated autologous oral mucosal epithelial transplantation. Am J Ophthalmol 2006; 141(2):267–275

[51] Basu S, Mohamed A, Chaurasia S, Sejpal K, Vemuganti GK, Sangwan VS. Clinical outcomes of penetrating keratoplasty after autologous cultivated limbal epithelial transplantation for ocular surface burns. Am J Ophthalmol 2011; 152(6):917–924.e1

[52] Rama P, Matuska S, Paganoni G, Spinelli A, De Luca M, Pellegrini G. Limbal stem-cell therapy and long-term corneal regeneration. N Engl J Med 2010; 363(2):147–155

[53] Marchini G, Pedrotti E, Pedrotti M, et al. Long-term effectiveness of autologous cultured limbal stem cell grafts in patients with limbal stem cell deficiency due to chemical burns. Clin Exp Ophthalmol 2012; 40(3):255–267

[54] Rama P, Bonini S, Lambiase A, et al. Autologous fibrin-cultured limbal stem cells permanently restore the corneal surface of patients with total limbal stem cell deficiency. Transplantation 2001; 72(9):1478–1485

[55] Fogla R, Padmanabhan P. Deep anterior lamellar keratoplasty combined with autologous limbal stem cell transplantation in unilateral severe chemical injury. Cornea 2005; 24(4):421–425

[56] Basu S, Sureka SP, Shanbhag SS, Kethiri AR, Singh V, Sangwan VS. Simple limbal epithelial transplantation: long-term clinical outcomes in 125 cases of unilateral chronic ocular surface burns. Ophthalmology 2016; 123(5): 1000–1010

[57] Basu S, Mohan S, Bhalekar S, Singh V, Sangwan V. Simple limbal epithelial transplantation (SLET) in failed cultivated limbal epithelial transplantation (CLET) for unilateral chronic ocular burns. Br J Ophthalmol 2018; 102(12):1640–1645

[58] Bhalekar S, Basu S, Sangwan VS. case report: successful management of immunological rejection following allogeneic simple limbal epithelial transplantation (SLET) for bilateral ocular burns. BMJ Case Rep [online]. 2013. https://www.ncbi.nlm.nih.gov/pmc/articles/PMC3618821/. Accessed September 4, 2018

[59] Vemuganti GK, Kashyap S, Sangwan VS, Singh S. Ex-vivo potential of cadaveric and fresh limbal tissues to regenerate cultured epithelium. Indian J Ophthalmol 2004; 52(2):113–120

[60] Singh D, Vanathi M, Gupta C, Gupta N, Tandon R. Outcomes of deep anterior lamellar keratoplasty following autologous simple limbal epithelial transplant in pediatric unilateral severe chemical injury. Indian J Ophthalmol 2017; 65(3):217–222

[61] Gupta N, Farooqui JH, Patel N, Mathur U. Early results of penetrating keratoplasty in patients with unilateral chemical injury after simple limbal epithelial transplantation. Cornea 2018; 37(10):1249–1254

[62] Hernández-Bogantes E, Amescua G, Navas A, et al. Minor ipsilateral simple limbal epithelial transplantation (mini-SLET) for pterygium treatment. Br J Ophthalmol 2015; 99(12):1598–1600

[63] Cárdenas-Cantú E, Zavala J, Valenzuela J, Valdez-García JE. Molecular basis of pterygium development. Semin Ophthalmol 2016; 31(6):567–583

[64] Chui J, Coroneo MT, Tat LT, Crouch R, Wakefield D, Di Girolamo N. Ophthalmic pterygium: a stem cell disorder with premalignant features. Am J Pathol 2011; 178(2):817–827

2 Penetrating Keratoplasty

Rachel H. Epstein, Ishani P. Majmudar, Parag A. Majmudar

Summary

The following chapter will provide background information as well as perioperative guidance essential for performing penetrating keratoplasty. A step-by-step depiction and description of the procedure should provide the reader with the knowledge and tools to successfully and safely perform this indispensable form of corneal transplantation.

Keywords: Cornea transplant, penetrating keratoplasty, surgical technique

2.1 Introduction

Corneal surgery has a long history marked by periods of innovation as well as long stretches of relative inactivity. The Greek physician Galen (130–200 AD) was one of the first to document the removal of superficial corneal scars in what might be considered the first corneal surgery. However, corneal transplantation would not be attempted until the 1800s. The first corneal transplants attempted in humans were xenografts; however, for reasons well known to us today, these proved to be unsuccessful. Eduard Zirm performed the first successful corneal allograft in 1905 on a 45-year-old male who had sustained alkali burns to both corneas. Although this rudimentary surgery allowed the patient to return to work, the modern era of cornea transplantation became possible only with advancements in antiseptic principles, anesthesia techniques and pharmacology, development of the operating microscope, Paton's work in the formation of the eye bank industry, and also improvement in suture technology, beginning in the mid-20th century. The 21st century has been marked by differentiation into anterior and posterior lamellar techniques, which has revolutionized the field of keratoplasty. The future of corneal transplantation will be limited by availability of donor tissue, especially in developing countries, and enhanced with better control of graft rejection and improved refractive outcomes. The development of femtosecond laser, as well as artificial, bioengineered, or three-dimensional-printed corneas may influence the future trajectory of corneal transplantation.[1,2,3,4]

2.2 Indications

Prior to the widespread use of lamellar techniques such as deep anterior lamellar keratoplasty (DALK) and Descemet's membrane endothelial keratoplasty (DMEK), in which only the diseased portion of the cornea are removed, penetrating keratoplasty (PK) was the only procedure for indications such as keratoconus and Fuchs. Conditions such as Fuchs' corneal dystrophy and pseudophakic corneal edema are now preferentially treated with posterior lamellar techniques such as Descemet's stripping automated endothelial keratoplasty (DSAEK) and DMEK. Even cases of prior failed PK can be treated with posterior lamellar techniques. For anterior corneal disorders like superficial scars or keratoconus, in which the endothelial layer is often unaffected, anterior lamellar techniques such as DALK are common; however, in cases of failure to complete the DALK procedure, the surgeon may need to convert to a PK

and therefore knowledge of this procedure is still mandatory. Currently, PK remains the procedure of choice when there is a combination of anterior and posterior corneal pathology. The major indications for PK include full-thickness corneal scars (due to trachoma, vitamin A deficiency, and infectious keratitis), but there is a geographic variation in the primary indications for PK. A recent systematic review revealed both chronological and regional variations in reported global PK indications. Specifically, prevailing reported indications for PK between 1980 and 2014 were keratoconus (Europe, Australia, the Middle East, Africa, and South America), pseudophakic bullous keratopathy/aphakic bullous keratopathy (North America), and keratitis (Asia).[5]

2.3 Preoperative Considerations

There is inconclusive data regarding the role of prophylactic preoperative antibiotics. Prophylactic use of antibiotics is considered to be a risk for development of multidrug-resistant organisms, allergic reactions, and increasing cost.

Several studies have demonstrated the patient's periocular flora to be the most common source of endophthalmitis. As such, preoperative management of blepharitis as well as intraoperative lid preparation are crucial. Any debris along the eyelid margin should be removed and care should be taken to adequately cover and retract the lashes out of the surgical field. A small Tegaderm cut in half, Steri-Strips, or an adapted surgical drape may be employed to this end.

2.3.1 Anesthesia

Koller used cocaine as the earliest anesthesia in ophthalmic surgery in 1884.[4] However, modern ophthalmic anesthesia involves local injection of medium- to long-acting anesthetic agents, often in conjunction with intravenous sedation. This is commonly known as monitored anesthesia care (MAC). However, in certain cases, it may be preferable to avoid periocular injections of anesthetic materials in order to reduce the volume in the retro-orbital space and the resultant increase in posterior pressure. In these cases, general anesthesia with endotracheal intubation or laryngeal mask airway may be preferable. The advantage of general anesthesia is that patient movement is completely minimized and the risk of expulsive choroidal hemorrhage is decreased during the open sky portion of the transplantation procedure. Wang et al[6] evaluated general versus local anesthesia in PK in a group of 141 patients and found that under general anesthesia, pupils remained more stable during PK and there was a decrease in the number of perioperative complications.

Riddle et al[7] reported a series of patients in whom neither local nor general anesthesia was possible as it presented too great a systemic risk. In these cases, topical anesthesia alone was used successfully without complications. While the majority of patients undergoing PK would not routinely be only given topical anesthesia, most surgeons would fall in the spectrum of local/MAC or general anesthesia, depending on the circumstances. In any case, complete eyelid and extraocular muscles akinesia are crucial as this can mitigate the potential for intraoperative pressure fluctuation resulting from muscle contraction.

2.4 Technique

- The eye is prepared in standard sterile fashion. The eyelid speculum should be optimized to maximize exposure while minimizing tension on the globe, which may complicate trephination or affect suture placement (▶Fig. 2.1).
- A scleral fixation ring may be placed to prevent scleral collapse in pediatric, aphakic, pseudophakic, or combination procedures. The diameter of the ring is sized to approximate the interpalpebral diameter, just inside the field delineated by the eyelid speculum. The ring is secured with four interrupted 8–0 Vicryl sutures placed at a partial scleral thickness depth. These sutures may be more comfortably passed from the periphery towards the limbus. While the ring should be securely fashioned to the sclera, it should be loose enough so that one could rotate it slightly employing a tying forceps (▶Fig. 2.2).
- Mark the geometric center of the host cornea; one may use the center of the pupil to capture the optical axis, which is generally nasally displaced. A midway point may be chosen should the center of the cornea and optical axis notably differ in location.
  - Use calipers to measure the corneal diameter from the center extending horizontally and vertically to determine the appropriate size for host and donor trephine as well as to demarcate the proposed area on the host for trephination. Using gentle pressure, the trephine may be used on a dry corneal surface to demarcate the proposed area prior to trephination (▶Fig. 2.3a, b).
  - The indication for which the transplant is being performed may alter the desired centration of the graft. For example, in a patient with keratoconus, care must be taken to avoid trephination in an area of thinning as well as account for the potential inferonasal predilection for the apex of ectasia.

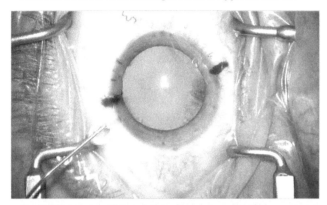

Fig. 2.1 Draping and lid speculum placement.

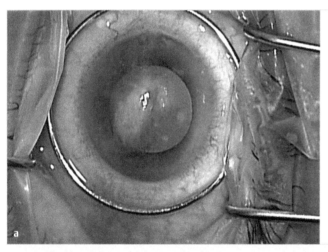
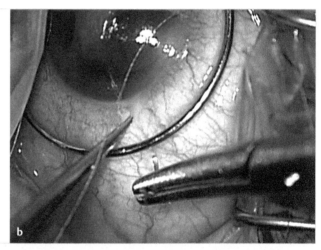

Fig. 2.2 (a, b) Selecting and suturing the Flieringa ring.

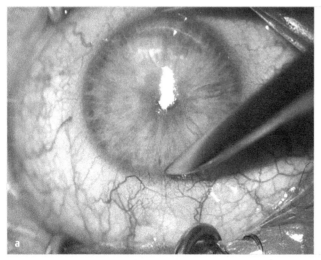
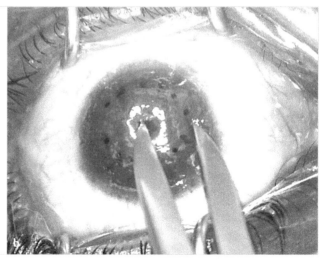

Fig. 2.3 (a) Measuring the vertical and horizontal white to white. **(b)** Marking the geometric center.

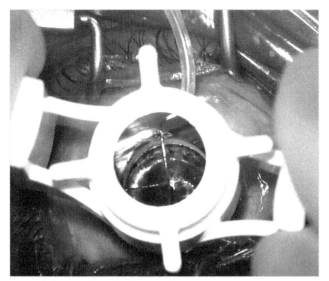

Fig. 2.4 Centration of the trephine.

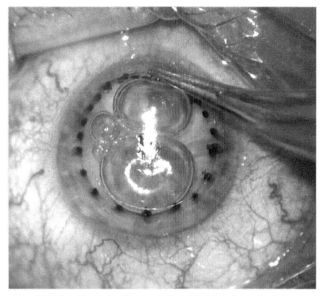

Fig. 2.5 Viscoelastic fill of the anterior chamber prior to host tissue resection.

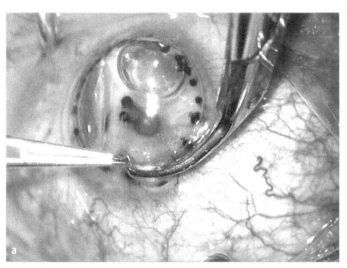

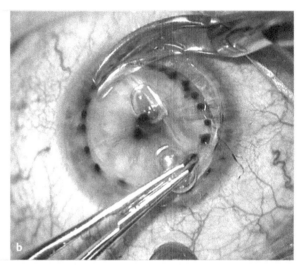

Fig. 2.6 (a, b) Curved corneal scissors to remove host cornea.

- At this juncture, surgeon preference may dictate whether donor or host trephination is pursued. It is advantageous to prepare the donor cornea prior to trephination of the host to minimize the amount of time spent "open sky."
  - Trephine the donor tissue, typically aiming for 0.25 or 0.5 mm larger than the planned host trephination; this allows for adequate apposition of tissue, minimizes tension on the wound, and minimizes narrowing of the anterior chamber angle. The exception is keratoconus and other ectatic disorders in which it is preferable to have an isometric graft (same size graft as the host trephination) to reduce myopia.
  - Trephination may be completed using a vacuumed or non-vacuumed trephine. Additionally, the femtosecond laser may be used to prepare both the donor and host tissues. However, this option is not very common due to its cost and availability factors (▶ Fig. 2.4).
- Once the donor cornea has been prepared, the host cornea is then trephined to near full-thickness depth; maintaining

a perpendicular position of trephine to cornea will optimize the symmetry of the cut for 360°. A near full-thickness trephine provides an additional amount of control as the anterior chamber may then be entered using a sharp blade, avoiding an abrupt shift in intraocular pressure, reducing the risk of suprachoroidal hemorrhage. At this juncture, a miotic agent may be injected to constrict the pupil and protect the crystalline lens if no lens procedures are planned or have been previously completed. Additionally, injection of a dispersive viscoelastic into the anterior chamber will encourage both iris and lens to remain posterior while the host cornea is excised (▶ Fig. 2.5).

- The host corneal tissue is excised using curved corneal scissors. It is advisable to have both right and left curved scissors to enhance maneuverability. Scissor tips should be visualized at all times and slight upward pressure during cutting may reduce undue iris trauma (▶ Fig. 2.6). Cuts made perpendicular to the host margin will reduce postoperative astigmatism, however cuts slightly beveled inwards may enhance a

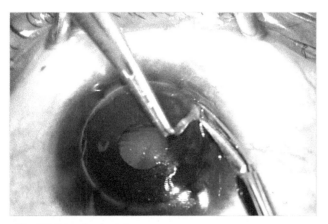

Fig. 2.7 Trimming host rim.

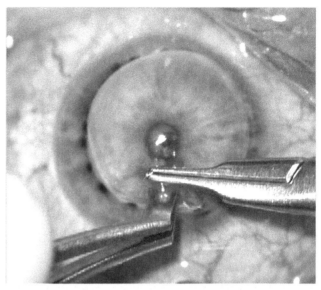

Fig. 2.8 First cardinal suture placement.

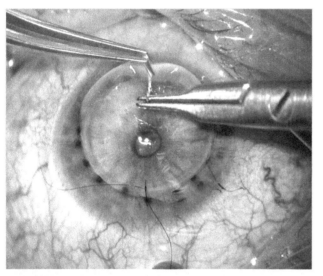

Fig. 2.9 Second cardinal suture placement.

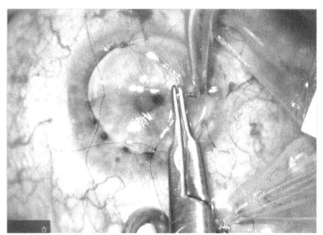

Fig. 2.10 Four cardinal sutures placed.

watertight seal by creating a posterior wound lip. It is also crucial to continue to refill the chamber with viscoelastic to prevent iris prolapse or trauma. Any remaining tissue tags may be judiciously removed (▶Fig. 2.7).

- The donor graft is then carefully grasped at the junction of epithelium and stroma with fine-toothed, two-pronged forceps, avoiding any contact of endothelium. The donor is carefully secured to the host corneal tissue with an interrupted 10–0 nylon suture at the 12 o'clock position. The needle may be adjusted once secured within the needle driver to optimize angulation and promote radial suture placement.

In order to get adequate depth bite of both tissues, it is helpful to approach the donor tissue nearly perpendicular with the needle emerging at the donor margin at about 90% depth. If necessary, the needle may be re-grasped prior to entering the host tissue similarly, just above the level of Descemet's membrane. A wrinkle in Descemet's membrane may be appreciated when the needle is at the recommended depth. The suture should enter the donor and emerge from the host equidistant from the wound. Interrupted suture may be tied using an initial triple loop followed by two additional single loops or a slip knot technique, which provides immediate stability to the wound while allowing for adjustment of tension as additional sutures are placed (▶Fig. 2.8).

- The second suture is placed 180° away from the first at the 6 o'clock position. Accurate placement of this suture is crucial for proper tissue alignment and minimizing postoperative astigmatism. It should be placed so that tissue is distributed equally on each side. As the tissue is engaged entering the donor, a linear fold around the level of Descemet's membrane emanating from the 12 o'clock suture running towards the 6 o'clock position suggests proper suture alignment. The suture placement may be further refined by rotating the inferior donor rim a few degrees in each direction prior to finishing the pass through the host. The suture is tied, the chamber is reformed, and if necessary, the suture may be replaced at that juncture or once the additional cardinal sutures have been placed (▶Fig. 2.9). To complete cardinal suture placement, the 3 o'clock suture followed by the 9 o'clock suture is placed and tied (▶Fig. 2.10).

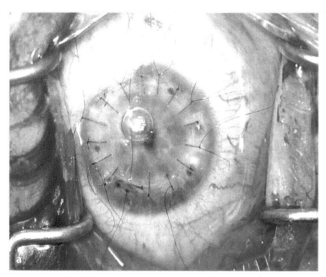 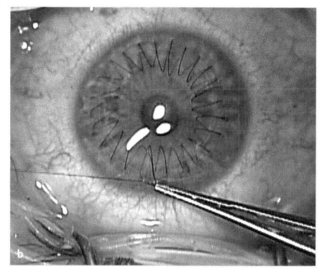

Fig. 2.11 (a) Additional interrupted suture placement. (b) Running suture placement.

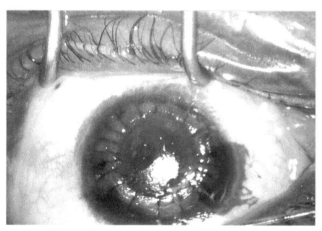

Fig. 2.12 Seidel assessment of wound.

- It is essential to continue to refill the anterior chamber periodically as this maneuver eases proper suture placement and tension as well as decreases the risk of iris incarceration within the wound.
- Generally, an additional 12 radial interrupted 10–0 nylon sutures and possibly a 10–0 nylon running suture with 90% stromal depth bites are placed to provide adequate wound apposition without gaping or override of tissue (▶ Fig. 2.11a, b). The decision to use running versus interrupted sutures is largely one of the surgeon preferences; however, interrupted sutures should be preferentially used when there is significant inflammation and vascularization as sutures in these areas will loosen earlier than others and if they are interrupted, these sutures may be selectively removed without compromising the wound integrity elsewhere.
- Once the sutures are at the desired tension, the ends are trimmed and rotated to bury the knots into either host or donor side, avoiding placement within the wound itself.
- The wound is assessed with a cellulose sponge and/or fluorescein staining (▶ Fig. 2.12). Leaks may be addressed by replacing the suture or placing additional 10–0 nylon interrupted suture to bolster weaker areas.
- The scleral fixation ring is removed.

- If there is concern for limbal stem cell deficiency, eyelid abnormalities, and/or neuropathic keratopathy, a medial and/or lateral tarsorrhaphy may be completed intraoperatively to enhance postoperative wound healing. Punctal occlusion, via punctal plugs or punctal cauterization, may be beneficial in these patients as well.
- No consensus for perioperative steroid or antibiotic administration prevails at this juncture. Betadine is applied at the conclusion of the case followed by a combination antibiotic/steroid ointment. The eye is patched and shielded.

2.5 Postoperative Management

Routine postoperative medication consists of topical prednisolone 1% combined with topical antibiotic four times daily. This regimen may include a nonsteroidal anti-inflammatory drug when done in combination with cataract surgery. Following discharge, patients are typically seen postoperative day 1 and pending stability, again at weeks 1, 3, and 7 followed by 3 months. It is imperative to educate patients on signs and symptoms suggestive of graft rejection and/or failure, specifically advising all to seek immediate follow-up with any of the RSVP signs:

- **R**edness.
- Extreme **S**ensitivity to light.
- Decreased **V**ision.
- **P**ain.

Typically, antibiotic is reduced over the subsequent postoperative month and 1% prednisolone is tapered down over several months, aiming to maintain a single daily dose interminably.

Corneal topography is performed at regular intervals to guide suture adjustment or removal. In the case of interrupted sutures, a period of 3 to 4 months is allowed to pass before removing sutures to preserve wound strength. Following suture removal, it is advisable to briefly increase topical steroid therapy to four times daily and reduce to once daily over 1 week with appropriate simultaneous antibiotic coverage.

- Recurrent epithelial ingrowth after laser-assisted in situ keratomileusis (LASIK).
- Limbal dermoid excision—eccentric SALK.

SALK can also be performed in various special ways:
- Microkeratome-assisted ALK: An automated microkeratome is used to cut the donor and the recipient corneas. The anterior cut stroma of the donor graft is then placed on the host cornea and sutured.[4,5,6]
- Femtosecond laser-assisted SALK: The femtosecond laser is used to create the lamellar cuts in both the donor and the recipient corneas.[7]
- Excimer laser-assisted ALK: Here, a deep excimer laser ablation is done on the host cornea with a plano configuration followed by suturing of a donor lamellar button on the recipient bed.

3.3.2 Deep Anterior Lamellar Kratoplasty

DALK refers to the procedure where all the layers of the cornea excluding the PDL, DM, and the endothelium are replaced.

Indications

- Corneal ectasias—keratoconus, pellucid marginal degeneration, and post-LASIK ectasia.
- Superficial and deep corneal scars not involving DM.
- Stromal dystrophies.
- Mucopolysaccharidosis.
- Therapeutic DALK.
- Tectonic DALK for descemetocele.
- Acute hydrops—primary stage with modifications in technique.

Contraindications

- Corneal dystrophies involving the endothelium.
- Deep scars involving the endothelium and overlying the pupillary axis.
- Keratoconic patients with coexisting Fuchs endothelial dystrophy.
- Cystinosis with endothelial involvement.
- Infective keratitis with Descemetic/endothelial involvement.
- Penetrating ocular trauma.

Surgical Technique

Anwar first proposed the most commonly used technique known as the "big bubble technique."[8,9,10] The cornea is trephined to partial thickness up to a depth of 80%. A 26-gauge needle attached to an air-filled syringe is inserted into the stromal lamellae from the depth of the trephined groove and air is injected into the corneal stroma. This leads to the formation of type 1 bubble, which separates the PDL, DM, and the endothelium on one side from the overlying stroma on the

other side. This big bubble is then expanded till the edge of the trephined groove. A small paracentesis may be created and a small bubble is injected into the anterior chamber to perform the big bubble—small bubble test. If the small bubble remains at the periphery of the anterior chamber, it indicates the creation of the big bubble, which is occupying space in the center of the anterior chamber. On the other hand, if the small bubble migrates to the center of the cornea, it indicates the absence of a big bubble. Once a big bubble has been confirmed by the small bubble test, superficial anterior keratectomy is done. This is followed by opening the big bubble space using a 15° blade and then using a curved Vannas scissor for cutting the remaining anterior stromal layers into quadrants, which are then excised along the trephined groove. The donor cornea from which the DM and the endothelium have been stripped is sutured over the recipient bed (▶ Fig. 3.1).

Various other techniques for performing DALK include:
- Fluid/viscoelastic dissection: For the separation of stroma from the underlying layers.[11,12]
- Manual dissection DALK: Anterior chamber is filled with an air bubble and the stroma is dissected layer by layer. The depth of the instrument in relation to the posterior corneal surface can be visualized using the Melles technique.
- Femtosecond laser-assisted DALK: The femtosecond laser is used to create lamellar cuts in both the donor and the recipient corneas. It can also be used to create side cuts, which can be vertical or in shaped patterns such as mushroom-shaped or zigzag cuts. The better apposition obtained between the graft and the recipient with these shaped cuts makes it possible to decrease the number of corneal sutures used, thus allowing a decrease in induced astigmatism. However, the amount of astigmatism that is induced finally will also depend on the suturing technique.
- Intraoperative optical coherence tomography (OCT)-assisted DALK: The intraoperative OCT (iOCT) can be used in various stages of surgery such as determining the depth of dissection of the initial groove, determining the depth at which the needle is passed into the deep stroma for creating a big bubble, confirming the formation of the big bubble, identifying micro- and macroperforations and their exact location as well as apposition of the perforation to the overlying stroma after suturing on the graft, determining the amount of residual stroma left in the case of pre-Descemetic DALK, detecting presence of interface fluid after suturing the donor graft, and so on.[13]

Complications of Deep Anterior Lamellar Kratoplasty

- Microperforations: These can happen during dissection and are generally not a reason for converting surgery into PK. Surgery can be continued as DALK by injecting air into the anterior chamber and fibrin glue can be used to close the microperforation.
- Macroperforations: These are large perforations and may result in inability to proceed with the DALK and having to

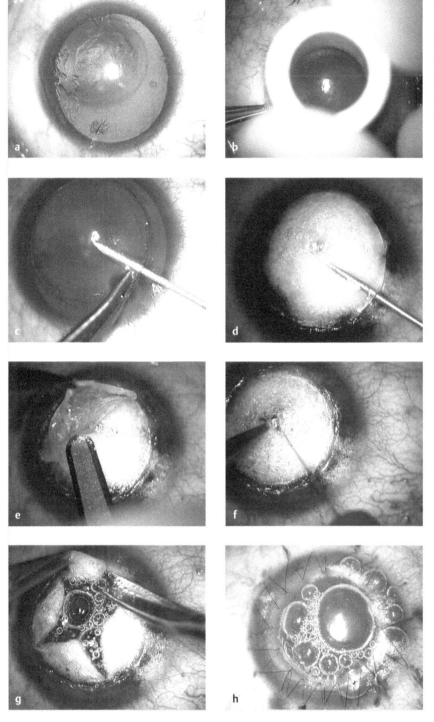

Fig. 3.1 (a) Preoperative photograph of advanced keratoconus. (b) Partial trephination of host cornea. (c) A 26-gauge needle with bevel down inserted into the stromal lamellae. (d) Formation of big bubble. (e) Superficial anterior keratectomy. (f) Opening the big bubble space using 15° blade. (g) Anterior stromal quadrants cut and excised along the trephined groove using Vannas scissors. (h) Donor cornea sutured over the host with a combination of continuous and interrupted sutures.

convert to PK. In this case, the PDL, DM, and endothelium are excised and a full-thickness graft is sutured in place.

• Double anterior chamber: This can happen either with or without microperforations when aqueous enters into the interface and creates a double anterior chamber. It may also occur with an improperly managed macroperforation.

Management depends on the cause. Microperforations may be closed with fibrin glue +/- air tamponade, the double anterior chamber drained, and the graft sutured in place. In case of macroperforations with double anterior chamber, it may be necessary to convert into a PK.

- Folds in the Descemet's membrane: A mismatch in the size between recipient bed and donor cornea can lead to folds in the DM, which can interfere with visual acuity. This can be avoided by using a slightly larger donor graft.
- Pupillary block: This can happen when the air bubble in the anterior chamber interferes with circulation of aqueous resulting in iris bombe, raised intraocular pressure, and peripheral anterior synechiae.
- Urrets-Zavalia syndrome: This refers to a fixed and dilated pupil after DALK and has sometimes been attributed to the use of atropine eye drops post surgery.

Disadvantages of Deep Anterior Lamellar Keratoplasty

Theoretically, DALK has a longer learning curve and is a technically more difficult surgery with additional time required for the procedure. However, with experience, these disadvantages can be overcome.

3.4 Jacob's Modified Technique of Pre-Descemetic DALK for Primary Treatment of Acute Hydrops

Acute corneal hydrops occurs secondary to a tear in the DM and results from aqueous seepage into the stroma, forming fluid clefts. Conventionally, this is managed medically with compression sutures or with intracameral gas or air injections followed in many cases by a secondary pre-Descemetic DALK at a later stage. However, this strategy results in healing with the formation of a scar, with the location of the scar depending on the area of the Descemetic tear. If the scar occurs in the visual axis, it can result in deterioration of vision and necessitates PK, thereby exposing the patient to all the risks associated with a PK such as rejection and secondary graft failure. Following conventional management, though some patients may undergo a secondary pre-Descemetic DALK at a later stage, this is possible only if the scarring is outside the visual axis. This approach is also associated with the morbidity and expense of a second surgery. Though contact lenses may fit better after resolution of hydrops, the patient can wear them only for a limited time per day and generally continues to have poor glass tolerance and poor vision during the remaining hours of the day. It also exposes the patients to all the risks associated with the contact lens wear. Patients who have suboptimal fit of the contact lens,

apical touch, and scarring will require special optical lenses, which are expensive.

One of the authors (Soosan Jacob) has described her technique of modified pre-Descemetic DALK in the primary stage during acute presentation of corneal hydrops.[14,15] This modified technique can be performed as a primary procedure for the treatment of acute hydrops and gives excellent results as well as safety and predictability. Surgery in the acute stage immediately after the occurrence of hydrops using this technique prevents healing by stromal scarring. It provides anatomical correction of ectasia and thinning. The procedure also simultaneously targets multiple pathologies that can be associated with advanced ectasia and results in topographic, pachymetric, biomechanical, visual, and structural improvement while allowing decreased contact lens dependence. It provides early and rapid visual rehabilitation, early anatomic rehabilitation, and optical correction by regaining corneal structure and transparency. It closes the Descemetic break while still maintaining transparency over the area of the break. As the host DM and endothelium are retained and scarring over the visual axis is avoided, it avoids the risks associated with a PK such as rejection and secondary graft failure. It has advantages of single-stage surgery and avoids costs and morbidities associated with two surgeries (▶ Fig. 3.2, ▶ Fig. 3.3, and ▶ Fig. 3.4).

Modifications in surgery include using a 26-gauge needle with bevel bent upward instead of down to avoid pressure buildup from air that is injected downward. The needle is tangentially directed away from the break and only small aliquots of air are injected slowly, at multiple sites again to avoid large pressure buildups. Air is injected only to create tissue emphysema, which is then used as a guide for the depth of dissection. Manual deep dissection is then proceeded centripetally using a blunt dissector leaving the area of the Descemetic tear or the break for the last. Deeper dissection can then be performed after gentle re-induction of emphysema or by using Melles technique of optical recognition. Minimal stroma is intentionally retained above the Descemetic tear to prevent the anterior chamber from collapsing. Finally, the donor graft with DM and endothelium stripped is sutured on to the host bed and the Descemet's tear is tamponaded with air in the anterior chamber. In eyes with extensive edema or with thin residual stroma, the initial groove can be created by manually deepening an ink trephine mark with a sharp crescent blade. This modified technique can also be used in keratoglobus and pellucid marginal degeneration but with a tuck in LK instead.

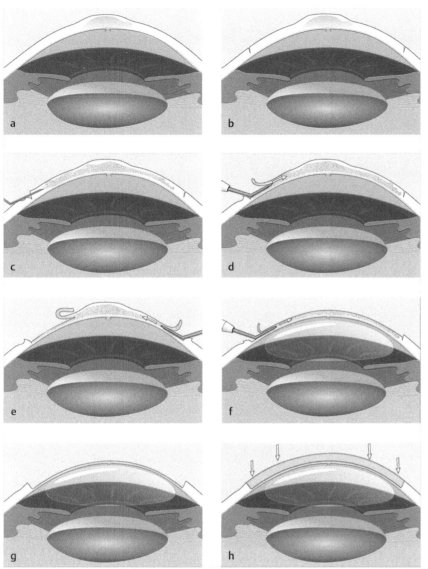

Fig. 3.2 Jacob's modified technique of pre-Descemetic DALK as primary treatment for acute hydrops. **(a)** Acute hydrops with a tear seen in the DM. **(b)** Partial trephination of the host cornea. **(c)** Induction of emphysema using a 26-gauge needle bevel up. **(d)** Manual dissection of host stroma using emphysematous cornea as a guide. **(e)** Centripetal dissection carried out from all around leaving the area over the DM tear for last. **(f)** Deeper dissection carried out using the Melles technique after introduction of air in the AC. **(g)** A few pre-Descemetic layers left intact to avoid opening up of the AC. The air in the AC tamponades the DM tear against overlying stroma. **(h)** Donor graft sutured over the host. AC, anterior chamber; DALK, deep anterior lamellar keratoplasty; DM, Descemet's membrane.

4 Descemet's Stripping Automated Endothelial Keratoplasty

Claudia Perez Straziota

Summary

This chapter provides an overview of Descemet's stripping automated endothelial keratoplasty (DSAEK) including surgical technique and pearls, reported outcomes, routine postoperative management, and diagnosis and management of postoperative complications. Throughout the chapter comparative data with other endothelial keratoplasty (EK) techniques are included to provide the reader with a full perspective of the different EK alternatives.

Keywords: Endothelial keratoplasty, DSAEK, corneal transplantation

4.1 Introduction

Endothelial keratoplasty (EK) has revolutionized the field of corneal transplantation for isolated endothelial disease by providing a safer procedure with more predictable refractive outcomes and lower risk of rejection compared to full-thickness penetrating keratoplasty (PK).[1] Since the first publications of posterior lamellar keratoplasty in 1956[2] and EK by Melles in 1998,[3] EK has evolved through deep lamellar endothelial keratoplasty (DLEK),[4] Descemet's stripping endothelial keratoplasty (DSEK),[5] Descemet's stripping automated endothelial keratoplasty (DSAEK),[6] and ultimately leading to the thinnest lenticule transplantations: ultrathin Descemet's stripping automated endothelial keratoplasty (UT-DSAEK) and Descemet's membrane endothelial keratoplasty (DMEK) (▶Fig. 4.1) (▶Video 4.1).[7,8] Among these technique variations, DSAEK remains the most widely used procedure for EK today; however, techniques that utilize thinner grafts, especially DMEK and pre-Descemet's endothelial keratoplasty (PDEK), are gaining acceptance worldwide. Those techniques are the focus of other chapters.

4.2 DSAEK Donor Tissue Preparation

The main objectives in the donor preparation for EK are to achieve a target lenticule thickness while obtaining the most planar surface possible to minimize postoperative refractive changes while inflicting minimal trauma to the endothelial cells in the graft. In some instances, despite a clear, well-centered DSAEK graft with no apparent irregularities, the final visual acuity is worse than expected. Two main factors have been proposed to explain this variability in results: graft thickness[9,10,11] (preoperative and postoperative) and the higher order aberrations (HOAs) induced by irregularities in the donor–host interface and tissue architecture.[6,12,13,14]

Initially, the donor preparation was performed using surgical manual techniques until microkeratome dissection

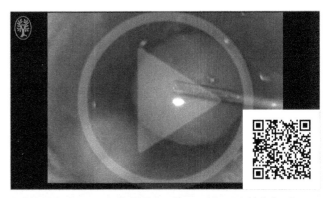

Video 4.1 Descemet's diaries. https://www.thieme.de/de/q.htm?p=opn/tp/311890101/9781684200979_video_04_01&t=video

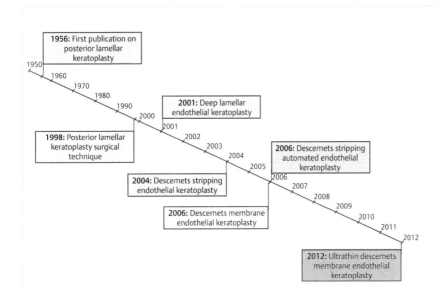

Fig. 4.1 Timeline of endothelial keratoplasty technique development.

1956: First publication on posterior lamellar keratoplasty

1998: Posterior lamellar keratoplasty surgical technique

2001: Deep lamellar endothelial keratoplasty

2004: Descemets stripping endothelial keratoplasty

2006: Descemets membrane endothelial keratoplasty

2006: Descemets stripping automated endothelial keratoplasty

2012: Ultrathin descemets membrane endothelial keratoplasty

of the donor tissue was proven to have advantages over hand dissection such as a reduced risk of donor perforation and faster visual recovery.[15]

Automated microkeratome dissection is the current standard for corneal tissue preparation for DSAEK lenticules, and since 2006, eye banks began to develop strategies to provide precut tissue to surgeons all over the nation for EK. No difference has been shown in terms of the quality of the tissue[16] or outcomes[17,18,19] using precut tissue prepared by the eye bank versus cutting the tissue in the operating room. Precut grafts save time and eliminate the additional stress of the additional step of cutting the donor tissue prior to the surgery.

4.2.1 Microkeratome-Assisted Lenticule Preparation

Different strategies have been suggested to consistently obtain thinner cuts with a single microkeratome pass, such as stromal dehydration,[20] development of a nomogram for microkeratome head setting based on central corneal thickness prior to the cut (▶Fig. 4.2),[21] and adjustment of the translational speed of the microkeratome in thicker donors, as slower translational speeds result in deeper cuts and thinner lenticules (▶Table. 4.1).[22]

With a single microkeratome cut, there is higher variability in thickness throughout the lenticule compared with two microkeratome passes (double pass).[23,24] This variability results in lenticules that are thinner in the center than in the periphery,[22] which has been related to the postoperative hyperopic shift observed after DSAEK.[25] The predictability of the final lenticule thickness decreases as the target thickness decreases, dropping from 78% of cuts within 10μm when the target is between 90 and 120 μm to 48% when the target falls below 90 μm.[26] Nevertheless, with the proper microkeratome head selection based on central corneal thickness, the majority of lenticules fall below 131 μm.[26]

In 2009, Busin et al[8] introduced the concept of UT-DSAEK at the European Society of Cataract and Refractive Surgery meeting and proposed the use of a preoperative lenticule thinner than 100 μm by using the "microkeratome double-pass technique" for donor preparation, which would standardize the preparation of grafts resulting in consistently thinner and more planar lenticules.[22,23]

In addition to a thinner lenticule, the double-pass microkeratome technique seems to provide better tissue architecture than a single-pass preparation, with comparable postoperative outcomes to DMEK without the steep learning curve,[27,28] or the specific anterior chamber fluid dynamics required for DMEK.

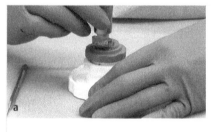
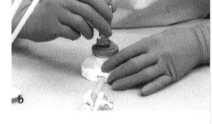
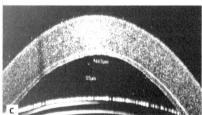

Fig. 4.2 Microkeratome double-pass technique for preparation of the UT-DSAEK lenticule. First pass (**a**), second pass (**b**), and OCT of the final lenticule cut (**c**). OCT, ocular coherence tomography; UT-DSAEK, ultrathin Descemet's stripping automated endothelial keratoplasty. (These images are provided courtesy of the Georgia Eye Bank.)

Table. 4.1 Translational speed of the microkeratome can be adjusted for thicker donors.[22] Nomogram for thin donor corneal disks for DSAEK performed using an automated microkeratome

Corneal thickness (μm)	Blade holder size (μm)	Advancement speed (mm/s)	Eyes (n)	Thickness (μm)	
				Mean ± SD	Range
475 to 500	450	3.0	3	97.00 ± 13.11	85,111
501 to 525	450	2.0	3	96.20 ± 19.56	67,117
526 to 550	450	1.5	5	99.11 ± 9.03	86,112
551 to 575	500	3.0	9	97.06 ± 13.72	74,117
576 to 600	500	2.0	15	97.00 ± 13.11	85,111
601 to 650	500	1.5	18	98.44 ± 13.56	73,119
≥ 651	Two passes: 140, then same nomogram for the RSB	1.5 for 140 μm blade handle	7	110.57 ± 15.61	88,130

Abbreviation: RSB, residual stromal bed.

The "double-pass microkeratome technique" consists an initial "de-bulking" pass of the microkeratome usually with a head between 300 and 350 μm and a second microkeratome pass that is adjusted to obtain a lenticule thickness below 100 to 130 μm. The second pass is started 180° away from the first pass and it is done in the opposite direction to obtain a more planar surface.

The head used for this step can be selected according to a nomogram developed by Busin (▶ Table 4.2),[8] targeting a residual bed with a central thickness below 100 μm. Other algorithms have also been suggested to adjust both the first pass in relationship to the initial corneal thickness and the second pass related to stromal bed thickness prior to the cut (▶ Fig. 4.3).[23] Lenticules created with the double-pass technique tend to be more planar, that is, with a more even distribution of thickness from the center to the periphery after the second pass of the microkeratome.[23]

Pressure in the system must be standardized by raising the infusion bottle to a height of 120 cm above the level of the artificial anterior chamber and then clamping the tubing 50 cm from the entrance. Attention must be given to maintain a uniform, slow movement of the hand-driven microkeratome,

requiring 4 to 6 seconds for each dissection, which will produce a planar surface that minimizes interface irregularities and hyperopic shift. ▶ Fig. 4.4 shows the optical coherence tomography (OCT) images of donor tissue before (▶ Fig. 4.4a, c) and after (▶ Fig. 4.4b, d) microkeratome double-pass tissue preparation for UT-DSAEK, and before (▶ Fig. 4.4e) and after (▶ Fig. 4.4f) regular single-pass microkeratome for DSAEK preparation.

Table 4.2 Busin nomogram for microkeratome double-pass UT-DSAEK lenticule preparation[8]

Residual stromal bed (μm)	Head selection for second microkeratome pass (μm)
<151	No second cut
151–190	50
191–210	90
211–230	110
>230	130

Abbreviation: UT-DSAEK, ultrathin Descemet's stripping automated endothelial keratoplasty.

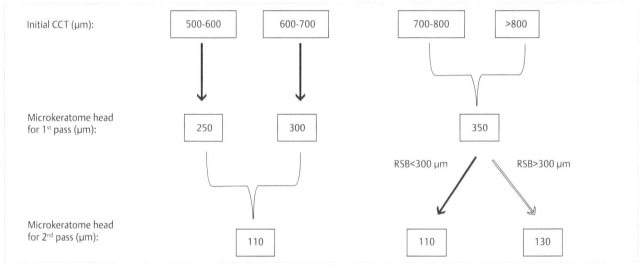

Fig. 4.3 Algorithm proposed by Sikder et al for microkeratome head selection.[23]

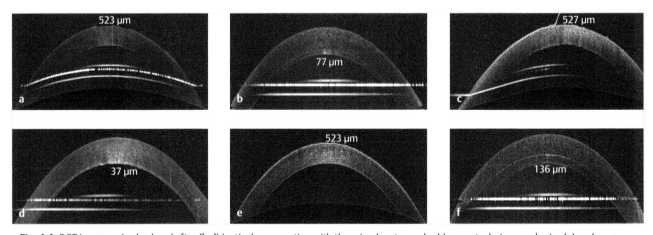

Fig. 4.4 OCT images prior **(a,c)** and after **(b,d)** lenticule preparation with the microkeratome double-pass technique and prior **(e)** and after **(f)** standard single microkeratome pass DSAEK lenticule preparation. DSAEK, Descemet's stripping automated endothelial keratoplasty. (These images are provided courtesy of Georgia Eye Bank.)

With the double-pass microkeratome technique, Busin reported 100% of the tissues with a postcut thickness below 151 μm, 95.6% below 131 μm, and 78.3% below 101 μm; and only 2.1% of the tissues were lost due to perforation.[29] Woodward et al.[30] obtained 65% of cuts below 100 μm and 92% below 131 μm with the double-pass technique and found no significant difference in rate of perforation when the second pass was done 180° from the first cut (23%) or at the thickest peripheral measurement in the residual bed (29%). Their higher perforation rate compared to the 7% reported by Busin[29] can be related to the larger chosen head size for the second cut.

4.2.2 Femtosecond Laser Ultrathin Lenticule Preparation

So far, despite the theoretical advantage of more predictable depth of cut and a faster recovery of visual acuity during the immediate postoperative period, femtosecond laser preparation of DSAEK donors has yielded worse long-term postoperative visual acuities and higher rate of re-grafting compared to microkeratome grafts.[31] This is due to the scattered laser emission and the high intraocular pressure (IOP) required during femtosecond applanation, which distorts the lenticule surface and creates ridges,[32] giving the femtosecond cuts a wavelike or concentric ring configuration in the stromal interface.[33,34] Additionally, the large cavitation bubbles increase the rate of endothelial cell loss to 50 to 65% by 12 months[32,35,36,37] and the graft detachments rates as high as 40%,[31,36,38] yielding overall inferior refractive outcomes compared to manual trephination.[31,32,33,36,38,39,40]

Docking the endothelial side of donor cornea on the applanation surface to decrease the laser emission path and scatter could result in a more predictable and regular cut; however, this comes at the cost of 30% less viable endothelial cells compared to epithelial side docking[35] even when ocular viscoelastic devices (OVDs) are used on the applanation surface.[41]

4.3 Surgical Procedure

The most important steps in DSAEK are corneal incision creation, descemetorrhexis, and lenticule insertion.

4.3.1 Main Corneal Incision

Several DSAEK graft insertion techniques and the use of DMEK tissue insertion devices have been developed in attempts to minimize tissue manipulation during the procedure and therefore minimize the loss of endothelial cells. Five-millimeter main incisions have been shown to have less endothelial cell loss compared to the 3.0 mm;[42,43] however, this difference does not appear to be clinically significant postoperatively.[42]

4.3.2 Descemetorrhexis

A deep anterior chamber facilitates complete descemetorrhexis. Filling of the anterior chamber with air, OVDs, or balanced salt solution is crucial to maintain an adequate depth that will not only facilitate removing Descemet's membrane but also prevent complications related to sudden anterior chamber collapse such as crystalline lens damage when apposed to the cornea, iris prolapse, or less frequently, suprachoroidal hemorrhage.

Descemetorrhexis is accomplished in most instances manually with the use of a reverse Sinsky hook under retroillumination of the cornea. After scoring Descemet's membrane, intraocular forceps are used to peel off Descemet's membrane from the host.

A retained fragment of Descemet's membrane can result in significant interface haze and irregularity, as well as postoperative lenticule detachment. Therefore, it is essential to assure complete descemetorrhexis, which can be confirmed by examination of the recipient's cornea with retroillumination or direct examination of the removed Descemet's membrane onto the recipient's cornea.

Femtosecond laser technology is currently being considered for host descemetorrhexis for DMEK by producing an 8- to 8.25-mm diameter cut 100 μm anterior to the thinnest measured point from the epithelial side and 100 μm posterior to the thinnest cut from the anterior chamber. Results have been promising, with lower detachment rates treated successfully with re-bubbling[44,45,46] and endothelial cell losses of 24% with femtosecond laser descemetorrhexis comparable to 29% with manual descemetorrhexis.[44,45,47]

The use of DSAEK Terry scrapers to scrape the periphery of the recipient stroma after descemetorrhexis has been shown to decrease the rate of postoperative graft dislocation from 50 to 4% in case series[48] and appears to be of help in the reattachment of partially detached lenticules.[49]

4.3.3 Lenticule Insertion

Suture pulling techniques do not seem to offer an advantage over the use of forceps in terms of endothelial cell loss,[50] and the Busin guide has shown less endothelial cell loss compared to forceps (25 vs. 34%, respectively), but no advantages in terms of final visual acuity outcomes or rate of graft failure;[51] therefore, the choice of insertion technique depends merely on surgeon's preference as long as the wound remains the appropriate size of 5 mm. Recently, tissue insertion devices have been designed to minimize tissue manipulation during insertion while using a smaller incision size, and endothelial cell loss appears to be less when these devices are used (average of 16% loss reported in 1 year)[52] compared to forceps folding techniques (35%) and sheets glide (35%).

The Busin glide and injection devices preserve the endothelium better compared to manual insertion with forceps;[51,53] however, this difference does not appear to be clinically relevant postoperatively neither in standard not in UT-DSAEK.[42] Therefore, insertion technique should be made by each individual surgeon to maximize the surgeon's performance and minimize iatrogenic tissue trauma through excessive manipulation.

Placing the sutures prior to viscoelastic removal will provide a pressurized eye to facilitate suture placement and reduce postoperative astigmatism. It is of equal or more importance to insert the tissue and then tie the sutures prior to unfolding, as not doing so increases the chances of tissue expulsion through the open main incision, especially when inserting ultrathin lenticules.

Transient interface fluid has been associated with transient interface opacities;[54] therefore, fluid and OVDs need to be

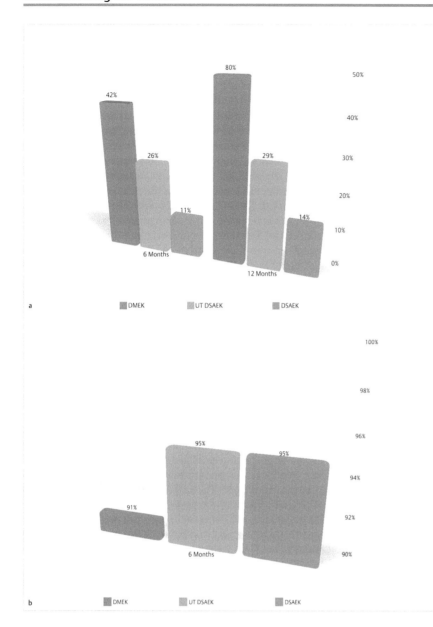

Fig. 4.5 Percentage of patients with DCVA better than 20/20 **(a)** and 20/40 **(b)** at 6 months postoperatively and of patients who achieve DCVA of 20/20 or better at 12 months postoperatively **(a)** after different EK techniques. DCVA, distance-corrected visual acuity; DMEK, Descemet's membrane endothelial keratoplasty; DSAEK, Descemet's stripping automated endothelial keratoplasty; EK, endothelial keratoplasty; UT-DSAEK ultrathin Descemet's stripping automated endothelial keratoplasty.

when the double-pass microkeratome technique is used.[29] After DMEK, there is still a hyperopic shift but it is considerably lower at +0.24 D (−1.50 to +2.25 D).[75]

Despite negligible changes in the anterior corneal topography after all types of EK,[13,25,81] there is an increase in posterior corneal HOAs after both DSAEK[11,13,83,92,93] and, to a lower degree, DMEK.[89] No studies are available in regards to HOAs after UT-DSAEK.

4.5.2 Endothelial Cell Loss

There is an expected endothelial cell loss density over time,[94,95,96] mostly during the first 6 postoperative months both after DSAEK and DMEK.[75,95] The main cause of endothelial cell loss after EK is excessive tissue manipulation during surgery. The introduction of the microkeratome, potentially femtosecond laser technology to assist in EK donor lenticule preparation, and new techniques to minimize the induction of horseshoe tears in DMEK lenticules[97] have decreased the degree of endothelial cell loss related to donor preparation. The consistent preparation of the tissue by an eye bank technician standardizes the procedure and decreases variability.

The reported rate of endothelial cell loss after DSAEK ranges 25 to 54% at 6 months, 24 to 61% at 1 year, and 53% at 5 years,[1,90,96,98] to which DMEK compares favorably, with 27 to 47% at 6 months,[99] 27% at 1 year, and 39% at 5 years.[100] Endothelial cell loss is not related to donor age, gender, or diagnosis nor it is related to death-to-use or death-to-preservation times. The correlation with donor endothelial cell count is controversial and appears to be more noticeable on 5-year postoperative cell counts.[100,101] In most cases, the graft can remain functional for many years despite this cell loss; however, as the endothelial cell density decreases below a critical threshold, corneal edema and visual degradation will occur.

4.6 Postoperative Complications

▶ Table 4.4 lists the most common postoperative complications and basic management options. The most common issues arising early include pupillary block, interface fluid, graft dislocation, immunologic graft rejection, graft failure, and epithelial ingrowth in the graft–host interface.

4.6.1 Pupillary Block

A large air bubble in front of the pupil or air migration posterior to the iris blocking aqueous flow through the pupil can lead to pupillary block, which is one of the most potentially devastating complications that may occur following DSAEK surgery (▶ Fig. 4.6a, b). Subsequent narrowing of the anterior chamber can lead to iridocorneal apposition with acute angle closure glaucoma and formation of peripheral anterior synechiae, and this prolonged elevated IOP can lead to irreversible optic nerve damage.

Patients and family members should be educated to the symptoms of pupillary block and encouraged to contact the surgeon's office immediately for concerns. If pupillary block occurs, the patient should be re-dilated in the office and placed in supine position to attempt to move the air onto the anterior chamber and break the block. If this does not suffice, immediate surgical exchange of air is warranted.

4.6.2 Interface Fluid

Interface fluid can be present in the early postoperative period, and it can be visualized with careful slit lamp examination with a thin slit beam. Interface fluid is usually accompanied by overlying recipient stromal edema, and in cases of persistent corneal edema with no apparent interface fluid, AS-OCT should be considered both for the diagnosis and quantification of interface fluid with partial graft–host separation that cannot be assessed clinically.

Retained viscoelastic in the donor–recipient interface has been reported to create a reticular-patterned haze in the interface (▶ Fig. 4.7a) that usually resolves during the postoperative period without consequences in final visual acuity[102] but,

in occasions, can be visually significant (▶ Fig. 4.7b, c).[103,104] Demonstration of interface fluid gaps with iOCT has been associated with interface textural haze and late postoperative graft–recipient gap closure.[54] Therefore, complete removal of viscoelastic with irrigation and aspiration prior to donor graft insertion is crucial for lenticule attachment.

Interface fluid can disappear spontaneously. Strict IOP control and, in some cases, prone position can be useful.[49] Even though some techniques have been described to remove the interface fluid in the slit lamp when venting incisions have been made,[105] most of surgeons prefer to observe and determine if spontaneous reattachment occurs. In some grafts that fail to re-attach, re-bubbling becomes necessary.

Re-bubbling can be done in many settings, either at the slit lamp, in a minor procedure room with a sterile field, or in the operating room. Recently, re-bubbling at the slit lamp using intravenous extension tubing has been described, improving the ergonomics and patient comfort during the procedure with successful anterior chamber air fill.[106] Regardless of the technique used, the majority of re-bubbling procedures are successful in re-apposing the graft, which, in most of cases, remains attached.[107] It is important to attempt to include only one large bubble when re-bubbling as there appears to be some endothelial damage when there are multiple bubbles (i.e, "fish eggs") in the anterior chamber. Should re-bubbling fail, a repeated re-bubbling procedure can be done, and in recalcitrant cases, repeated EK should be considered. Repeat grafting will also eliminate possible biologic tissue dysfunction that could be interfering with the reattachment of the lenticule.

4.6.3 Graft Dislocation

Graft dislocation (▶ Fig. 4.8a) and graft detachment (▶ Fig. 4.8b, c) have been reported as the most common postoperative complications both in DSAEK and DMEK series.[55,107,108] The most common causes include interface fluid or viscoelastic and remnants of Descemet's membrane. Other causes of graft dislocation can be eye rubbing, failure to maintain supine position as instructed, and abnormal IOP, with both intraocular hypertension and hypotony reported.[49]

Despite the use of intraoperative strategies to maximize postoperative graft adhesion, risk factors inherent to the donor graft tissue or the recipient have not been clearly identified[101,109] and graft dislocation can still occur. The rates of postoperative graft detachment and dislocation in large DSAEK case series

Table 4.4 Common postoperative complications after DSAEK

First postoperative week	Postoperative month 1	After postoperative month 6
• Pupillary block (usually postoperative day 1) • Interface fluid • Graft detachment	• Ocular hypertension due to steroid response • Primary graft failure: failure of cornea to clear despite of graft attachment • Epithelial downgrowth	• Immunologic graft rejection • Secondary graft failure: endothelial cell decompensation or due to immunologic graft rejection • Epithelial downgrowth

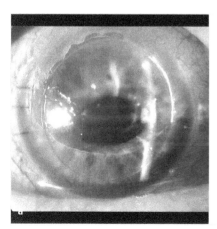
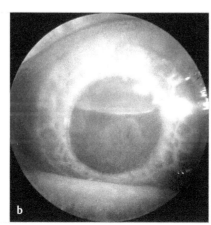

Fig. 4.6 Postoperative anterior **(a)** and posterior **(b)** pupillary block after DSAEK. DSAEK, Descemet's stripping automated endothelial keratoplasty. (These images are provided courtesy of W. Barry Lee, MD.)

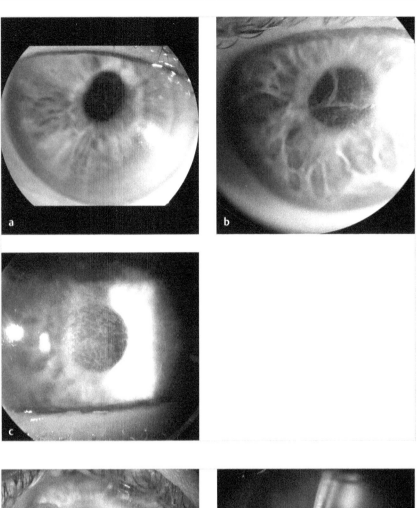

Fig. 4.7 Mild **(a)**, moderate **(b)**, and severe, visually significant **(c)** reticular interface haze from retained viscoelastic after Descemet's stripping automated endothelial keratoplasty. (These images are provided courtesy of W. Barry Lee, MD.)

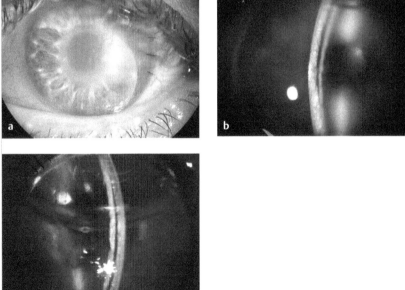

Fig. 4.8 Graft dislocation **(a)**, and partial **(b)** and total **(c)** lenticule detachment after Descemet's stripping automated endothelial keratoplasty. (These images are provided courtesy of [a] W. Barry Lee, MD and [b,c] Anthony Aldave, MD.)

range from 2[58] to 82%,[6,90,107,109,110] depending on intraoperative techniques used to promote attachment and the surgeon's level of expertise; whereas the published series after UT-DSAEK have reported 4 to 5%[8,29,88] and DMEK case series a wide range between 4 and 40%, probably related to surgeon's learning curves, tissue manipulation,[28,111,112,113] and larger amount of partial detachments.[47,111,113,114]

The vast majority of these detachments resolve after air reinjection procedures (or "re-bubbling") in up to 35% in large DSAEK series and a meta-analyses,[68,90,115] 3.9% after UT-DSAEK,[29] and as high as the 62% after DMEK.[47,75,115] (▶ Fig. 4.9)

In contrast, the rate of graft detachment in DMEK patients has been reported to be as high as 34.6[99] and 62%.[75] The majority

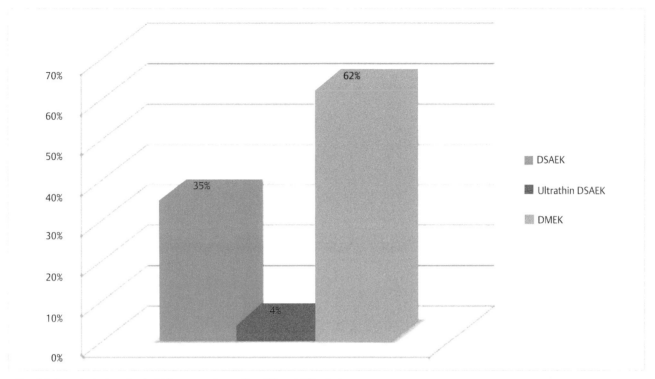

Fig. 4.9 Reported rates of re-bubbling procedures after different EK techniques.

of these detachments are peripheral and less than one-third of the graft, with complete detachment happening only in few cases. AS-OCT can be a good predictor of graft attachment, especially when performed during the first hour postoperatively. Full attachment, less than one-third graft detachment during the first postoperative hour, and complete attachment 1 week postoperatively have all been shown to be good predictors of attachment at 6 months.[116]

When a graft is detached, careful slit lamp examination must be performed until the lenticule is located. Trypan blue can be administered to stain the DMEK lenticule if not visible. If the lenticule is not located in the anterior chamber, pupillary dilation is necessary as it may have descended into the posterior pole, in which case, pupil dilation followed by prone positioning is needed to bring the lenticule into the anterior chamber. Anterior chamber depth, position of the iris, and assessment of the residual air bubble, if applicable, are also important features to note in these cases.

Once a graft detachment is diagnosed, the decision of re-bubbling versus observation for spontaneous reattachment should be done on a case-by-case basis, following a discussion between the surgeon and the patient. Even DSAEK cases that have been completely detached and dislocated into the posterior pole have been reported to reattach fully after persistent-prone position.[117]

4.6.4 Graft Failure

▸Table 4.5 summarizes the two types of graft failure, their frequency, etiology, clinical manifestations, and management. Two forms of graft failure can compromise success and visual outcomes: primary and secondary graft failure.

Primary Graft Failure

Primary graft failure (▸Fig. 4.10) refers to failure of corneal edema to resolve postoperatively due to persistent endothelial decompensation with or without graft detachment. According to the eye bank association, a primary graft failure is "reasonably likely" attributable to biologic tissue dysfunction if all three of the following criteria are present: corneal edema present from the time of surgery that does not clear after 8 weeks, no known intraoperative complications or postoperative complications, and no recipient conditions that would explain the biologic dysfunction. Endothelial cell loss or decompensation from surgical trauma and excessive tissue manipulation, that is, *iatrogenic graft failure*, is a very common cause of primary graft failure, especially in DMEK cases. Therefore, adequate wound size (5 mm), minimizing graft manipulation and avoiding traumatic graft insertion, will decrease the risk of primary graft failure.

The rate of primary graft failure has been reported from 0.86 to 5% after standard DSAEK,[90,118,119] 0.76 to 1.4% after UT-DSAEK,[29,88] and 4 to 8% after DMEK cases,[75,114] the latter likely from iatrogenic failure due to complexity in tissue manipulation.[120]

The histopathologic findings of removed failed DSAEK lenticules show, in most cases, a significant degree of endothelial cell attenuation, evidence of retained material either on the interface stromal side or in the endothelial side, retained host Descemet's membrane or presence of full-thickness cornea from eccentric trephination,[121,122] and electronic microscopy of DMEK failed grafts, most commonly shows a decreased density of endothelial cells and thickened Descemet's membrane with diffuse abnormal collagen inclusions. This demonstrates that the main causes of primary graft failure in all EK cases are related to the procedure and tissue manipulation and a possible pre-existing endothelial cell dysfunction prior to transplantation.[120]

Secondary Graft Failure

Secondary graft failure ▶ Fig. 4.11a, b), reported in up to 3.5% of cases[119,123] of DSAEK and 0.7% in 1-year follow-up of DMEK cases,[75] occurs after there had been an initial postoperative improvement of corneal edema with visual rehabilitation, followed by a later decompensation of the endothelial cells.

Overall, the average 5-year DSAEK graft survival has been reported to be 94% in patients without glaucoma, 93% in patients with prior medically treated glaucoma, and 40% in patients with prior filtering procedures.[98] The common denominator for secondary graft failure is endothelial cell loss after DSAEK and immunologic rejection in DMEK cases.[75]

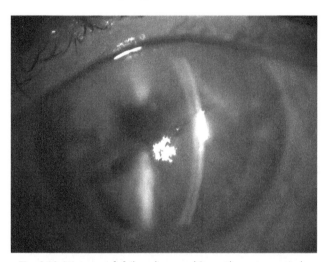

Fig. 4.10 Primary graft failure diagnosed 3 months postoperatively (L mark created by eye bank). (These images are provided courtesy of Anthony Aldave, MD.)

Histopathologic examination of failed DSAEK grafts has shown hypocellularity in both the stromal or the endothelial cell layer in most of the cases (▶ Fig. 4.12a–d), persistent fetal Descemet's membrane, retained fragments of Descemet's membrane, partial donor Descemet's membrane detachment, blood in the graft–host interface, retrocorneal fibrous membrane, epithelial downgrowth, and eccentric trephination of donor.[124,125] Comparatively, analyses of DMEK failed grafts mostly show loss of endothelial cell layer, and it is of note that in upside down grafts, not only the endothelial cell layer remains intact but there appears to be some metabolic activity in the endothelial cells.[126]

The treatment of a failed DSAEK graft is a repeated procedure, either with the same initial technique than the primary procedure (except from descemetorrhexis) or with a different EK technique with careful attention to peripheral stromal scrapping with the Terry scraper and complete removal of interface air and fluid during DSAEK procedures. Postoperative management is also the same as the primary procedure, with strict topical steroid treatment over the first 2 to 3 months, followed by a slow monthly taper and potentially indefinite treatment with a low-potency topical steroid.

4.6.5 Immunologic Graft Rejection

The rate of immunologic graft rejection of 2.1% after UT-DSAEK[29] compared to 7.6%[127] after DSAEK is likely explained to be the reduction of transplanted stromal tissue, decreasing the antigenic load associated with the stromal tissue and reducing the chances of immune reaction. This is further demonstrated by the even lower rate of rejection after DMEK, reported as inexistent by 6 months,[114] and as low as 0.7 to 0.8% after 1 and 2 years, respectively.[115,128]

The Kaplan–Meier predictions of probability of rejection at 12 and 24 months are also lower after UT-DSAEK compared to DSAEK (▶ Fig. 4.13)[29,70,115,129] and both comparable to the projected risk of rejection after PK of 5 to 14% and 15 to 29% within the first and second year, respectively.[115,123,129,130,131] In contrast,

Table 4.5 Features of primary and secondary DSAEK graft failure

	Primary	Secondary
Etiology	Endothelial cell failure	Immunologic rejection Failure to improve visual acuity despite of clear graft (no clinical manifestations)
Frequency	DSAEK: 5% DMEK: 8%	Immunologic graft rejection in 1 year: DSAEK: 4–9% DMEK: 0.7–5% Failure to improve vision: DSAEK: 2.3%
Clinical manifestations	Symptoms: painless. Failure to improve visual acuity after surgery Findings: failure to clear corneal edema postoperatively. Stromal edema, stromal folds, attached graft	Symptoms: pain, irritation, photophobia, decline in visual acuity Findings: immunologic rejection: keratic precipitates, stromal edema, stromal folds, anterior chamber inflammation
Management	Repeat procedure	Aggressive treatment with topical steroid: pred. acetate 1% every hour until resolution, then taper monthly up to one drop more than when rejected. Repeat procedure if rejection progresses to graft failure

Abbreviations: DSAEK, Descemet's stripping automated endothelial keratoplasty; DMEK, Descemet's membrane endothelial keratoplasty; pred., prednisolone.

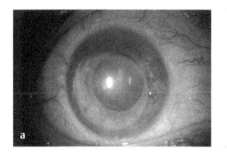
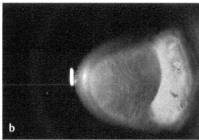

Fig. 4.11 (a,b) Secondary graft failure. (These images are provided courtesy of J. Bradley Randleman, MD.)

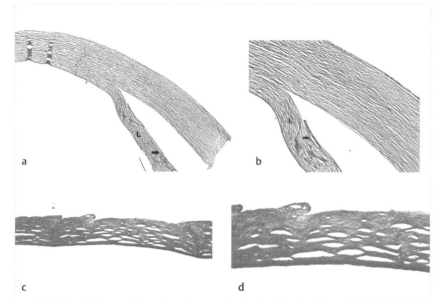

Fig. 4.12 Histopathology of failed Descemet's stripping automated endothelial keratoplasty lenticules 10 × (a), 25 × (b), 40 × (c), and 100 × (d). (These images are provided courtesy of H. Grossniklauss, MD.)

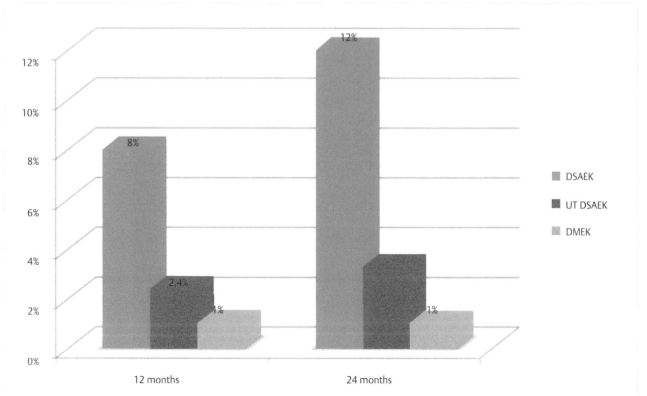

Fig. 4.13 Kaplan–Meier predictions of probability of rejection 1 and 2 years after DSAEK,[129] ultrathin DSAEK,[132] and DMEK.[115]
DMEK, Descemet's membrane endothelial keratoplasty; DSAEK, Descemet's stripping automated endothelial keratoplasty; UT DSAEK, ultrathin Descemet's stripping automated endothelial keratoplasty.

the projected probabilities of immunologic graft rejection after DMEK are significantly lower at 1% both at the first and second years,[49,115] providing a significant advantage from the immune reaction standpoint and an alternative in patient with higher risk or immune graft rejection prior to transplantation. Intensive topical steroid treatment remains the standard treatment for immune graft rejection, and the resolution of graft rejection with any of these strategies has been reported as 73.3 to 94% of cases within 6 months.[70,129]

The overall risk of rejection in the postoperative course increases with time from 6% on year 1 to 14% on year 2 and up to 22% on year 3.[70,94,138] This risk has been reported to be higher in African Americans, younger patients, patients with diagnoses different from Fuchs' dystrophy, and patients with history of glaucoma and prior glaucoma surgeries.[70,119] The most common etiology, however, is sudden cessation of steroid treatment.[70]

Immunologic rejection of DSAEK grafts ranges between 4 and 9%.[1,70,94,127,133,134] Thinner EK lenticules, such as in UT-DSAEK

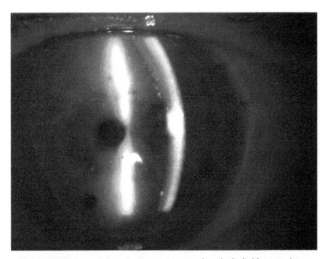

Fig. 4.14 Descemet's stripping automated endothelial keratoplasty raft rejection with diffuse keratic precipitates. (These images are provided courtesy of Anthony Aldave, MD.)

and DMEK, have a lower rejection rate,[29,135] likely due to less stromal tissue transplanted, ranging from 0.7 to 5.1% after DMEK.[75,99,115]

All keratoplasty patients should be well educated to recognize the symptoms of rejection and be asked to contact the surgeon's office should any of these symptoms arise, as early initiation of aggressive treatment increases the chances of graft recovery. Common symptoms of rejection are decreased vision, ocular injection, photophobia, and pain. Detectable signs at the slit lamp include diffuse keratic precipitates (▶Fig. 4.14), occasionally presenting as an endothelial rejection line, corneal edema with stromal folds, anterior chamber cells, and conjunctival injection.[70]

Graft rejection should be treated aggressively with frequent topical steroids, such as prednisolone acetate 1% every hour or difluprednate four to six times daily. Furthermore, in recalcitrant cases, 4-mg oral steroids or subconjunctival triamcinolone can be considered.

Ongoing assessment of IOP is essential during treatment of acute graft rejection, because IOP elevation due to high dose steroid treatment is not infrequent. Once the initial episode of rejection has resolved, a slow extended taper of steroids will decrease the risk of recurrent rejection. Occasionally, these patients will need long-term treatment with a dosage slightly above the dosage that precipitated the rejection.

4.6.6 Epithelial Downgrowth

The source of epithelial cells can be host epithelial cells implanted into the anterior chamber during the insertion of the donor graft, donor retained epithelial cells implanted following eccentric trephination (▶Fig. 4.15a),[136] or host epithelial cell migration most commonly from the corneal epithelium but also potentially from conjunctival epithelium.[124]

The point of entrance for host epithelium can be a poorly constructed or closed wound, disrupted wound architecture,

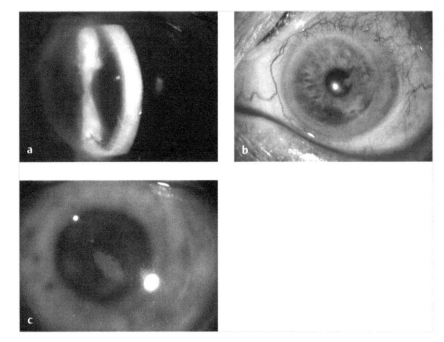

Fig. 4.15 Epithelial downgrowth in Descemet's stripping automated endothelial keratoplasty due to full peripheral trephination (**a**), venting incision (**b**), and occasionally forming epithelial pearls (**c**). (These images are provided courtesy of Anthony Aldave, MD.)

either by vitreous prolapse, iris prolapse, or debris within the corneal incision or through venting incisions (▶Fig. 4.15b). DSAEK with stromal puncture is a risk factor for epithelial ingrowth,[137] which is why most surgeons have abandoned intraoperative stromal puncture technique for interface fluid drainage.

Epithelial downgrowth can appear in the stromal interface as an irregular flat haze. The epithelial pearls then become confluent and homogenously white with a sharp demarcation (▶Fig. 4.15c). Immediate surgery is not necessary if the patient is asymptomatic. Peripheral epithelial pearls not affecting the visual axis can be monitored closely for progression. Some reports have shown the improvement in interface haze with intracameral administration of 0.1 mL of 5-fluoroacil (400 µg/mL) and the elimination of membranes with argon laser treatments in recalcitrant, recurrent cases.[136,138] Moreover, repeat EK can be performed if it becomes necessary.

4.6.7 Interface Haze and Irregularity

One of the biggest challenges in DSAEK, more than in DMEK, is to achieve good postoperative uncorrected distance visual acuity and quality of vision. Scarring and irregularities of the graft–host interface can cause interface haze that can compromise visual quality.[103]

Aside of irregularities in the lenticule resulting from donor preparation, another cause of postoperative interface haze and irregularity is incomplete removal of Descemet's membrane, which can induce light scatter as well as interfere with complete lenticule attachment.

Management of interface haze initially involves observation, as in most cases, it will resolve spontaneously or persist without affecting final visual acuity. However, in cases of limited visual acuity due to interface haze or lenticule folds in the central axis, a repeated DSAEK can be performed with good outcomes.

4.6.8 Posterior Surface Astigmatism

One of the greatest advantages of EK over PK is the significantly less induction of postoperative anterior corneal irregular astigmatism, because EK eliminates corneal suture-related irregularities. The anterior corneal curvature remains relatively stable after DSAEK; however, the posterior corneal curvature changes drastically when the donor tissue is inserted into the posterior recipient cornea. DSAEK grafts classically induce a hyperopic shift of 0.8 to 1.5 D,[6,110,135] and the suboptimal final visual acuity and relatively slow visual rehabilitation seen in DSAEK may be related to the irregularities of the donor graft and posterior surface astigmatism. New techniques including UT-DSAEK, PDEK, and DMEK have been introduced to allow faster visual rehabilitation and to improved visual outcomes.[103,135] Posterior HOAs after DMEK are significantly less compared to DSAEK and PK.[13]

Occasionally, patients with significant lenticule folds located in the visual axis can experience distortion in visual acuity. These patients usually do rather well with a repeated DSAEK or DMEK procedure.[119]

4.7 Repeat DSAEK

In a report by Letko et al, 76% of repeated DSAEK were due to dissatisfaction with visual acuity, despite of the absence of other corneal abnormalities on examination, compared to 24% due to endothelial decompensation and corneal edema.[119]

Regardless of the indication to repeat the procedure, repeated DSAEK results in improvement of visual acuity in 97% of cases; therefore, in patients without clinical findings, who undergo DSAEK only due to dissatisfaction with final visual acuity, the majority experience improvement in visual acuity, and essentially 100% of patients, who undergo repeated DSAEK due to graft failure from endothelial decompensation, also experience improvement in visual acuity after the repeated procedure.[119]

4.8 Conclusion

The development of EK has revolutionized the field of keratoplasty by offering a less invasive transplantation alternative to patients with corneal pathology confined to the endothelium. Despite conflicting evidence, lenticule thickness does appear to play a role in postoperative outcomes and immunologic rejection, as thinner lenticule transplantation procedures such as DMEK offer potentially better outcomes and lower risk of rejection. However, the learning curve for DMEK is quite steep and it requires specific conditions for lenticule unfolding that make some patients poor candidates. DSAEK remains a solid alternative for these patients and remains the standard EK technique in many surgeons' hands.

References

[1] Price MO, Gorovoy M, Price FW, Jr, Benetz BA, Menegay HJ, Lass JH. Descemet's stripping automated endothelial keratoplasty: three-year graft and endothelial cell survival compared with penetrating keratoplasty. Ophthalmology 2013;120(2):246–251

[2] Tillett CW. Posterior lamellar keratoplasty. Am J Ophthalmol. 1956;41(3): 530–533

[3] Melles GR, Eggink FA, Lander F, et al. A surgical technique for posterior lamellar keratoplasty. Cornea 1998;17(6):618–626

[4] Terry MA, Ousley PJ. Deep lamellar endothelial keratoplasty in the first United States patients: early clinical results. Cornea 2001;20(3):239–243

[5] Melles GR, Wijdh RH, Nieuwendaal CP. A technique to excise the descemet membrane from a recipient cornea (descemetorhexis). Cornea 2004;23(3):286–288

[6] Gorovoy MS. Descemet-stripping automated endothelial keratoplasty. Cornea 2006;25(8):886–889

[7] Melles GR, Ong TS, Ververs B, van der Wees J. Descemet membrane endothelial keratoplasty (DMEK). Cornea 2006;25(8):987–990

[8] Busin M, Patel AK, Scorcia V, Ponzin D. Microkeratome-assisted preparation of ultrathin grafts for descemet stripping automated endothelial keratoplasty. Invest Ophthalmol Vis Sci 2012;53(1):521–524

[9] Chen ES, Shamie N, Terry MA. Descemet-stripping endothelial keratoplasty: improvement in vision following replacement of a healthy endothelial graft. J Cataract Refract Surg 2008;34(6):1044–1046

[10] Chen ES, Shamie N, Terry MA, Hoar KL. Endothelial keratoplasty: improvement of vision after healthy donor tissue exchange. Cornea 2008;27(3):279–282

[11] Hindman HB, Huxlin KR, Pantanelli SM, et al. Post-DSAEK optical changes: a comprehensive prospective analysis on the role of ocular wavefront aberrations, haze, and corneal thickness. Cornea 2013;32(12):1567–1577

[12] Koenig SB, Covert DJ, Dupps WJ, Jr, Meisler DM. Visual acuity, refractive error, and endothelial cell density six months after Descemet stripping and automated endothelial keratoplasty (DSAEK). Cornea 2007;26(6):670–674

[13] Rudolph M, Laaser K, Bachmann BO, Cursiefen C, Epstein D, Kruse FE. Corneal higher-order aberrations after Descemet's membrane endothelial keratoplasty. Ophthalmology 2012;119(3):528–535

[14] Muftuoglu O, Prasher P, Bowman RW, McCulley JP, Mootha VV. Corneal higher-order aberrations after Descemet's stripping automated endothelial keratoplasty. Ophthalmology 2010;117(5):878–884.e6

[15] Price MO, Price FW, Jr. Descemet's stripping with endothelial keratoplasty: comparative outcomes with microkeratome-dissected and manually dissected donor tissue. Ophthalmology 2006;113(11):1936–1942

[16] Rose L, Briceño CA, Stark WJ, Gloria DG, Jun AS. Assessment of eye bank-prepared posterior lamellar corneal tissue for endothelial keratoplasty. Ophthalmology 2008;115(2):279–286

[17] Price MO, Baig KM, Brubaker JW, Price FW, Jr. Randomized, prospective comparison of precut vs surgeon-dissected grafts for descemet stripping automated endothelial keratoplasty. Am J Ophthalmol 2008;146(1):36–41

[18] Chen ES, Terry MA, Shamie N, Hoar KL, Friend DJ. Precut tissue in Descemet's stripping automated endothelial keratoplasty donor characteristics and early postoperative complications. Ophthalmology 2008;115(3):497–502

[19] Terry MA. Endothelial keratoplasty: a comparison of complication rates and endothelial survival between precut tissue and surgeon-cut tissue by a single DSAEK surgeon. Trans Am Ophthalmol Soc 2009;107:184–191

[20] Thomas PB, Mukherjee AN, O'Donovan D, Rajan MS. Preconditioned donor corneal thickness for microthin endothelial keratoplasty. Cornea 2013; 32(7):e173–e178

[21] Nahum Y, Leon P, Busin M. Postoperative graft thickness obtained with single-pass microkeratome-assisted ultrathin Descemet stripping automated endothelial keratoplasty. Cornea 2015;34(11):1362–1364

[22] Villarrubia A, Cano-Ortiz A. Development of a nomogram to achieve ultrathin donor corneal disks for Descemet-stripping automated endothelial keratoplasty. J Cataract Refract Surg 2015;41(1):146–151

[23] Sikder S, Nordgren RN, Neravetla SR, Moshirfar M. Ultra-thin donor tissue preparation for endothelial keratoplasty with a double-pass microkeratome. Am J Ophthalmol 2011;152(2):202–208.e2

[24] Nieuwendaal CP, van Velthoven ME, Biallosterski C, et al. Thickness measurements of donor posterior disks after descemet stripping endothelial keratoplasty with anterior segment optical coherence tomography. Cornea 2009;28(3):298–303

[25] Dupps WJ, Jr, Qian Y, Meisler DM. Multivariate model of refractive shift in Descemet-stripping automated endothelial keratoplasty. J Cataract Refract Surg 2008;34(4):578–584

[26] Choulakian MY, Li JY, Ramos S, Mannis MJ. Single-pass microkeratome system for eye bank DSAEK tissue preparation: is stromal bed thickness predictable and reproducible? Cornea 2016;35(1):95–99

[27] Terry MA. Endothelial keratoplasty: why aren't we all doing Descemet membrane endothelial keratoplasty? Cornea 2012;31(5):469–471

[28] Dapena I, Ham L, Droutsas K, van Dijk K, Moutsouris K, Melles GR. Learning curve in Descemet's membrane endothelial keratoplasty: first series of 135 consecutive cases. Ophthalmology 2011;118(11):2147–2154

[29] Busin M, Madi S, Santorum P, Scorcia V, Beltz J. Ultrathin descemet's stripping automated endothelial keratoplasty with the microkeratome double-pass technique: two-year outcomes. Ophthalmology 2013;120(6):1186–1194

[30] Woodward MA, Titus MS, Shtein RM. Effect of microkeratome pass on tissue processing for Descemet stripping automated endothelial keratoplasty. Cornea 2014;33(5):507–509

[31] Heinzelmann S, Maier P, Bohringer D, Auw-Hadrich C, Reinhard T. Visual outcome and histological findings following femtosecond laser-assisted versus microkeratome-assisted DSAEK. Graefe's archive for clinical and experimental ophthalmology/Albrecht Von Graefes Arch Klin Exp Ophthalmol 2013;251(8):1979–1985

[32] Vetter JM, Butsch C, Faust M, et al. Irregularity of the posterior corneal surface after curved interface femtosecond laser-assisted versus microkeratome-assisted descemet stripping automated endothelial keratoplasty. Cornea 2013;32(2):118–124

[33] Soong HK, Mian S, Abbasi O, Juhasz T. Femtosecond laser-assisted posterior lamellar keratoplasty: initial studies of surgical technique in eye bank eyes. Ophthalmology 2005;112(1):44–49

[34] Phillips PM, Phillips LJ, Saad HA, et al. "Ultrathin" DSAEK tissue prepared with a low-pulse energy, high-frequency femtosecond laser. Cornea 2013;32(1):81–86

[35] Bernard A, He Z, Gauthier AS, et al. Femtosecond laser cutting of endothelial grafts: comparison of endothelial and epithelial applanation. Cornea 2015;34(2):209–217

[36] Cheng YY, Schouten JS, Tahzib NG, et al. Efficacy and safety of femtosecond laser-assisted corneal endothelial keratoplasty: a randomized multicenter clinical trial. Transplantation 2009;88(11):1294–1302

[37] Feng Y, Qu HQ, Ren J, Prahs P, Hong J. Corneal endothelial cell loss in femtosecond laser-assisted Descemet's stripping automated endothelial keratoplasty: A 12-month follow-up study. Chin Med J (Engl) 2017;130(24):2927–2932

[38] Ivarsen A, Hjortdal J. Clinical outcome of Descemet's stripping endothelial keratoplasty with femtosecond laser-prepared grafts. Acta Ophthalmol 2018;96(5):e655–e656

[39] Mootha VV, Heck E, Verity SM, et al. Comparative study of descemet stripping automated endothelial keratoplasty donor preparation by Moria CBm microkeratome, horizon microkeratome, and Intralase FS60. Cornea 2011;30(3):320–324

[40] Jones YJ, Goins KM, Sutphin JE, Mullins R, Skeie JM. Comparison of the femtosecond laser (IntraLase) versus manual microkeratome (Moria ALTK) in dissection of the donor in endothelial keratoplasty: initial study in eye bank eyes. Cornea 2008;27(1):88–93

[41] Liu YC, Teo EP, Adnan KB, et al. Endothelial approach ultrathin corneal grafts prepared by femtosecond laser for descemet stripping endothelial keratoplasty. Invest Ophthalmol Vis Sci 2014;55(12):8393–8401

[42] Price MO, Bidros M, Gorovoy M, et al. Effect of incision width on graft survival and endothelial cell loss after Descemet stripping automated endothelial keratoplasty. Cornea 2010;29(5):523–527

[43] Terry MA, Saad HA, Shamie N, et al. Endothelial keratoplasty: the influence of insertion techniques and incision size on donor endothelial survival. Cornea 2009;28(1):24–31

[44] Pilger D, von Sonnleithner C, Bertelmann E, Joussen AM, Torun N. Femtosecond laser-assisted descemetorhexis: a novel technique in Descemet membrane endothelial keratoplasty. Cornea 2016;35(10):1274–1278

[45] Einan-Lifshitz A, Sorkin N, Boutin T, et al. Comparison of femtosecond laser-enabled descemetorhexis and manual descemetorhexis in Descemet membrane endothelial keratoplasty. Cornea 2017;36(7):767–770

[46] Einan-Lifshitz A, Sorkin N, Boutin T, et al. Descemet membrane endothelial keratoplasty for failed deep anterior lamellar keratoplasty: a case series. Cornea 2018;37(6):682–686

[47] Price MO, Giebel AW, Fairchild KM, Price FW, Jr. Descemet's membrane endothelial keratoplasty: prospective multicenter study of visual and refractive outcomes and endothelial survival. Ophthalmology 2009;116(12):2361–2368

[48] Terry MA, Hoar KL, Wall J, Ousley P. Histology of dislocations in endothelial keratoplasty (DSEK and DLEK): a laboratory-based, surgical solution to dislocation in 100 consecutive DSEK cases. Cornea 2006;25(8):926–932

[49] Hayes DD, Shih CY, Shamie N, et al. Spontaneous reattachment of Descemet stripping automated endothelial keratoplasty lenticles: a case series of 12 patients. Am J Ophthalmol 2010;150(6):790–797

[50] Kaiserman I, Bahar I, McAllum P, Slomovic AR, Rootman DS. Suture-assisted vs forceps-assisted insertion of the donor lenticula during Descemet stripping automated endothelial keratoplasty. Am J Ophthalmol 2008;145(6):986–990

[51] Bahar I, Kaiserman I, Sansanayudh W, Levinger E, Rootman DS. Busin guide vs forceps for the insertion of the donor lenticule in Descemet stripping automated endothelial keratoplasty. Am J Ophthalmol 2009;147(2): 220–226.e1

[52] Khor WB, Han SB, Mehta JS, Tan DT. Descemet stripping automated endothelial keratoplasty with a donor insertion device: clinical results and complications in 100 eyes. Am J Ophthalmol 2013;156(4):773–779

[53] Foster JB, Swan KR, Vasan RA, Greven MA, Walter KA. Small-incision Descemet stripping automated endothelial keratoplasty: a comparison of small-incision tissue injector and forceps techniques. Cornea 2012;31(1):42–47

[54] Juthani VV, Goshe JM, Srivastava SK, Ehlers JP. Association between transient interface fluid on intraoperative OCT and textural interface opacity after DSAEK surgery in the PIONEER study. Cornea 2014;33(9):887–892

[55] Price FW Jr, Price MO. Descemet's stripping with endothelial keratoplasty in 200 eyes: Early challenges and techniques to enhance donor adherence. J Cataract Refract Surg 2006;32(3):411–418

[56] Miyakoshi A, Ozaki H, Otsuka M, Hayashi A. Efficacy of intraoperative anterior segment optical coherence tomography during Descemet's stripping automated endothelial keratoplasty. ISRN Ophthalmol 2014;2014:562062

[57] Knecht PB, Kaufmann C, Menke MN, Watson SL, Bosch MM. Use of intraoperative fourier-domain anterior segment optical coherence tomography during descemet stripping endothelial keratoplasty. Am J Ophthalmol 2010;150(3):360–365.e2

[58] Terry MA, Shamie N, Chen ES, Hoar KL, Friend DJ. Endothelial keratoplasty a simplified technique to minimize graft dislocation, iatrogenic graft failure, and pupillary block. Ophthalmology 2008;115(7):1179–1186

[59] Acar BT, Muftuoglu O, Acar S. Comparison of sulfur hexafluoride and air for donor attachment in Descemet stripping endothelial keratoplasty in patients with pseudophakic bullous keratopathy. Cornea 2014;33(3):219–222

[60] Güell JL, Morral M, Gris O, Elies D, Manero F. Bimanual technique for insertion and positioning of endothelium-Descemet membrane graft in Descemet membrane endothelial keratoplasty. Cornea 2013;32(12):1521–1526

[61] Rickmann A, Szurman P, Jung S, et al. Impact of 10% SF6 gas compared to 100% air tamponade in Descemet's membrane endothelial keratoplasty. Curr Eye Res 2018;43(4):482–486

[62] Siebelmann S, Lopez Ramos S, Scholz P, et al. Graft detachment pattern after Descemet membrane endothelial keratoplasty comparing air versus 20% SF6 tamponade. Cornea 2018;37(7):834–839

[63] Marques RE, Guerra PS, Sousa DC, et al. Sulfur hexafluoride 20% versus air 100% for anterior chamber tamponade in DMEK: a meta-analysis. Cornea 2018;37(6):691–697

[64] Botsford B, Vedana G, Cope L, Yiu SC, Jun AS. Comparison of 20% sulfur hexafluoride with air for intraocular tamponade in Descemet membrane endothelial keratoplasty (DMEK). Arq Bras Oftalmol 2016;79(5):299–302

[65] Schaub F, Enders P, Snijders K, et al. One-year outcome after Descemet membrane endothelial keratoplasty (DMEK) comparing sulfur hexafluoride (SF6) 20% versus 100% air for anterior chamber tamponade. Br J Ophthalmol 2017;101(7):902–908

[66] Güell JL, Morral M, Gris O, Elies D, Manero F. Comparison of sulfur hexafluoride 20% versus air tamponade in Descemet membrane endothelial keratoplasty. Ophthalmology 2015;122(9):1757–1764

[67] von Marchtaler PV, Weller JM, Kruse FE, Tourtas T. Air versus sulfur hexafluoride gas tamponade in Descemet membrane endothelial keratoplasty: a fellow eye comparison. Cornea 2018;37(1):15–19

[68] Schaub F, Simons HG, Roters S, et al. [Influence of 20% sulfur hexafluoride (SF6) on human corneal endothelial cells: An in vitro study] Ophthalmologe 2016;113(1):52–57

[69] Steven P, Le Blanc C, Velten K, et al. Optimizing descemet membrane endothelial keratoplasty using intraoperative optical coherence tomography. JAMA Ophthalmol 2013;131(9):1135–1142

[70] Wu EI, Ritterband DC, Yu G, Shields RA, Seedor JA. Graft rejection following descemet stripping automated endothelial keratoplasty: features, risk factors, and outcomes. Am J Ophthalmol 2012;153(5):949–957.e1

[71] Shimazaki J, Iseda A, Satake Y, Shimazaki-Den S. Efficacy and safety of long-term corticosteroid eye drops after penetrating keratoplasty: a prospective, randomized, clinical trial. Ophthalmology 2012;119(4):668–673

[72] Price MO, Price FW Jr, Kruse FE, Bachmann BO, Tourtas T. Randomized comparison of topical prednisolone acetate 1% versus fluorometholone 0.1% in the first year after descemet membrane endothelial keratoplasty. Cornea 2014;33(9):880–886

[73] Li JY, Terry MA, Goshe J, Davis-Boozer D, Shamie N. Three-year visual acuity outcomes after Descemet's stripping automated endothelial keratoplasty. Ophthalmology 2012;119(6):1126–1129

[74] van Dijk K, Ham L, Tse WH, et al. Near complete visual recovery and refractive stability in modern corneal transplantation: Descemet membrane endothelial keratoplasty (DMEK). Cont Lens Anterior Eye 2013;36(1):13–21

[75] Guerra FP, Anshu A, Price MO, Giebel AW, Price FW. Descemet's membrane endothelial keratoplasty: prospective study of 1-year visual outcomes, graft survival, and endothelial cell loss. Ophthalmology 2011;118(12):2368–2373

[76] Terry MA, Straiko MD, Goshe JM, Li JY, Davis-Boozer D. Descemet's stripping automated endothelial keratoplasty: the tenuous relationship between donor thickness and postoperative vision. Ophthalmology 2012;119(10):1988–1996

[77] Woodward MA, Raoof-Daneshvar D, Mian S, Shtein RM. Relationship of visual acuity and lamellar thickness in descemet stripping automated endothelial keratoplasty. Cornea 2013;32(5):e69–e73

[78] Van Cleynenbreugel H, Remeijer L, Hillenaar T. Descemet stripping automated endothelial keratoplasty: effect of intraoperative lenticule thickness on visual outcome and endothelial cell density. Cornea 2011;30(11):1195–1200

[79] Phillips PM, Phillips LJ, Maloney CM. Preoperative graft thickness measurements do not influence final BSCVA or speed of vision recovery after descemet stripping automated endothelial keratoplasty. Cornea 2013;32(11):1423–1427

[80] Ahmed KA, McLaren JW, Baratz KH, Maguire LJ, Kittleson KM, Patel SV. Host and graft thickness after Descemet stripping endothelial keratoplasty for Fuchs endothelial dystrophy. Am J Ophthalmol 2010;150(4):490–497.e2

[81] Lombardo M, Terry MA, Lombardo G, Boozer DD, Serrao S, Ducoli P. Analysis of posterior donor corneal parameters 1 year after Descemet stripping automated endothelial keratoplasty (DSAEK) triple procedure. Graefes Arch Clin Exp Ophthalmol 2010;248(3):421–427

[82] Acar BT, Akdemir MO, Acar S. Visual acuity and endothelial cell density with respect to the graft thickness in Descemet's stripping automated endothelial keratoplasty: one year results. Int J Ophthalmol 2014;7(6):974–979

[83] Dickman MM, Cheng YY, Berendschot TT, van den Biggelaar FJ, Nuijts RM. Effects of graft thickness and asymmetry on visual gain and aberrations after descemet stripping automated endothelial keratoplasty. JAMA Ophthalmol 2013;131(6):737–744

[84] Daoud YJ, Munro AD, Delmonte DD, et al. Effect of cornea donor graft thickness on the outcome of Descemet stripping automated endothelial keratoplasty surgery. Am J Ophthalmol 2013;156(5):860–866.e1

[85] Shinton AJ, Tsatsos M, Konstantopoulos A, et al. Impact of graft thickness on visual acuity after Descemet's stripping endothelial keratoplasty. Br J Ophthalmol 2012;96(2):246–249

[86] Wacker K, Bourne WM, Patel SV. Effect of graft thickness on visual acuity after Descemet stripping endothelial keratoplasty: a systematic review and meta-analysis. Am J Ophthalmol 2016;163:18–28

[87] Di Pascuale MA, Prasher P, Schlecte C, et al. Corneal deturgescence after Descemet stripping automated endothelial keratoplasty evaluated by Visante anterior segment optical coherence tomography. Am J Ophthalmol 2009;148(1):32–37.e1

[88] Roberts HW, Mukherjee A, Aichner H, Rajan MS. Visual outcomes and graft thickness in microthin DSAEK—one-year Results. Cornea 2015;34(11):1345–1350

[89] van Dijk K, Droutsas K, Hou J, Sangsari S, Liarakos VS, Melles GR. Optical quality of the cornea after Descemet membrane endothelial keratoplasty. Am J Ophthalmol 2014;158(1):71–79.e1

[90] Lee WB, Jacobs DS, Musch DC, Kaufman SC, Reinhart WJ, Shtein RM. Descemet's stripping endothelial keratoplasty: safety and outcomes: a report by the American Academy of Ophthalmology. Ophthalmology 2009;116(9):1818–1830

[91] Esquenazi S, Rand W. Effect of the shape of the endothelial graft on the refractive results after Descemet's stripping with automated endothelial keratoplasty. Can J Ophthalmol/Journal Canadien d'ophtalmologie 2009;44(5):557–561

[92] Clemmensen K, Ivarsen A, Hjortdal J. Changes in corneal power after Descemet stripping automated endothelial keratoplasty. J Refract Surg 2015;31(12):807–812

[93] Newman LR, Rosenwasser GO, Dubovy SR, Matthews JL. Clinicopathologic correlation of textural interface opacities in descemet stripping automated endothelial keratoplasty: a case study. Cornea 2014;33(3):306–309

[94] Li JY, Terry MA, Goshe J, Shamie N, Davis-Boozer D. Graft rejection after Descemet's stripping automated endothelial keratoplasty: graft survival and endothelial cell loss. Ophthalmology 2012;119(1):90–94

[95] Terry MA, Chen ES, Shamie N, Hoar KL, Friend DJ. Endothelial cell loss after Descemet's stripping endothelial keratoplasty in a large prospective series. Ophthalmology 2008;115(3):488–496.e3

[96] Price MO, Price FW Jr. Endothelial cell loss after descemet stripping with endothelial keratoplasty influencing factors and 2-year trend. Ophthalmology 2008;115(5):857–865

[97] Tenkman LR, Price FW, Price MO. Descemet membrane endothelial keratoplasty donor preparation: navigating challenges and improving efficiency. Cornea 2014;33(3):319–325

[98] Price MO, Fairchild KM, Price DA, Price FW, Jr. Descemet's stripping endothelial keratoplasty five-year graft survival and endothelial cell loss. Ophthalmology 2011;118(4):725–729

[99] Monnereau C, Quilendrino R, Dapena I, et al. Multicenter study of descemet membrane endothelial keratoplasty: first case series of 18 surgeons. JAMA Ophthalmol 2014;132(10):1192–1198

[100] Feng MT, Price MO, Miller JM, Price FW Jr. Air reinjection and endothelial cell density in Descemet membrane endothelial keratoplasty: five-year follow-up. J Cataract Refract Surg 2014;40(7):1116–1121

[101] Terry MA, Shamie N, Chen ES, Hoar KL, Phillips PM, Friend DJ. Endothelial keratoplasty: the influence of preoperative donor endothelial cell densities on dislocation, primary graft failure, and 1-year cell counts. Cornea 2008;27(10):1131–1137

[102] Vira S, Shih CY, Ragusa N, et al. Textural interface opacity after descemet stripping automated endothelial keratoplasty: a report of 30 cases and possible etiology. Cornea 2013;32(5):e54–e59

[103] Anshu A, Planchard B, Price MO, da R Pereira C, Price FW, Jr. A cause of reticular interface haze and its management after descemet stripping endothelial keratoplasty. Cornea 2012;31(12):1365–1368

[104] Chhadva P, Cabot F, Ziebarth N, Kymionis GD, Yoo SH. Persistent corneal opacity after descemet stripping automated endothelial keratoplasty suggesting inert material deposits into the interface. Cornea 2013;32(11):1512–1513

[105] Srinivasan S, Rootman DS. Slit-lamp technique of draining interface fluid following Descemet's stripping endothelial keratoplasty. Br J Ophthalmol 2007;91(9):1202–1205

[106] Sáles CS, Straiko MD, Terry MA. Novel technique for rebubbling DMEK grafts at the slit lamp using intravenous extension tubing. Cornea 2016;35(4):582–585

[107] Suh LH, Yoo SH, Deobhakta A, et al. Complications of Descemet's stripping with automated endothelial keratoplasty: survey of 118 eyes at One Institute. Ophthalmology 2008;115(9):1517–1524

[108] Droutsas K, Ham L, Dapena I, Geerling G, Oellerich S, Melles G. [Visual acuity following Descemet-membrane endothelial keratoplasty (DMEK): first 100 cases operated on for Fuchs endothelial dystrophy] Klin Monatsbl Augenheilkd 2010;227(6):467–477

[109] Hood CT, Woodward MA, Bullard ML, Shtein RM. Influence of preoperative donor tissue characteristics on graft dislocation rate after Descemet stripping automated endothelial keratoplasty. Cornea 2013;32(12): 1527–1530

[110] Koenig SB, Covert DJ. Early results of small-incision Descemet's stripping and automated endothelial keratoplasty. Ophthalmology 2007;114(2):221–226

[111] Gorovoy IR, Gorovoy MS. Descemet membrane endothelial keratoplasty postoperative year 1 endothelial cell counts. Am J Ophthalmol 2015;159(3): 597–600.e2

[112] Brockmann T, Brockmann C, Maier AK, et al. Clinicopathology of graft detachment after Descemet's membrane endothelial keratoplasty. Acta Ophthalmol 2014;92(7):e556–e561

[113] Green M, Wilkins MR. Comparison of early surgical experience and visual outcomes of DSAEK and DMEK. Cornea 2015;34(11):1341–1344

[114] Hamzaoglu EC, Straiko MD, Mayko ZM, Sáles CS, Terry MA. The first 100 eyes of standardized Descemet stripping automated endothelial keratoplasty versus standardized Descemet membrane endothelial keratoplasty. Ophthalmology 2015;122(11):2193–2199

[115] Anshu A, Price MO, Price FW Jr. Risk of corneal transplant rejection significantly reduced with Descemet's membrane endothelial keratoplasty. Ophthalmology 2012;119(3):536–540

[116] Yeh RY, Quilendrino R, Musa FU, Liarakos VS, Dapena I, Melles GR. Predictive value of optical coherence tomography in graft attachment after Descemet's membrane endothelial keratoplasty. Ophthalmology 2013;120(2): 240–245

[117] Kam KW, Young AL. Spontaneous reattachment of a posteriorly dislocated endothelial graft: a case report. Case Rep Transplant 2013;2013:631702

[118] Mojica G, Padnick-Silver L, Macsai MS. Incidence of presumed iatrogenic graft failure in Descemet stripping automated endothelial keratoplasty. Cornea 2012;31(8):872–875

[119] Letko E, Price DA, Lindoso EM, Price MO, Price FW Jr. Secondary graft failure and repeat endothelial keratoplasty after Descemet's stripping automated endothelial keratoplasty. Ophthalmology 2011;118(2):310–314

[120] Ćirković A, Schlötzer-Schrehardt U, Weller JM, Kruse FE, Tourtas T. Clinical and ultrastructural characteristics of graft failure in DMEK: 1-year results after repeat DMEK. Cornea 2015;34(1):11–17

[121] Suh LH, Dawson DG, Mutapcic L, et al. Histopathologic examination of failed grafts in descemet's stripping with automated endothelial keratoplasty. Ophthalmology 2009;116(4):603–608

[122] Oster SF, Ebrahimi KB, Eberhart CG, Schein OD, Stark WJ, Jun AS. A clinicopathologic series of primary graft failure after Descemet's stripping and automated endothelial keratoplasty. Ophthalmology 2009;116(4):609–614

[123] Price MO, Gorovoy M, Benetz BA, et al. Descemet's stripping automated endothelial keratoplasty outcomes compared with penetrating keratoplasty from the Cornea Donor Study. Ophthalmology 2010;117(3):438–444

[124] Phillips PM, Terry MA, Kaufman SC, Chen ES. Epithelial downgrowth after Descemet-stripping automated endothelial keratoplasty. J Cataract Refract Surg 2009;35(1):193–196

[125] Zhang Q, Randleman JB, Stulting RD, et al. Clinicopathologic findings in failed descemet stripping automated endothelial keratoplasty. Arch Ophthalmol 2010;128(8):973–980

[126] Yoeruek E, Hofmann J, Bartz-Schmidt KU. Histological and ultrastructural findings of corneal tissue after failed descemet membrane endothelial keratoplasty. Acta Ophthalmol 2014;92(3):e213–e216

[127] Jordan CS, Price MO, Trespalacios R, Price FW Jr. Graft rejection episodes after Descemet stripping with endothelial keratoplasty: part one: clinical signs and symptoms. Br J Ophthalmol 2009;93(3):387–390

[128] Dapena I, Ham L, Netuková M, van der Wees J, Melles GR. Incidence of early allograft rejection after Descemet membrane endothelial keratoplasty. Cornea 2011;30(12):1341–1345

[129] Price MO, Jordan CS, Moore G, Price FW, Jr. Graft rejection episodes after Descemet stripping with endothelial keratoplasty: part two: the statistical analysis of probability and risk factors. Br J Ophthalmol 2009;93(3):391–395

[130] Alldredge OC, Krachmer JH. Clinical types of corneal transplant rejection. Their manifestations, frequency, preoperative correlates, and treatment. Arch Ophthalmol 1981;99(4):599–604

[131] Claesson M, Armitage WJ, Fagerholm P, Stenevi U. Visual outcome in corneal grafts: a preliminary analysis of the Swedish Corneal Transplant Register. Br J Ophthalmol 2002;86(2):174–180

[132] Price FW Jr, Price MO. Descemet's stripping with endothelial keratoplasty in 50 eyes: a refractive neutral corneal transplant. J Refract Surg 2005;21(4):339–345

[133] Pedersen IB, Ivarsen A, Hjortdal J. Graft rejection and failure following endothelial keratoplasty (DSAEK) and penetrating keratoplasty for secondary endothelial failure. Acta ophthalmologica. 2015;93(2):172–177

[134] Ezon I, Shih CY, Rosen LM, Suthar T, Udell IJ. Immunologic graft rejection in descemet's stripping endothelial keratoplasty and penetrating keratoplasty for endothelial disease. Ophthalmology 2013;120(7):1360–1365

[135] Busin M, Albé E. Does thickness matter: ultrathin Descemet stripping automated endothelial keratoplasty. Curr Opin Ophthalmol 2014;25(4):312–318

[136] Itty S, Proia AD, DelMonte DW, Santaella RM, Carlson A, Allingham RR. Clinical course and origin of epithelium in cases of epithelial downgrowth after Descemet stripping automated endothelial keratoplasty. Cornea 2014;33(11):1140–1144

[137] Bansal R, Ramasubramanian A, Das P, Sukhija J, Jain AK. Intracorneal epithelial ingrowth after descemet stripping endothelial keratoplasty and stromal puncture. Cornea 2009;28(3):334–337

[138] Wong RK, Greene DP, Shield DR, Eberhart CG, Huang JJ, Shayegani A. 5-Fluorouracil for epithelial downgrowth after Descemet stripping automated endothelial keratoplasty. Cornea 2013;32(12):1610–1612

5 Corneal Endothelial Reconstruction: Current and Future Approaches

Hon Shing Ong, Jodhbir S. Mehta

Summary

Visual loss from corneal endothelial failure is a leading indication for corneal transplantation. The concept of selective replacement of damaged or lost endothelial cells using lamellar keratoplasty techniques has revolutionized the treatment of corneal endothelial failure over the past two decades. Current endothelial keratoplasty techniques, Descemet's stripping endothelial keratoplasty (DSEK), Descemet's stripping automated endothelial keratoplasty (DSAEK), and Descemet's membrane endothelial keratoplasty (DMEK), are associated with improved visual outcomes, lower risks of graft rejection, and superior graft survival rates compared to full-thickness penetrating keratoplasty (PK) procedures. With continual refinements and advancements in such endothelial keratoplasty techniques, these procedures are getting more effective in reversing corneal blindness caused by corneal endothelial failure. However, being donor-dependent, access to corneal transplantation is limited by a global shortage of available donor tissue. The difference between donor cornea availability and demand for corneal transplants has, therefore, driven a search for alternative treatment modalities for corneal endothelial replacement. Research into such alternative therapies currently focuses on two main areas: regenerative medicine and cell-based approaches. This chapter aims to provide an overview of current transplantation techniques used to treat endothelial failure and the limitations of each of these procedures. Novel therapies that are on the horizon for the treatment of corneal endothelial failure will also be introduced.

Keywords: Cornea, endothelial failure, keratoplasty, DSAEK, DSEK, DMEK, regenerative medicine, cell-based therapies

5.1 Introduction

Visual loss from corneal endothelial failure is a leading indication for corneal transplantation. A shift towards lamellar keratoplasty techniques for the treatment of corneal blindness have resulted in faster visual rehabilitation and lower rates of graft complications. This chapter describes the surgical techniques currently used to treat endothelial failure, the limitations of such procedures, and potential future approaches to replace the diseased corneal endothelium.

5.2 The Corneal Endothelium in Health

The corneal endothelium is the innermost single-cell layer of the cornea. It plays an important role in the dynamic maintenance of corneal hydration. Corneal endothelial cells are connected by intercellular junctions, which are tight but leaky, allowing passive diffusion of fluid from the anterior chamber across the corneal endothelium into the corneal stroma.[1] Conversely, active ionic pumps, such as the Na$^+$/K$^+$ adenosinetriphosphatase transporter, move fluid against an osmotic gradient from the corneal stroma back into the anterior chamber.[2,3,4] Such "pump-leak" mechanisms maintain corneal aqueous content at an ideal level—78% water. This supports optimal interlamellar spacing of collagen fibrils within the corneal stroma and corneal transparency.[5,6]

At birth, the average human corneal endothelial cell density is approximately 6,000 cells/mm^2.[7] This falls to about 3,500 cells/mm^2 by 5 years of age, as a result of physiological cell loss and concurrent corneal growth. Throughout life, there is a gradual decline of endothelial cell density of approximately 0.6% per year. This natural loss in endothelial cells with age does not usually result in any clinically significant impairment in corneal structure and function.

5.3 The Corneal Endothelium in Disease

Diseases of the corneal endothelium, such as Fuchs' endothelial corneal dystrophy (FECD) or ocular insults including intraocular surgeries, anterior segment laser therapies, ocular trauma, or inflammation, can result in an accelerated loss of corneal endothelial cells. When the corneal endothelial cell density falls below a certain level, the ability of the corneal endothelium to regulate corneal hydration becomes impaired.[8,9,10] In corneal endothelial failure, the cornea becomes edematous, resulting in loss of corneal transparency and eventually blindness.

Human corneal endothelial cells are thought not to regenerate *in vivo*.[11,12] At approximately 6 weeks of human gestation, corneal endothelial cells are arrested in the quiescent, nonproliferative G1 phase of the cell cycle.[13,14] Studies have shown that the lack of ability for human corneal endothelial cells to proliferate *in vivo* is attributed to a combination of factors such as cell–cell contact-dependent inhibition,[15,16] a lack of effective growth factor stimulation,[16,17] and the presence of rich mitotic inhibitors such as transforming growth factor (TGF-β) isoforms present in the aqueous humour.[15,16,17,18,19] Both TGF-β1 and -β2 isoforms have been shown to block endothelial cell proliferation by suppressing an entry into the S phase of the cell cycle, perhaps via an upregulation of the G1-phase inhibitor, p27(Kip1).[20,21]

As corneal endothelial cells are unable to spontaneously regenerate *in vivo* when the corneal endothelial cell density falls to a pathological level (typically <500–600 cells/mm^2), the restoration of physiological corneal endothelial function depends on: (1) replenishment with an exogenous source of cells (corneal transplantation or cell-based therapies); (2) repair of damaged cells (regenerative medicine), or (3) redistribution of remaining cells to replace lost cells (regenerative medicine).

5.4 Corneal Endothelial Replacement: Current Approaches

In current clinical practice, corneal transplantation is the predominant treatment for corneal blindness caused by endothelial dysfunction. For more than half a century, penetrating keratoplasty (PK) has been the main procedure for the treatment of most causes of corneal blindness. This is a full-thickness transplant; all layers of the cornea are replaced with a donor PK graft fixed with sutures.

Over the past 15 to 20 years, there has been a fundamental shift in the treatment of corneal diseases towards replacing only diseased parts of the cornea.[22,23] Indeed, the concept of selective replacement of damaged endothelial cells has revolutionized the treatment of corneal endothelial failure.[23] In the late 1990s, Melles et al first described an intrastromal approach for posterior lamellar keratoplasty.[24] This selectively replaced only diseased corneal endothelium and avoided full-thickness surgery. Subsequent modifications of this technique have since led to more advanced endothelial keratoplasty techniques with improved visual outcomes and graft survival rates. These procedures have now replaced PK as mainstay techniques for treating endothelial dysfunction.[25] In current clinical practice worldwide, there are two leading techniques for endothelial keratoplasty: (1) Descemet's stripping automated endothelial keratoplasty (DSAEK) or Descemet's stripping endothelial keratoplasty (DSEK), depending on how the donor graft is cut, and (2) Descemet's membrane endothelial keratoplasty (DMEK).[22,23,26]

In this chapter, we aim to provide an overview of DSAEK/DSEK and DMEK. We will also introduce novel therapies that are on the horizon for the treatment of corneal endothelial failure.

5.4.1 Descemet's Stripping Automated Endothelial Keratoplasty or Descemet's Stripping Endothelial Keratoplasty

In DSAEK/DSEK, transplanted donor endothelial grafts consist of donor endothelium, Descemet's membrane (DM), and some posterior stroma. In DSAEK, an automated microkeratome is used to cut donor grafts.[27] In institutions where automated microkeratomes are not available, a lamellar dissection technique can be used to cut the endothelial graft.[28] This manual technique is termed DSEK.

In DSAEK/DSEK, the central DM is stripped from the recipient's stroma with its diseased endothelium (descemetorhexis). Through a small corneal or scleral incision, the cut donor endothelial graft is transferred into the patient's anterior chamber. It is then made to attach to the posterior cornea without sutures, by the use of air or gas tamponade (▶ Fig. 5.1).

DSAEK/DSEK procedures have several advantages over PK. Unlike PK, they are minimally invasive, avoiding full-thickness central corneal trephination and intraoperative "open sky" situations, thereby reducing the risk of sight-threatening complications like expulsive hemorrhage. DSAEK/DSEK also offer better mechanical integrity and globe strength. In the event of ocular trauma, the risk of sight-threatening open-globe injuries is higher in eyes that had undergone PK compared to eyes

that had undergone DSAEK/DSEK because PK is associated with inherent weakness at the graft–host junction. Furthermore, DSAEK/DSEK are less likely to induce postoperative corneal astigmatism as central corneal sutures are not needed. This allows faster visual rehabilitation.[29] Corneal suture-related problems and ocular surface disorders, seen commonly following PK, occur less frequently after DSAEK/DSEK. As less donor tissue is transplanted in DSAEK/DSEK than in PK, studies have also shown that DSAEK/DSEK procedures are associated with a lower risk of rejection.[30] Lastly, DSAEK/DSEK allow more accurate intraocular lens (IOL) power calculations when combined with cataract extraction, as they do not change the corneal profile as much as PK.

Given the advantages over PK, DSAEK/DSEK have overtaken PK as primary procedures for the treatment of corneal endothelial failure in many centers worldwide. With the increasing popularity of DSAEK/DSEK among corneal surgeons, research has focused on methods to improve the postoperative outcomes of these surgical techniques. One example of a significant advance is in the techniques used to insert donor endothelial grafts. When DSAEK/DSEK were first performed, donor endothelial graft insertion was carried out using a "folding" technique. [25] The donor tissue was folded into a 60/40 "taco" shape and inserted into the anterior chamber using forceps. The donor tissue was then unfolded in the eye. The problem with the folding technique is that it was associated with significant endothelial cell loss. Specular microscopy and scanning electron microscopy studies have reported up to 30 to 40% endothelial cell loss with the folding technique.[31]

Newer methods of graft insertion that are less traumatic to the endothelial cells have since been introduced. Some examples are the use of modified lens cartridges or an IOL sheet glide to push or pull the endothelial graft into the anterior chamber.[32] Furthermore, customized endothelial graft insertion devices have also been developed. Examples of these devices include the Busin glide (Asico, USA),[33] the EndoGlide (Network Medical Products, UK),[34] the Endosaver (Ocular Systems Inc, USA), among various others. These newer methods and devices maintain graft orientation stromal side up during graft insertion and are less traumatic to the endothelium as they minimize the need for intraocular manipulation when unfolding the graft. They also prevent endothelial cell to endothelial cell touch during donor insertion. The risk of cell loss is thus reduced.

▶ Fig. 5.2 shows the technique of graft loading and insertion using the EndoGlide. The harvested graft is loaded and made to scroll in the EndoGlide with minimal contact and trauma to donor endothelial cells. The insertion technique using the EndoGlide maintains anterior chamber stability and orientation of the donor endothelial graft, avoiding excessive intraocular manipulation and thus preventing endothelial cell loss.

Another key development in DSAEK surgery relates to the thickness of the transplanted endothelial graft. The transplantation of ultrathin DSAEK grafts, defined as grafts of less than 100-μm thickness, has been reported to have improved visual outcomes compared to the transplantation of thicker grafts.[35,36] To consistently create thin endothelial grafts, various strategies have been proposed. One of these strategies includes a "double-pass technique."[37,38] In this technique, an initial debulking cut is performed with a 300-μm head microkeratome; this is followed by a second refinement cut, depending

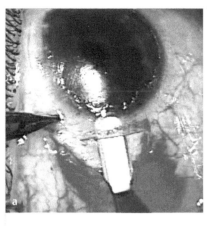

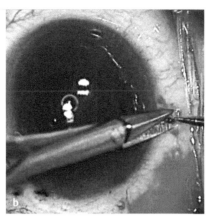

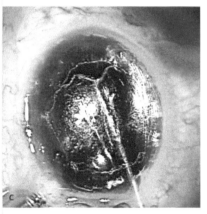

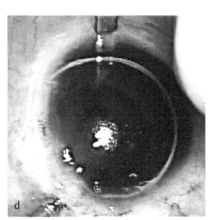

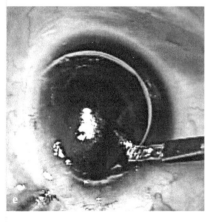

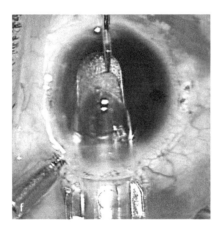

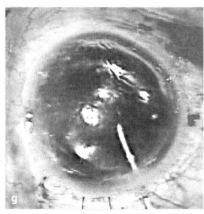

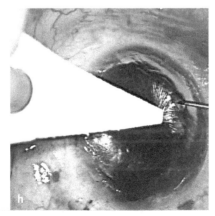

Fig. 5.1 Surgical technique of Descemet's stripping automated endothelial keratoplasty. (a) Epithelium debridement, conjunctival peritomy, and scleral tunneled incision. (b) Inferior peripheral iridectomy. (c) Descemetorhexis under air. (d) Pull-through incision. (e) Venting incisions. (f) DSAEK graft is pulled into the eye. (g) Air bubble injected into anterior chamber to provide tamponade of the DSAEK graft. (h) Venting incisions are opened to release interface fluid. DSAEK, Descemet's stripping automated endothelial keratoplasty.

Vital dyes such as trypan blue 0.06% (VisionBlue, D.O.R.C., the Netherlands) can be used to aid visualization of the DM during harvesting. Other longer lasting dyes, such as combinations of 0.15% trypan blue, 0.025% brilliant blue, and 4% polyethylene glycol (MembraneBlue-Dual, D.O.R.C., the Netherlands), may be used for intraocular graft visualization. However, recent studies have showed a time-dependent corneal endothelial cell toxicity following dye exposure.[52]

In DMEK, correct graft orientation is important to avoid graft failure. After insertion of the graft into the eye, it can be difficult to assess the orientation of the graft. Asymmetrical marks, such as S-stamps[53] or peripheral scalene triangles,[54] made on the graft may be helpful.

As DM is highly fragile, it can be a challenge to harvest a DMEK graft without damage and wastage of donor tissue. As a result, various strategies have been employed in attempts to simplify the DMEK harvesting technique and improve its success. Examples of some techniques include the use of a fluid blister or air dissection to cleave a plane between DM and corneal stroma.[55,56]

Customized surgical instruments have also been developed to improve the success of harvesting DMEK grafts. ▶ Fig. 5.4a, b shows the Tan-Jod DMEK block (AE-1570, Asico, USA) designed for harvesting DMEK grafts. This instrument has a rotating base, which allows easier scoring and loosening of the peripheral DM by the surgeon. In contrast to standard graft preparation blocks, this block is made of a transparent material with a reflective base. The reflection of light from a standard operating microscope allows better visualization of the DM. Stripping under conventional cornea preservation media such as Optisol/McCarey-Kaufman media or organ culture imparts a pink–red glow, which simulates a "red reflex," similar to performing a capsulorhexis during cataract surgery. This allows visualization of the DM without the need of vital dyes. Any aberrant tags can be detected early to ensure a smooth graft edge. This reduces the risk of radial tears. Another instrument designed to facilitate DMEK graft preparation is the Tan DMEK stripper (AE-2336, Asico) (▶ Fig. 5.4c). This instrument has two ends. The double-tipped end is designed for circumferential scoring of the peripheral margins of DM to avoid radial tears. The curved single-tipped end is designed for lamellar separation of the DM from the stroma. This is useful in situations where the DM is particularly fragile and tears easily when peeled with forceps.

Donor Insertion

The insertion and unfolding of the scrolled graft within the eye are arguably the most difficult steps in DMEK surgery (▶ Fig. 5.5). One of the challenges of DMEK comes from the fact that the DM, once separated from the stroma, has an innate tendency to form a tight scroll with the endothelium on the outer surface. This is especially so for tissues from younger donors.

Current techniques of transferring the DMEK graft into the anterior chamber involve the injection of the graft through a small incision. Various instruments have been used for DMEK graft insertion. These include glass injectors[57,58] and the use of IOL cartridges,[59,60] among various others. All these techniques protect the DM scroll from the wound. However, the endothelium of the DMEK graft remains on the outside ("endothelium-out"). The graft is, thus, susceptible to endothelial cell loss caused by contact of its endothelium with the lumen of the injector. More recently, the concept of "endothelium-in" instruments for graft insertion has been described. An example is a novel pull-through approach using the EndoGlide for DMEK.[61] In this technique, a stromal carrier (in the form of a customized sheet or anterior stromal cap) is used to support and stabilize the donor DM. This prevents the harvested DM from naturally scrolling endothelial side outward and enables an "endothelium-in" coiling into the EndoGlide chamber similar to DSAEK. For donor graft insertion, the EndoGlide is introduced into the anterior chamber and a pair of microforceps is used to pull the DMEK graft in, leaving the stromal carrier behind in the EndoGlide cartridge. This maintains the orientation of the graft and allows the surgeon more control during insertion. A new

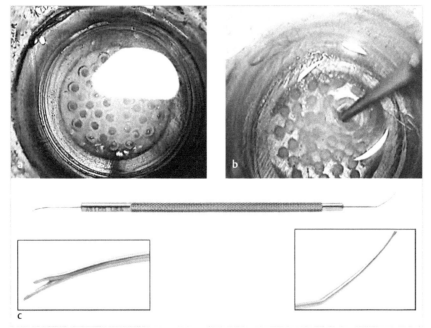

Fig. 5.4 Customized surgical instruments for DMEK donor preparation. **(a)** Tan-Jod DMEK block (AE-1570, Asico, USA) designed for harvesting DMEK grafts; this block is made of a transparent material with a reflective base—reflection of light from a standard operating microscope allows better visualization of the DM. **(b)** Stripping under cornea preservation media imparts a pink–red glow which simulates a "red reflex" similar to performing a capsulorhexis during cataract surgery. **(c)** Tan DMEK stripper (AE-2336, Asico, USA); this instrument has two ends: a double-tipped end for circumferential scoring of the peripheral margins of DM and a curved single-tipped end designed for lamellar separation of DM from the stroma. DM, Descemet's membrane; DMEK, Descemet's membrane endothelial keratoplasty.

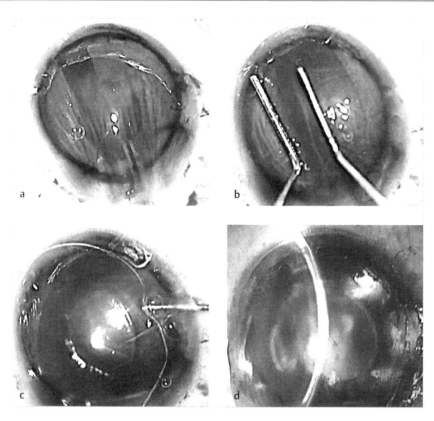

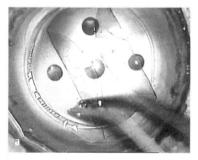

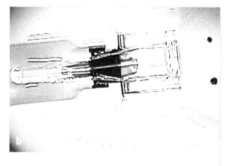

Fig. 5.5 Surgical technique of DMEK. **(a)** Insertion of the DMEK graft into the anterior chamber using a glass injector through a clear corneal incision. **(b)** Unfolding of the DM graft by tapping on the recipient's corneal surface. **(c)** Gas bubble injected into anterior chamber to provide tamponade of the DMEK graft. **(d)** Intraoperative slit lamp showing full attachment of the DMEK graft. DM, Descemet's membrane; DMEK, Descemet's membrane endothelial keratoplasty.

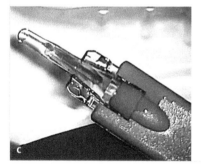

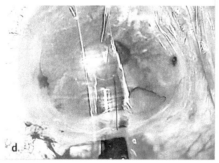

Fig. 5.6 Technique of DMEK graft loading using the DMEK EndoGlide (Network Medical Products, UK). **(a)** Endothelium of the DMEK graft is protected with viscoelastic and folded "endothelium-in." **(b)** DMEK graft pulled and loaded into the DMEK EndoGlide. **(c)** Clip is fixed to the back of the EndoGlide to create of "closed system" during graft insertion and thus maintains anterior chamber stability. **(d)** Graft is pulled into the anterior chamber with microforceps; the orientation of the graft is maintained. DMEK, Descemet's membrane endothelial keratoplasty.

modified version of the EndoGlide, known as the DMEK Endo-Glide (Network Medical Products, UK), has also recently been introduced. It is specifically designed to provide controlled DMEK graft unfolding following insertion into the anterior chamber and can be inserted through a small 2.65-mm corneal incision. No carrier is required for graft loading (▶Fig. 5.6).

A variant of DMEK that has been introduced is pre-Descemet's endothelial keratoplasty (PDEK).[62] In PDEK, the pre-Descemet's layer (Dua's layer) together with DM and endothelium is transplanted. To obtain a PDEK graft, it involves an intrastromal injection of air in a donor cornea to create a type 1 big bubble. The presence of the pre-Descemet's layer in a PDEK graft prevents the scrolling of the DM. A PDEK graft is, thus, easier to handle and avoids difficulties of intraocular unfolding of tightly scrolled DMEK grafts. The main limitation of PDEK is the consistency of obtaining a type 1 big bubble during donor harvest; in addition, the maximum possible diameter of a PDEK graft is approximately 7.5 to 8.5 mm, depending on the extent of the big bubble.

References

[1] Srinivas SP. Dynamic regulation of barrier integrity of the corneal endothelium. Optom Vis Sci 2010;87(4):E239–E254

[2] Carlson KH, Bourne WM, McLaren JW, Brubaker RF. Variations in human corneal endothelial cell morphology and permeability to fluorescein with age. Exp Eye Res 1988;47(1):27–41

[3] Maurice DM. The location of the fluid pump in the cornea. J Physiol 1972;221(1):43–54

[4] Bourne WM. Clinical estimation of corneal endothelial pump function. Trans Am Ophthalmol Soc 1998;96:229–239, discussion 239–242

[5] Bonanno JA. Molecular mechanisms underlying the corneal endothelial pump. Exp Eye Res 2012;95(1):2–7

[6] Edelhauser HF. The balance between corneal transparency and edema: the Proctor Lecture. Invest Ophthalmol Vis Sci 2006;47(5):1754–1767

[7] Bourne WM. Biology of the corneal endothelium in health and disease. Eye (Lond) 2003;17(8):912–918

[8] Tuft SJ, Coster DJ. The corneal endothelium. Eye (Lond) 1990;4(Pt 3):389–424

[9] McCartney MD, Wood TO, McLaughlin BJ. Freeze-fracture label of functional and dysfunctional human corneal endothelium. Curr Eye Res 1987;6(4):589–597

[10] Mahdy MA, Eid MZ, Mohammed MA, Hafez A, Bhatia J. Relationship between endothelial cell loss and microcoaxial phacoemulsification parameters in noncomplicated cataract surgery. Clin Ophthalmol 2012;6:503–510

[11] Murphy C, Alvarado J, Juster R, Maglio M. Prenatal and postnatal cellularity of the human corneal endothelium. A quantitative histologic study. Invest Ophthalmol Vis Sci 1984;25(3):312–322

[12] Edelhauser HF. The resiliency of the corneal endothelium to refractive and intraocular surgery. Cornea 2000;19(3):263–273

[13] Joyce NC, Meklir B, Joyce SJ, Zieske JD. Cell cycle protein expression and proliferative status in human corneal cells. Invest Ophthalmol Vis Sci 1996;37(4):645–655

[14] Joyce NC, Navon SE, Roy S, Zieske JD. Expression of cell cycle-associated proteins in human and rabbit corneal endothelium in situ. Invest Ophthalmol Vis Sci 1996;37(8):1566–1575

[15] Joyce NC, Harris DL, Mello DM. Mechanisms of mitotic inhibition in corneal endothelium: contact inhibition and TGF-beta2. Invest Ophthalmol Vis Sci 2002;43(7):2152–2159

[16] Joyce NC. Proliferative capacity of corneal endothelial cells. Exp Eye Res 2012;95(1):16–23

[17] Lu J, Lu Z, Reinach P, et al. TGF-beta2 inhibits AKT activation and FGF-2-induced corneal endothelial cell proliferation. Exp Cell Res 2006;312(18):3631–3640

[18] Joyce NC, Harris DL, Zies, ke JD. Mitotic inhibition of corneal endothelium in neonatal rats. Invest Ophthalmol Vis Sci 1998;39(13):2572–2583

[19] Harris DL, Joyce NC. Transforming growth factor-beta suppresses proliferation of rabbit corneal endothelial cells in vitro. J Interferon Cytokine Res 1999;19(4):327–334

[20] Kim TY, Kim WI, Smith RE, Kay ED. Role of p27(Kip1) in cAMP- and TGF-beta 2-mediated antiproliferation in rabbit corneal endothelial cells. Invest Ophthalmol Vis Sci 2001;42(13):3142–3149

[21] Kikuchi M, Zhu C, Senoo T, Obara Y, Joyce NC. p27kip1 siRNA induces proliferation in corneal endothelial cells from young but not older donors. Invest Ophthalmol Vis Sci 2006;47(11):4803–4809

[22] Park CY, Lee JK, Gore PK, Lim CY, Chuck RS. Keratoplasty in the United States: A 10-Year Review from 2005 through 2014. Ophthalmology 2015;122(12):2432–2442

[23] Tan DT, Dart JK, Holland EJ, Kinoshita S. Corneal transplantation. Lancet 2012;379(9827):1749–1761

[24] Melles GR, Eggink FA, Lander F, et al. A surgical technique for posterior lamellar keratoplasty. Cornea 1998;17(6):618–626

[25] Güell JL, El Husseiny MA, Manero F, Gris O, Elies D. Historical review and update of surgical treatment for corneal endothelial diseases. Ophthalmol Ther 2014;3(1)(–)(2):1–15

[26] Price FW, Jr, Feng MT, Price MO. Evolution of endothelial keratoplasty: where are we headed? Cornea 2015;34(Suppl 10):S41–S47

[27] Gorovoy MS. Descemet-stripping automated endothelial keratoplasty. Cornea 2006;25(8):886–889

[28] Melles GR, Wijdh RH, Nieuwendaal CP. A technique to excise the descemet membrane from a recipient cornea (descemetorhexis). Cornea 2004;23(3):286–288

[29] Koenig SB, Covert DJ, Dupps WJ Jr, Meisler DM. Visual acuity, refractive error, and endothelial cell density six months after Descemet stripping and automated endothelial keratoplasty (DSAEK). Cornea 2007;26(6):670–674

[30] Ang M, Soh Y, Htoon HM, Mehta JS, Tan D. Five-year graft survival comparing Descemet stripping automated endothelial keratoplasty and penetrating keratoplasty. Ophthalmology 2016;123(8):1646–1652

[31] Mehta JS, Por YM, Poh R, Beuerman RW, Tan D. Comparison of donor insertion techniques for descemet stripping automated endothelial keratoplasty. Arch Ophthalmol 2008;126(10):1383–1388

[32] Ang M, Saroj L, Htoon HM, Kiew S, Mehta JS, Tan D. Comparison of a donor insertion device to sheets glide in Descemet stripping endothelial keratoplasty: 3-year outcomes. Am J Ophthalmol 2014;157(6):1163–1169.e3

[33] Busin M, Bhatt PR, Scorcia V. A modified technique for descemet membrane stripping automated endothelial keratoplasty to minimize endothelial cell loss. Arch Ophthalmol 2008;126(8):1133–1137

[34] Khor WB, Mehta JS, Tan DT. Descemet stripping automated endothelial keratoplasty with a graft insertion device: surgical technique and early clinical results. Am J Ophthalmol 2011;151(2):223–32.e2

[35] Neff KD, Biber JM, Holland EJ. Comparison of central corneal graft thickness to visual acuity outcomes in endothelial keratoplasty. Cornea 2011;30(4):388–391

[36] Shinton AJ, Tsatsos M, Konstantopoulos A, et al. Impact of graft thickness on visual acuity after Descemet's stripping endothelial keratoplasty. Br J Ophthalmol 2012;96(2):246–249

[37] Busin M, Madi S, Santorum P, Scorcia V, Beltz J. Ultrathin descemet's stripping automated endothelial keratoplasty with the microkeratome double-pass technique: two-year outcomes. Ophthalmology 2013;120(6):1186–1194

[38] Busin M, Patel AK, Scorcia V, Ponzin D. Microkeratome-assisted preparation of ultrathin grafts for descemet stripping automated endothelial keratoplasty. Invest Ophthalmol Vis Sci 2012;53(1):521–524

[39] Thomas PB, Mukherjee AN, O'Donovan D, Rajan MS. Preconditioned donor corneal thickness for microthin endothelial keratoplasty. Cornea 2013;32(7):e173–e178

[40] Rosa AM, Silva MF, Quadrado MJ, Costa E, Marques I, Murta JN. Femtosecond laser and microkeratome-assisted Descemet stripping endothelial keratoplasty: first clinical results. Br J Ophthalmol 2013;97(9):1104–1107

[41] Kurji KH, Cheung AY, Eslani M, et al. Comparison of visual acuity outcomes between nanothin descemet stripping automated endothelial keratoplasty and Descemet membrane endothelial keratoplasty. Cornea 2018;37(10):1226–1231

[42] Patel SV, Baratz KH, Hodge DO, Maguire LJ, McLaren JW. The effect of corneal light scatter on vision after descemet stripping with endothelial keratoplasty. Arch Ophthalmol 2009;127(2):153–160

[43] Droutsas K, Lazaridis A, Giallouros E, Kymionis G, Chatzistefanou K, Sekundo W. Scheimpflug densitometry after DMEK versus DSAEK-two-year outcomes. Cornea 2018;37(4):455–461

[44] Melles GR, Ong TS, Ververs B, van der Wees J. Descemet membrane endothelial keratoplasty (DMEK). Cornea 2006;25(8):987–990

[45] Singh A, Zarei-Ghanavati M, Avadhanam V, Liu C. Systematic review and meta-analysis of clinical outcomes of descemet membrane endothelial keratoplasty versus Descemet stripping endothelial keratoplasty/Descemet stripping automated endothelial keratoplasty. Cornea 2017;36(11):1437–1443

[46] Droutsas K, Lazaridis A, Papaconstantinou D, et al. Visual outcomes after Descemet membrane endothelial keratoplasty versus Descemet stripping automated endothelial keratoplasty-comparison of specific matched pairs. Cornea 2016;35(6):765–771

[47] Tourtas T, Laaser K, Bachmann BO, Cursiefen C, Kruse FE. Descemet membrane endothelial keratoplasty versus descemet stripping automated endothelial keratoplasty. Am J Ophthalmol 2012;153(6):1082–90.e2

[48] Guerra FP, Anshu A, Price MO, Price FW. Endothelial keratoplasty: fellow eyes comparison of Descemet stripping automated endothelial keratoplasty and Descemet membrane endothelial keratoplasty. Cornea 2011;30(12):1382–1386

[49] Marques RE, Guerra PS, Sousa DC, Gonçalves AI, Quintas AM, Rodrigues W. DMEK versus DSAEK for Fuchs' endothelial dystrophy: a meta-analysis. Eur J Ophthalmol 2019;29(1):15-22

[50] Pavlovic I, Shajari M, Herrmann E, Schmack I, Lencova A, Kohnen T. Meta-analysis of postoperative outcome parameters comparing Descemet membrane endothelial keratoplasty versus Descemet stripping automated endothelial keratoplasty. Cornea 2017;36(12):1445–1451

[51] Brissette A, Conlon R, Teichman JC, Yeung S, Ziai S, Baig K. Evaluation of a new technique for preparation of endothelial grafts for descemet membrane endothelial keratoplasty. Cornea 2015;34(5):557–559

[52] Weber IP, Rana M, Thomas PBM, Dimov IB, Franze K, Rajan MS. Effect of vital dyes on human corneal endothelium and elasticity of Descemet's membrane. PLoS One 2017;12(9):e0184375

[53] Veldman PB, Dye PK, Holiman JD, et al. The S-stamp in Descemet membrane endothelial keratoplasty safely eliminates upside-down graft implantation. Ophthalmology 2016;123(1):161–164

[54] Bhogal M, Maurino V, Allan BD. Use of a single peripheral triangular mark to ensure correct graft orientation in Descemet membrane endothelial keratoplasty. J Cataract Refract Surg 2015;41(9):2022–2024

[55] Muraine M, Gueudry J, He Z, Piselli S, Lefevre S, Toubeau D. Novel technique for the preparation of corneal grafts for descemet membrane endothelial keratoplasty. Am J Ophthalmol 2013;156(5):851–859

[56] Zarei-Ghanavati S, Zarei-Ghanavati M, Ramirez-Miranda A. Air-assisted donor preparation for DMEK. J Cataract Refract Surg 2011;37(7):1372–, author reply 1372

[57] Dapena I, Moutsouris K, Droutsas K, Ham L, van Dijk K, Melles GR. Standardized "no-touch" technique for descemet membrane endothelial keratoplasty. Arch Ophthalmol 2011;129(1):88–94

[58] Arnalich-Montiel F, Muñoz-Negrete FJ, De Miguel MP. Double port injector device to reduce endothelial damage in DMEK. Eye (Lond) 2014;28(6):748–751

[59] Kruse FE, Laaser K, Cursiefen C, et al. A stepwise approach to donor preparation and insertion increases safety and outcome of Descemet membrane endothelial keratoplasty. Cornea 2011;30(5):580–587

[60] Kim EC, Bonfadini G, Todd L, Zhu A, Jun AS. Simple, inexpensive, and effective injector for descemet membrane endothelial keratoplasty. Cornea 2014;33(6):649–652

[61] Ang M, Mehta JS, Newman SD, Han SB, Chai J, Tan D. Descemet membrane endothelial keratoplasty: preliminary results of a donor insertion pull-through technique using a donor mat device. Am J Ophthalmol 2016;171:27–34

[62] Agarwal A, Dua HS, Narang P, et al. Pre-Descemet's endothelial keratoplasty (PDEK). Br J Ophthalmol 2014;98(9):1181–1185

[63] Gain P, Jullienne R, He Z, et al. Global survey of corneal transplantation and eye banking. JAMA Ophthalmol 2016;134(2):167–173

[64] Kinoshita S, Koizumi N, Ueno M, et al. Injection of cultured cells with a ROCK inhibitor for bullous keratopathy. N Engl J Med 2018;378(11):995–1003

[65] Peh GSL, Ong HS, Adnan K, Ang HP, Lwin CN, Seah XY, Lin SJ, Mehta JS. Functional evaluation of two corneal endothelial cell-based therapies: tissue-engineered construct and cell injection. Sci Rep 2019;9(1):6087

[66] Peh GSL, Ang HP, Lwin CN, et al. Regulatory compliant tissue-engineered human corneal endothelial grafts restore corneal function of rabbits with bullous keratopathy. Sci Rep 2017;7(1):14149

[67] Coster DJ, Lowe MT, Keane MC, Williams KA; Australian corneal graft registry contributors. A comparison of lamellar and penetrating keratoplasty outcomes: a registry study. Ophthalmology 2014;121(5):979–987

[68] Braunstein RE, Airiani S, Chang MA, Odrich MG. Corneal edema resolution after "descemetorhexis". J Cataract Refract Surg 2003;29(7):1436–1439

[69] Borkar DS, Veldman P, Colby KA. Treatment of fuchs endothelial dystrophy by Descemet stripping without endothelial keratoplasty. Cornea 2016;35(10):1267–1273

[70] Soh YQ, Peh GS, Mehta JS. Evolving therapies for Fuchs' endothelial dystrophy. Regen Med 2018;13(1):97–115

[71] Bhogal M, Lwin CN, Seah XY, Peh G, Mehta JS. Allogeneic Descemet's membrane transplantation enhances corneal eendothelial monolayer formation and restores functional integrity following Descemet's stripping. Invest Ophthalmol Vis Sci 2017;58(10):4249–4260

[72] Soh YQ, Mehta JS. Regenerative therapy for fuchs endothelial corneal dystrophy. Cornea 2018;37(4):523–527

[73] Jullienne R, Manoli P, Tiffet T, et al. Corneal endothelium self-healing mathematical model after inadvertent descemetorhexis. J Cataract Refract Surg 2015;41(10):2313–2318

[74] Soh YQ, Peh G, George BL, et al. Predicative factors for corneal endothelial cell migration. Invest Ophthalmol Vis Sci 2016;57(2):338–348

6 Pre-Descemet's Endothelial Keratoplasty

Priya Narang, Amar Agarwal

Summary

Pre-Descemet's endothelial keratoplasty (PDEK) involves the separation of pre-Descemet's layer along with Descemet's membrane and endothelium that is transferred to the recipient's eye. The advantage with PDEK is that young and infant donor tissue can also be employed for harvesting the graft unlike the usage of donor corneas above 40 years of age for Descemet's membrane endothelial keratoplasty.

Keywords: PDEK, endothelial keratoplasty, pre-Descemet's layer, pre-Descemet's membrane, DMEK, DSAEK

6.1 Introduction

Endothelial keratoplasty (EK) comprises Descemet's membrane endothelial keratoplasty (DMEK) and Descemet's stripping endothelial keratoplasty (DSEK) as the major variants, whereas many surgeons have also employed their automated version of DMAEK and DSAEK across the globe. In terms of visual output, DMEK as an EK procedure has always scored in spite of it being technically challenging as compared to other subtypes. Melles et al described DMEK that represents the perfect anatomic replacement of the diseased Descemet's membrane (DM)–endothelium complex with a healthy donor DM–endothelium.[1,2]

Pre-Descemet's endothelial keratoplasty (PDEK),[3] being a new variant in the field of EK, further extends the lexicon of EK that mainly comprises the separation of pre-Descemet's membrane (PDL) along with DM–endothelium complex from the residual donor stroma by the formation of a type 1 bubble.[4] The feasibility of the PDEK procedure with both an adult and infant donor tissue[3,5] makes it highly acceptable in the era of shortage of donor tissue.

6.2 Importance of Air Dissection and Types of Bubbles

Air dissection is a well-established entity that relegates the use of microforceps or a microkeratome for dissection of the corneal stroma. An air-filled syringe is used to inject air into the stroma with the endothelial side up and is advanced under direct observation at a required depth beneath the endothelium. The advantage with air dissection is that it is cost effective as it is done manually by the surgeon and the major drawback with it is that it requires a certain amount of surgical skill set on behalf of the surgeon as the needle that is employed to inject air must be introduced at the correct depth below the DM–endothelium complex (▶ Video 6.1).

- Type 1 bubble: This is the kind of bubble that is essential to obtain for performing a PDEK procedure. This bubble typically spreads from center to periphery and is dome-shaped. The diameter of the bubble usually varies from 7.5 to 8.5 mm; this bubble never extends to extreme periphery due to adhesions between the PDL and the residual stroma. The injection of air leads to separation of the PDL–DM–endothelium complex in toto from the residual stromal bed (▶ Fig. 6.1a–d).

- Type 2 bubble: This type of bubble is typically formed when the air enters the plane between the PDL and the DM–endothelium complex. Type 2 bubble typically spreads from periphery to center and is around 10 to 11 mm in diameter. It extends up to extreme periphery as there are no adhesions between the PDL and the DM (▶ Fig. 6.2a–d). With the formation of this bubble, it becomes essential to perform a DMEK instead of a PDEK procedure. Immense care should be taken when a type 2 bubble is formed as it has a thin wall and if it is subjected to excessive air push, then the bubble can rupture, leading to perforation of graft and eventually transcending into donor tissue wastage.

- Mixed bubble: When both type 1 and type 2 bubbles are formed and they coexist, mixed bubble is said to have been achieved. These types of bubbles pose a surgical challenge to the surgeon as it requires delicate handling and manipulation to avoid the rupture of the bubble.

During the process of bubble formation, the tip of the needle may rupture the endothelium (▶ Fig. 6.3a, b), which is completely an undesirable event as it may often lead to a situation where the corneal tissue can no longer be used and needs to be discarded as neither a type 1 nor a type 2 bubble can be created either for a PDEK or a DMEK procedure, respectively. However, if the DM perforation occurs and if it is recognized, the surgeon can withhold the injection of air. The surgeon can again withdraw and re-enter at a deeper plane as compared to the previous one and again attempt at making a bubble. Alternatively, a cannula attached to a syringe filled with viscoelastic can also be taken and can be reintroduced to make a bubble, although the use of viscoelastic is not recommended. The advantage with the use of viscoelastic is that it seems to plug the small hole in the DM and facilitates the creation of the type 1 bubble (▶ Fig. 6.3a–d). Eventually, if the hole in the DM is big enough, then it cannot be sealed with the help of viscoelastic,

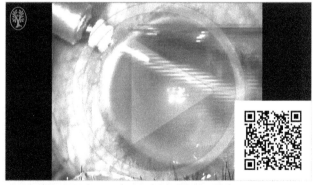

Video 6.1 Pre-Descemet's endothelial keratoplasty in 15 steps. https://www.thieme.de/de/q.htm?p=opn/tp/311890101/9781684200979_video_06_01&t=video

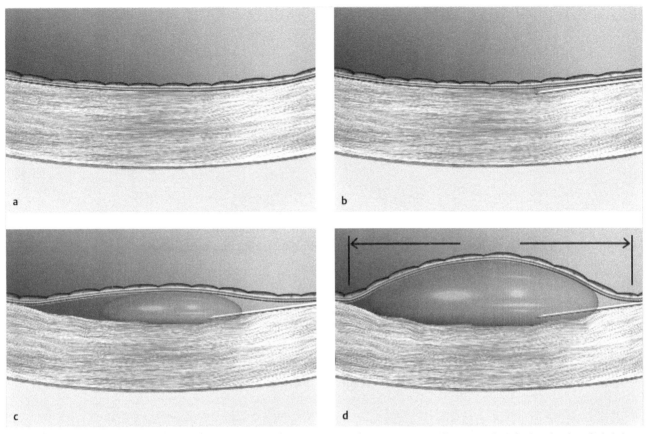

Fig. 6.1 Graphical display of creation of type 1 bubble. **(a)** The image demonstrates all the layers of cornea with graft placed with endothelial side up. **(b)** An air-filled 30-G needle introduced from the periphery beneath the pre-Descemet's layer (PDL). The PDL–Descemet's membrane (DM)–endothelium complex is seen lying above the bevel of the needle. **(c)** Further injection of air lifts the entire PDL–DM–endothelium complex that comprises PDEK graft above the residual stroma. **(d)** Fully formed type 1 bubble formed. PDEK, pre-Descemet's endothelial keratoplasty.

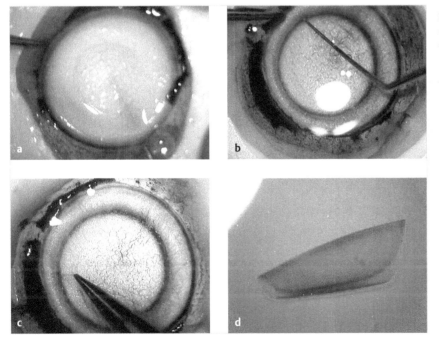

Fig. 6.2 Accidental creation of type 2 bubble. **(a)** Air being injected to form a type 1 bubble. **(b)** Type 2 bubble is formed that extends up to extreme periphery. **(c)** DM–endothelium complex being separated from above the surface of the bubble. **(d)** DMEK graft placed in the storage media. DM, Descemet's membrane; DMEK, Descemet's membrane endothelial keratoplasty.

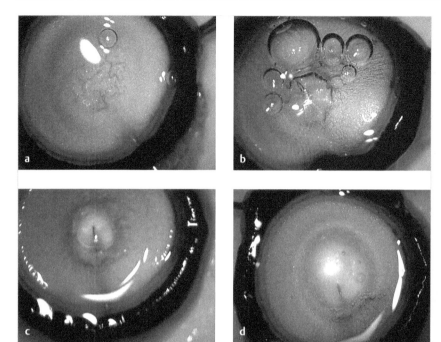

Fig. 6.3 Plugging the DM–endothelium hole with viscoelastic. **(a)** Air being injected into the donor tissue to create a type 1 bubble. **(b)** Perforation of the DM is noted with leakage of small air bubbles from the endothelium side. **(c)** Further injection of air is withheld. The needle is withdrawn and 30-G needle attached to a syringe filled with viscoelastic is introduced. Viscoelastic is injected as it helps to plug the small perforation. **(d)** Type 1 bubble created with the help of viscoelastic. DM, Descemet's membrane.

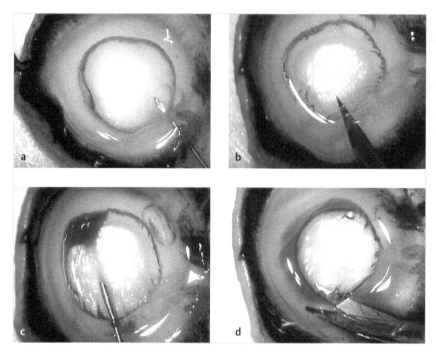

Fig. 6.4 Donor graft preparation. **(a)** An air-filled 30-G needle is introduced from the corneoscleral rim up to the mid-periphery and air is injected to create a type 1 bubble. **(b)** The bubble is punctured at the extreme periphery with the help of a side-port blade. **(c)** Trypan blue is injected to stain the bubble. **(d)** The graft is cut along the peripheral edge of the bubble with the corneoscleral scissor.

and sequentially despite various efforts, only a type 2 bubble will be formed that necessitates the conversion to a DMEK procedure.

Occasionally, a very small bubble is formed after injection of air. In such a scenario, viscoelastic can come to the rescue of the surgeon as the injection of viscoelastic facilitates the breakdown of superficial adhesions between the PDL and the stromal layer, as it tends to overcome resistance offered by the collagenous layer better than air.

Despite all the surgical challenges that a surgeon comes across in the creation of a bubble, the surgical competence and the correct art of handling the corneal tissue effectively saves the loss of corneal tissue, renders economic practicality and enhances the productivity by retaining the clinical merits of the PDEK procedure.

6.3 Surgical Technique

6.3.1 Donor Graft Preparation

Bubble Creation

The donor button with the corneoscleral rim is dissected from the whole cornea and is placed with the endothelial side up. For the process of bubble creation, a 30-G needle is used that is attached to an air-filled 5-mL syringe. The needle is introduced with a bevel-up position from the periphery up to the mid-peripheral area at a considerable depth from the DM so as to create a plane of separation between the PDL and the residual stroma (▶ Fig. 6.4a). Air is injected and a type 1 bubble is formed that is dome-shaped and is around 8 mm in diameter.

Graft Staining

Staining of the graft is done with trypan blue that allows a considerable clear visualization of the graft. The bubble is penetrated with a side-port blade at the extreme periphery (▶Fig. 6.4b) and trypan blue is injected inside (▶Fig. 6.4c). The bubble is then cut all across the periphery with a corneoscleral scissors (▶Fig. 6.4d) and is placed in the storage media.

6.3.2 Recipient Bed Preparation

The procedure is performed under local anesthesia; supplemental anesthesia is administered as necessary.

In cases of bullous keratopathy, the initial step comprises scrapping and debridement of epithelium. This facilitates enhanced intraoperative view during the surgical procedure. An anterior chamber maintainer (ACM) or a Trocar ACM[6] is introduced into the eye that is connected to the air pump. This helps to maintain adequate depth of anterior chamber (AC) at all times and it also ensures appropriate shift between air and fluid infusion as and when required (▶Fig. 6.5a–f). A 2.8-mm corneal tunnel is made and two side-port incisions are framed. With the AC completely inflated with air, DM is scored and stripped using a reverse Sinskey hook (▶Fig. 6.6a–d). Inferior iridectomy is performed with a vitrectomy probe introduced from the corneal incision (▶Fig. 6.6e). This maneuver ensures prevention of pupillary block at a later stage.

6.3.3 Donor Graft Insertion

The graft is held gently with a nontoothed forceps and is placed into the cartridge of a foldable intraocular lens (IOL) that is filled with balanced salt solution (▶Fig. 6.6f).[7] Air infusion is stopped and the graft is gently injected into the AC through a clear corneal incision, avoiding wound-assisted implantation (▶Fig. 6.7a). Graft orientation is verified and the graft is gently unfolded using air and fluidics. Corneal indentation and massaging are also performed to facilitate the graft unrolling. Once the graft has partly unrolled, a small air bubble is injected beneath the graft that helps it to adhere to the corneal surface (▶Fig. 6.7b, c). The peripheral edges of the graft can be unrolled by gently manipulating it with reverse Sinskey hook (▶Fig. 6.7d). Once the graft has fully unrolled, air infusion is started (▶Fig. 6.7e, f). This facilitates total adherence of the graft to the recipient bed. Corneal sutures are taken and a complete closure of all wounds is achieved to get the well-formed AC in the postoperative period (▶Fig. 6.8a, b).

6.3.4 Postoperative Care

In the immediate postoperative period, the patient is advised to lie in supine position for approximately 3 hours and continue doing so for most part of the day. Slit lamp examination is done to confirm the graft centration and location. On the second postoperative day, intraocular pressure is checked and the patency of inferior iridectomy is confirmed. Topical antibiotics and steroids are prescribed that are slowly tapered over a period of 4 months (▶Fig. 6.9, ▶Fig. 6.10, ▶Fig. 6.11, ▶Fig. 6.12, ▶Fig. 6.13, and ▶Fig. 6.14).

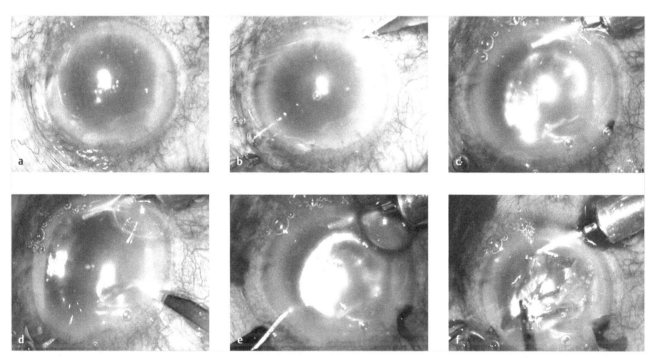

Fig. 6.5 Recipient bed preparation. **(a)** Preoperative status of the recipient eye. **(b)** Side-port incision being made to introduce an ACM. **(c)** ACM is placed in position and is connected to an air pump for continuous air infusion. **(d)** Inferotemporal side-port incision being made. **(e)** Inferonasal side-port incision made. **(f)** Epithelium debridement done to facilitate intraoperative view. ACM, anterior chamber maintainer.

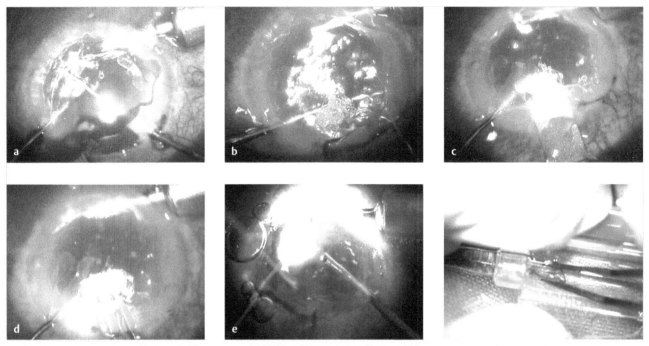

Fig. 6.6 Recipient bed preparation. **(a)** Descemetorhexis initiated with reverse Sinskey hook. **(b)** Descemetorhexis is completely performed at 360°. **(c)** A 2.8-mm corneal tunnel incision is made. **(d)** The recipient's diseased DM–endothelium complex being removed. **(e)** Inferior iridectomy being performed with vitrectomy probe. **(f)** Donor graft is loaded on to the cartridge of the foldable intraocular lens.

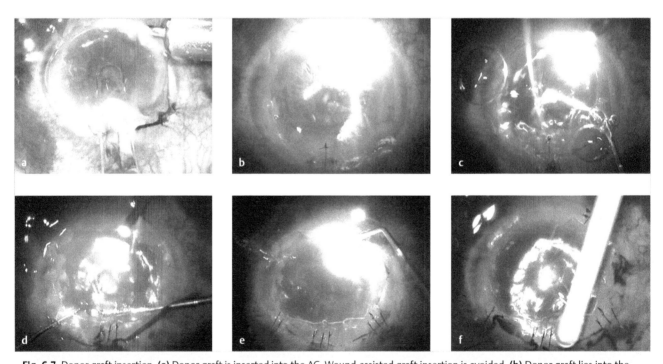

Fig. 6.7 Donor graft insertion. **(a)** Donor graft is inserted into the AC. Wound-assisted graft insertion is avoided. **(b)** Donor graft lies into the AC. **(c)** Graft unrolling is attempted with air and fluidics. Endoilluminator is used to enhance the graft visualization and also to check the correct orientation. **(d)** The periphery of the unrolled graft is gently manipulated with reverse Sinskey hook. **(e)** After proper centration and unrolling of the graft, air is injected beneath and all the corneal wounds are sutured. **(f)** The tautness of the globe is confirmed. AC, anterior chamber.

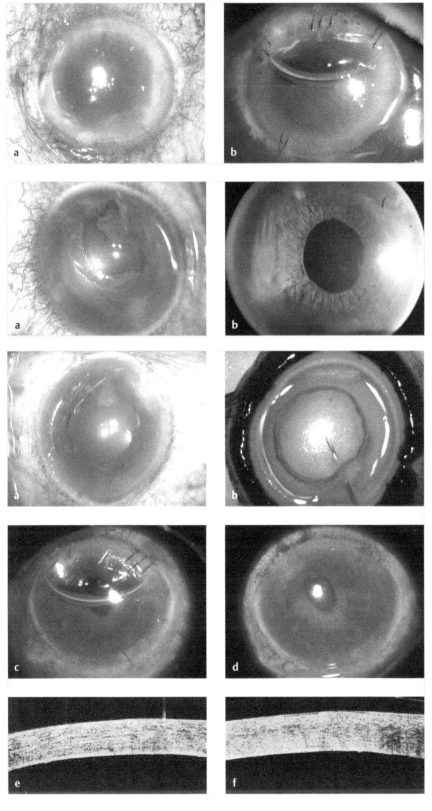

Fig. 6.8 Preoperative and postoperative image. (a) Preoperative image of the patient. (b) One-week postoperative image of the patient.

Fig. 6.9 Preoperative and postoperative image. (a) Preoperative pseudophakic bullous keratopathy. (b) Three months postoperative vision 20/20.

Fig. 6.10 PDEK using a 1-year-old donor. (a) Pseudophakic bullous keratopathy. (b) Type 1 big bubble prepared for PDEK graft. (c) Postoperative day 1 after PDEK. (d) Postoperative 1 week after PDEK. (e) Anterior segment OCT postoperative day 1. (f) Anterior segment OCT postoperative 1 week. OCT, optical coherence tomography; PDEK, Pre-Descemet's endothelial keratoplasty.

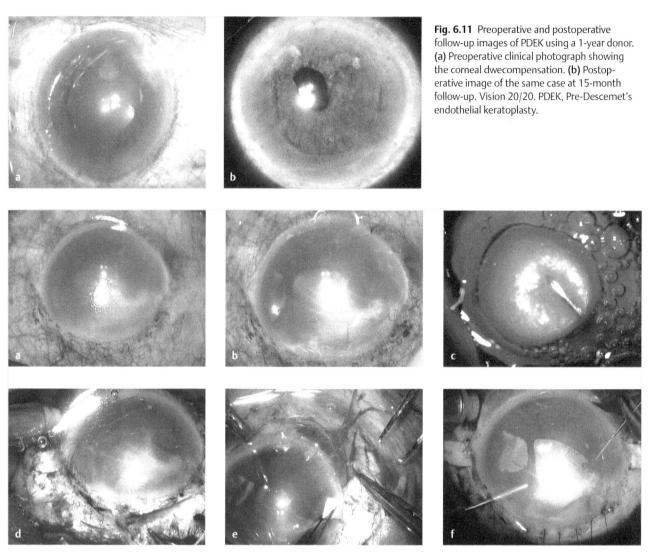

Fig. 6.11 Preoperative and postoperative follow-up images of PDEK using a 1-year donor. **(a)** Preoperative clinical photograph showing the corneal dwecompensation. **(b)** Postoperative image of the same case at 15-month follow-up. Vision 20/20. PDEK, Pre-Descemet's endothelial keratoplasty.

Fig. 6.12 Surgical procedure of PDEK with an infant 9-month-old donor cornea—Step 1. **(a)** Pseudophakic bullous keratopathy with decentered IOL. **(b)** Epithelium removed. Note corneal vascularization and corneal haze. **(c)** Type 1 big bubble prepared for PDEK graft. **(d)** IOL explanted. **(e)** Glued IOL. **(f)** Pupilloplasty. IOL, intraocular lens; PDEK, Pre-Descemet's endothelial keratoplasty.

6.3.5 Discussion

EK as a technique has evolved from deep lamellar endothelial keratoplasty and transitioned to DSEK/DSAEK and further to DMEK (▶Table 6.1). PDEK, being a latest entry into this horizon, is expected to have a broad acceptance due to its similar characteristics of rapid visual recovery, predictable wound strength, and a significant greater optical predictability similar to a DMEK procedure with an added advantage of less chances of donor tissue loss due to tearing away of the DM and also of better graft maneuverability due to extra strength and splinting effect of the PDL to the DM–endothelium complex (▶Video 6.2). Like DMEK, the preparation of PDEK graft does not require large investment in addition to all the other benefits of a DMEK procedure. PDEK involves the addition of the PDL in the donor graft that increases the thickness of the graft to approx-imately 30 to 35 µm as measured with an optical coherence tomography. The graft is comparatively thicker than that of the DMEK but thinner as compared to DSEK/DSAEK or an ultrathin DSAEK (UT-DSAEK). Visual rehabilitation after PDEK is comparatively faster as compared to other EK techniques, except DMEK that involves pure DM transplantation.

Clinically, in our series, we have observed that the incidence of graft dislocation and rebubbling rate are comparatively less in PDEK as compared to DMEK and that can probably be attributed to the addition of the PDL to the donor graft that enhances the graft sustainability. Although, the validation of the PDEK procedure by other surgeons would enhance the acceptability of the technique before it is widely emulated and performed across the globe taking into consideration the complications and feasibility of the technique. The risk of donor tissue loss can be minimized by the eye banks if they supply premade ready-to-use donor graft tissue.

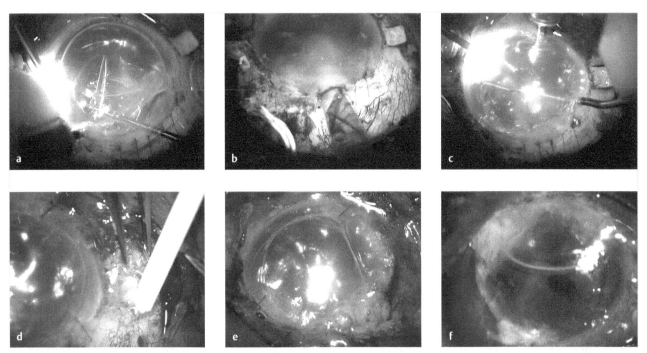

Fig. 6.13 Surgical procedure of PDEK with an infant 9-month-old donor cornea—Step 2. **(a)** Descemetorhexis being performed under air. The endoilluminator helps to enhance the visualization. **(b)** The infant donor graft is loaded onto the cartridge of a foldable IOL injector (the spring is removed to prevent any damage to the graft), and is slowly injected into the eye. **(c)** The donor graft is unrolled, and the endoilluminator helps to identify the correct graft orientation. **(d)** Fibrin glue being applied beneath the scleral flaps (for case 3). **(e)** Corneal incisions closed with 10–0 nylon suture and the AC is filled with air. **(f)** Postoperative image of the case on the fourth postoperative day. AC, anterior chamber; IOL, itraocular lens; PDEK, Pre-Descemet's endothelial keratoplasty.

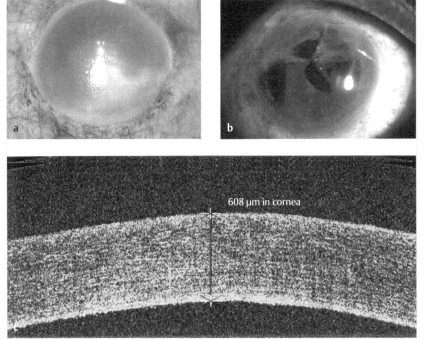

Fig. 6.14 Preoperative and postoperative follow-up images using a 9-month-old donor. **(a)** Preoperative image of decentered IOL with bullous keratopathy with anterior stromal haze. **(b)** Postoperative image of at 6-month follow-up. Vision 20/30. **(c)** Anterior segment OCT showing attached graft. IOL, intraocular lens; OCT, optical coherence tomography.

608 µm in cornea

Table 6.1 Comparison of the different endothelial keratoplasty techniques

	DSEK	DMEK	PDEK
Surgical layers	Stroma + DM + Endo	DM + Endo	Pre-Descemet's + DM + Endo
Technical difficulty	Easy	Difficult	Moderate
Type of procedure	Tissue additive	Tissue neutral	Minimal tissue additive
Artificial anterior chamber	Required	NR	NR
Microkeratome	Required (DSAEK)	NR	NR
Induced hyperopia	Yes	No	No
Corneal thickness	Increased	Normal	Minimal
Intrastromal interface	Yes	No	Minimal
Cost	Costly	Cost-effective	Cost-effective
Eye bank prepared donor tissue	Available	No	Can be made available
Graft unrolling	Easy	Difficult	Moderate
Tissue handling	Good	Difficult	Good
Visual recovery	Slow	Fast	Fast

Abbreviations: DM, Descemet's membrane; DSAEK, Descemet's stripping automated endothelial keratoplasty; Endo, endothelium; NR, not required.

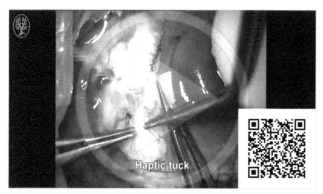

Video 6.2 Double infusion cannula technique. https://www.thieme.de/de/q.htm?p=opn/tp/311890101/9781684200979_video_06_02&t=video

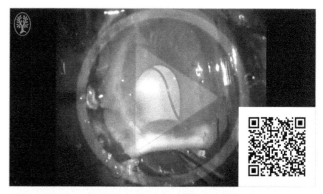

Video 6.3 Infant young donor keratoplasty. https://www.thieme.de/de/q.htm?p=opn/tp/311890101/9781684200979_video_06_03&t=video

6.4 Infant Donor Cornea for Pre-Descemet's Endothelial Keratoplasty

There is a substantial shortage of donor tissue for EK worldwide (▶ Video 6.3). The feasibility of using infant donor graft for PDEK has been highlighted before and doing so potentially increase the pool of suitable donor tissue for PDEK.[5]

The upper age limit for donor tissue usage is considered to be around 75 years but there is still not a clear-cut consensus on the lower age limit of donor tissue usage. Under such circumstances, most centers accept tissue from pediatric donors over 6 months of age. Infant donor tissue has not been used in the past due to various reasons involved with the fear of implanting an immature tissue, although it runs high on endothelial cell density (ECD) count along with the technical reason of implanting a tissue with greater corneal curvature and also increased antigenicity that would increase the risk of immune reaction. Increased steepness, elasticity, and flexibility of the infant donor tissue have limited its application for graft replacement, especially for a penetrating keratoplasty. The same criteria also applies for EK where difficulty in unrolling the graft is observed more so in a DMEK. Harvesting a donor tissue for DMEK with young donors below 40 years of age is believed and considered to be difficult and should be avoided due to presumed strong adhesions between the DM and stroma that can lead to tearing of the DM during harvesting of donor tissue.

The utilization of young donor tissue with favorable outcomes has been reported for DSEK[8] and of an infant donor tissue for DSAEK.[9] Sun et al have reported conflicting results with neonate corneas in DSEK procedure,[10] whereas in our study, we reported the feasibility of an infant donor tissue in PDEK.[5]

6.5 Discussion

Posterior lamellar keratoplasty has the benefit of transferring the healthy endothelium from the donors with or without the addition of the stromal tissue.

Surgeons have performed DSEK with neonate corneas where they have reported achieving the maximum size of lenticule as 8 mm along with the thinner central lenticule as compared to a thicker peripheral rim of the lenticule. This can be attributed to the increased corneal curvature in newborns as compared to adults. They also observed that due to increased flexibility of the cornea, the unrolling of the graft was a bit difficult and that due to this, there were increased chances of graft dislocation and lenticule contraction in the postoperative period.[10]

Other group of surgeons has performed DSEK with pediatric donor tissue and has reported good outcomes. The employment of young donor tissue for EK has a theoretical advantage of transferring a donor lenticule with high ECD that could compensate the issue of ECD loss that eventually occurs post surgery. In EK, a frequent concern among surgeons is potential tissue loss as a result of DM graft preparation failure, which is minimized with the PDEK procedure, as failure to get a type 1 bubble may be associated with the formation of type 2 bubble. Under such scenario, the surgeon can perform a DMEK instead of PDEK procedure.

In conclusion, a stepwise approach to donor preparation and donor insertion makes PDEK a standardized and reproducible procedure with a successful outcome in terms of usage of young donor corneas with high ECD. The procedure of PDEK also involves skill set on behalf of the surgeon to create a type 1 bubble but this limitation is totally circumvented by the fact that PDEK does not require the employment of costly microkeratome as in a DSAEK, DMAEK, or UT-DSEK, thereby cutting the cost of surgical procedure and also inculcating the procedure of the use of infant donor cornea with a graft thickness of around 35 µm that is eventually less as compared to DSAEK or UT-DSEK tissue.

6.6 Complications of Pre-Descemet's Endothelial Keratoplasty

Complications are an inherent and an integral part of any intraocular surgery and they act as a source of continuous refinement in the surgical procedure taking into consideration the technicality of the surgery and also of the surgical skill of the surgeon.

- Tissue loss in graft preparation: This complication can occur when the surgeon dissects in a wrong plane, creating either a type 2 bubble or perforation of the DM–endothelium complex. In the previously mentioned situation, the surgeon can switch over from PDEK to DMEK, whereas in case of latter situation, the donor tissue is totally lost and is rendered useless.

A fresh donor tissue is then needed to complete the surgical procedure.

- Air reinjection and rebubbling: In cases of partial graft detachment where there is an inadequate air fill, rebubbling is often needed to place the graft back in position. Air leakage can occur due to either inappropriate wound closure or due to loss of air in the posterior chamber in pseudophakic and aphakic eyes. In such cases, performing pupilloplasty helps to adequately maintain the AC air fill. Graft repositioning and centration need to be done properly and the patient should be regularly followed up at periodic intervals to detect any incidence of reoccurrence.
- Graft failure and resurgery: Graft failure can occur following a complete graft detachment from the recipient bed. Relocation of the same graft is attempted initially, and in case if it is extremely reticent, then resurgery is preferred.
- Pupillary block: This can occur due to blockage of the iridectomy leading to rise in intraocular pressure. If the AC is overfilled with air, then slight decompression should be attempted by pressing the corneal tunnel.

References

[1] Melles GR, Eggink FA, Lander F, et al. A surgical technique for posterior lamellar keratoplasty. Cornea 1998;17(6):618–626

[2] Melles GR, Ong TS, Ververs B, van der Wees J. Descemet membrane endothelial keratoplasty (DMEK). Cornea 2006;25(8):987–990

[3] Agarwal A, Dua HS, Narang P, et al. Pre-Descemet's endothelial keratoplasty (PDEK). Br J Ophthalmol 2014;98(9):1181–1185

[4] Dua HS, Faraj LA, Said DG, Gray T, Lowe J. Human corneal anatomy redefined: a novel pre-Descemet's layer (Dua's layer). Ophthalmology 2013;120(9): 1778–1785

[5] Agarwal A, Agarwal A, Narang P, Kumar DA, Jacob S. Pre-Descemet endothelial keratoplasty with infant donor corneas: a prospective analysis. Cornea 2015;34(8):859–865

[6] Agarwal A, Narang P, Kumar DA, Agarwal A. Trocar anterior chamber maintainer (T-ACM): Improvised technique of infusion. J Cataract Refract Surg Article in Press

[7] Price FW, Jr, Price MO. Descemet's stripping with endothelial keratoplasty in 200 eyes: Early challenges and techniques to enhance donor adherence. J Cataract Refract Surg 2006;32(3):411–418

[8] Huang T, Wang Y, Hu A, Luo Y, Chen J. Use of paediatric donor tissue in Descemet stripping endothelial keratoplasty. Br J Ophthalmol 2009;93(12):1625–1628

[9] Kim P, Yeung SN, Lichtinger A, Amiran MD, Rootman DS. Descemet stripping automated endothelial keratoplasty using infant donor tissue. Cornea 2012;31(1):52–54

[10] Sun YX, Hao YS, Hong J. Descemet membrane stripping endothelial keratoplasty with neonate donors in two cases. Br J Ophthalmol 2009;93(12): 1692–1693

the intrinsic (cornea and lens) refractive elements of the eye. The entire complex is grafted onto the anterior corneoscleral surface by surrounding periosteum. The ocular surface is reconstructed using buccal mucosa, which encases the lamina offering physical protection in addition to nourishment to the osseous part of the lamina.[86]

7.5.1 Patient Selection

Owing to the complexity of the surgery, the OOKP is reserved for end-stage ocular surface disease with a high likelihood of failure with other treatment modalities such as traditional keratoplasty and limbal stem cell transplantation.[87] Indications include bilateral corneal blindness resulting from severe end-stage SJS, ocular cicatricial pemphigoid, chemical burns, trachoma, severe ocular trauma, severe LSCD, or multiple failed grafts. The procedure is generally only for bilaterally blind patients; the better or only eye should be at best counting fingers but better than NPL. Only one eye is operated with the other eye held as insurance against device failure or future developments. A list of indications and contraindications is provided in ▶ Table 7.5.

Similar to the Boston KPro, the success of the OOKP device begins with appropriate patient selection. Suitable candidates must be highly motivated and possess the cognitive and psychological wherewithal to commit to lifelong treatment and follow-up. The procedure is laborious and time-consuming and is not suitable for patients who are well habituated to blindness. It is, therefore, important to determine that the patient is desirous of surgery and not proceeding out of a sense of obligation to family and/or health professionals. Patients should have a realistic understanding of the benefits and limitations of the device and should be prepared for a mercurial postoperative course, including a lifelong risk of vision loss, serious complications, and further surgery. Patients should be aware that there is a risk of loss of light perception, which is not only devastating emotionally but may also impair circadian rhythms and mood.[88] The presence of positive social and family support is of paramount importance.[86]

Absolute contraindications include pediatric patients (increased bone resorption and absence of permanent teeth), phthisis bulbi, NPL, irreversible vision loss from concomitant pathology, and inability to accept the cosmetic burden of the device.[87]

The OOKP should not be performed in cases where there is a high risk of failure or where the presence of concomitant pathology renders the procedure futile. Inappropriate surgery is harmful as the psychopathological picture is worse for those with unfulfilled expectations and persistent false hope.[88,89] For patients with an irreversible handicap, the acceptance of blindness is an important basis for approaching rehabilitation and obtaining a positive mental equilibrium.[89]

Finally, the OOKP is generally considered the "very last and disfiguring resort."[87] Therefore, other surgical attempts at ocular surface reconstruction are frequently performed prior to consideration of OOKP.[87] However, visual acuity outcomes with the OOKP are inversely related to the number of previous anterior segment surgeries.[87] In patients with a high risk of

Table 7.5 Indications and contraindications of the OOKP

Indications
Patients should fulfill all of the following criteria: • Severe visual loss (<6/60 in better or only eye) because of corneal opacity (uncorrectable with scleral contact lens)   • Poor prognosis of conventional keratoplasty because of high risk of rejection or limbal stem cell deficiency   • Severe dry eye and/or severe irreparable lid damage
Common indications: • Stevens–Johnson syndrome   • Mucous membrane pemphigoid   • Chemical injury   • Thermal injury   • Trachoma
Absolute contraindications
Age under 18
Phthisical eye
Vision ≥ 6/60
No light perception in candidate eye
Eyes with inoperable retinal detachment or other pathologies of the posterior segment that severely interfere with potential visual acuity
Advanced glaucoma or severe optic nerve damage (relative contraindications)
Unrealistic expectations
Patient is unable to accept: • Multistaged operations and possible further surgery   • Cosmetic burden   • Lifelong follow-up   • Risk of severe complications or permanent visual loss

Abbreviation: OOKP, osteo-odonto-keratoprosthesis.
Source: Adapted from the Rome–Vienna protocol[87] and Zarei-Ghanavati et al.[86]

failure with other surgical modalities, it is better to proceed directly to OOKP rather than delay the inevitable with temporizing procedures.

7.5.2 Preoperative Assessment

The preoperative evaluation is performed by a multidisciplinary team, including ophthalmologists, maxillofacial surgeons, anesthetists, and a clinical psychologist.[86] Many of the principles are similar to that for other KPro. Specific features include a careful evaluation of the oral cavity to rule out dental and oral mucosal pathology.[90] A list of investigations is provided in ▶ Table 7.6.

Ophthalmic Assessment

The ocular history, clinical examination, and ancillary investigations should be carefully reviewed to ascertain that the visual potential justifies device implantation. The visual potential should be assessed using the same techniques as for the Boston KPro, including detailed history, ocular examination, serial IOP measurements, confrontational visual fields, automated visual field testing, OCT of the optic nerve and retina, B-scan ultrasonography, and electrophysiology. Many of these techniques will be precluded by media opacity and poor preoperative visual acuity. Fundus visualization through opaque media with endoscopic vitrectomy may be performed in eyes where the viability of the optic nerve and/or retina is uncertain.[91]

Accurate light projection in conjunction with a normal B-scan is encouraging, but its absence does not preclude visual rehabilitation as the ocular surface may interfere with transmission.[87] However, the candidate eye must have good light perception.[87] A- and B-scans are performed to determine the following: axial length, lens status, and exclusion of retinal detachment, gross glaucomatous cupping, and prephthisis.[88] MRI scans are performed in eyes where ultrasonography

Table 7.6 List of preoperative investigations for patients who are under consideration for osteo-odonto-keratoprosthesis

Preoperative assessment

Preoperative ophthalmological assessment:
- VA (intact light perception): Essential
- Entoptic phenomena: Not mandatory
- Electrodiagnosis (flash VEP, flash ERG): Not mandatory
- Ultrasonography (no pathologic findings): Essential
- A-scan biometry: Essential
- Digital estimation of intraocular pressure: Essential
- Examination for dry eye: Not mandatory

Preoperative oral assessment:
- Orthopantomography: Essential
- X-ray of tooth: Essential
- Spiral CT: Not mandatory

Other:
- Preoperative psychological assessment: Essential
- Preoperative anesthesia assessment: Essential

Abbreviations: CT, computed tomography; ERG, electroretinogram; VA, visual acuity; VEP, visual evoked potential.
Source: Adapted from the Rome–Vienna protocol[87] and Zarei-Ghanavati et al.[86]

is precluded by the presence of a silicone oil tamponade.[91] Knowledge of the lens status is important for surgical planning. Areas of corneal thinning or previous perforation should be noted and preparations made for a concomitant lamellar corneal graft during the stage 1 procedure. Other features that will influence the complexity of surgery include anterior chamber depth, and areas of iris adhesion, symblepharon, and ankyloblepharon. Documentation of the severity of the ocular surface disease is useful in qualifying the selection of an OOKP over other treatment modalities.[88]

Complete closure of the lids is not mandatory, but feasible efforts should be made to reconstruct the eyelids to protect the buccal mucous membrane graft.[87] In the absence of eyelids, OOKP can be performed through the palpebral skin following removal of the tarsal plate, but with slightly diminished outcomes likely secondary to faster bone absoprtion.[87]

Oral Assessment

The oral assessment has two components: evaluation of the buccal mucosal graft donor site and selection of an appropriate tooth to form a dentine/bone lamina.[88]

- Buccal mucosal assessment: The attributes of buccal mucous membrane include physiological properties, proliferative capability, and adaptation to high bacterial load.[88] In many patients, the underlying mucocutaneous disease precipitating OOKP may also cause cicatrizing changes to the oral mucosa, thereby compromising the harvest site.[88] Typically, a 3-cm diameter graft is required. If sufficient buccal membrane is not available, other mucous membranes such as palatal and labial can be considered.[87] Smoking cessation is strongly encouraged to improve the chance of graft revascularization.[88] Betel nut chewing is detrimental to tissue quality.[88]
- Dental assessment: The procedure involves harvesting a monoradicular tooth and surrounding intact alveolar bone to fashion a biological skirt to support the PMMA optical cylinder. The ideal tooth should possess a number of characteristics. First, the tooth must be single-rooted and has not undergone previous root treatment. The ideal tooth is usually a canine, although other single-rooted teeth can be used. Second, the tooth must be of adequate shape and size with a good covering of alveolar bone. Third, there should be adequate surrounding space to avoid collateral damage to its neighbor during extraction. Pathologies of the dental crown (e.g., fillings) are not a contraindication but periodontal disease should be assessed and treated. Where possible, the tooth should be selected to minimize cosmetic defect.[88] In edentulous patients, alternative sources of laminae can be considered such as tibial bone (tibial KPro) and human leukocyte antigen (HLA)-matched allograft teeth of living donors.

Clinical assessment must be substantiated with radiological assessment. Essential views are orthopantomograms and intraoral periapical radiographs. These images are sufficient in the majority of cases. Assessment may be augmented with computed tomography (CT) scans.[88]

7.5.3 Surgical Technique

The OOKP is performed in two stages separated by an interval of 2 to 4 months, in accordance with the Rome–Vienna protocol.[87] Both stages are performed under general anesthesia and require the administration of intravenous antibiotics at induction. The first stage involves harvesting of the mucous membrane graft, and preparation of the globe and osteo-odonto-acrylic lamina. The second stage involves retrieval of the lamina and its insertion into the eye. The intervening period allows fibrovascular investment of the lamina and bone tissue recovery from surgical trauma. Furthermore, any infection introduced from the oral cavity will manifest while the lamina is submuscular rather than in the eye.[88]

Stage 1

- Step 1a: Preparation of the mucous membrane graft: A full-thickness buccal membrane graft is harvested below the parotid duct and should be large enough to cover the globe from medial to lateral canthi and from upper to lower fornices. This typically translates to a 3-cm diameter graft.[88] The graft is trimmed of muscle and excess fat and soaked in an antibiotic solution (usually cefuroxime) until required.
- Step 1b: Preparation of the globe: After a 360° limbal peritomy, a superficial keratectomy is performed and all corneal epithelium and Bowman's membrane are removed. If preoperative assessment of the optic nerve and retina was prohibited by corneal opacification, indirect fundoscopy should be attempted at this stage to assess the visual potential for future intervention.[92] The conjunctiva and tenons are recessed to form the underlying sclera. The rectus muscles are isolated with stay sutures. Cautery is performed judiciously so as to preserve the episcleral vessels.[87] Areas of severe corneal thinning or tectonic compromise are reinforced with a lamellar corneal graft. The mucous membrane graft is anchored to the sclera and rectus insertions (for vascular supply) with interrupted 6–0 Vicryl sutures.[88] A plastic conformer is placed on the globe at the end of the procedure and is left in situ for a month to prevent adhesions.[86] A postoperative spike in IOP occurs as the mucous membrane graft compromises uveoscleral outflow and this is managed with acetazolamide supplemented with intravenous mannitol.[93]

The stage 1 procedure may be divided into two separate procedures in patients at risk of mucous membrane graft failure. Preparation of the mucous membrane graft and globe is performed first and the patient is readmitted for tooth harvesting and formation of the OOKP lamina once graft survival has been established.[88]

- Step 2a: Preparation of the osteo-odonto-acrylic lamina: A monoradicular tooth (usually a canine) complete with surrounding alveolar bone is harvested en bloc. Care is taken to conserve periosteum as it is subsequently required

to cover the bone of the implant.[87] A dental flywheel under continuous irrigation is used to mold the tooth and surrounding bone to an approximately 3-mm-thick rectangular lamella. A central aperture is drilled perpendicularly through the lamina to accommodate a biconvex PMMA optical cylinder of appropriate power (based on A-scan biometry). The aperture should be large enough to allow the cylinder to be inserted without excessive force, but small enough to ensure a snug fit.[87] Cement is placed around the optic and acts as a filler rather than an adhesive.[86]

The entire complex is embedded in a subcutaneous pouch for biointegration, usually under the lower lid of the contralateral eye.[85] Alternatively, a submuscular pouch underneath the orbicularis oculi may be used.[94] The lamina is removed after 2 or 3 months in preparation from transplantation. Delay beyond this period may result in partial absorption.[87]

In edentulous patients, laminae can be prepared from tibial bone or allograft tooth from HLA-matched living donors.

Stage 2

The tooth–optic complex is explanted for inspection and further surgery is only contemplated if the lamina is of sufficient size with adequate vascularization.[87] The soft tissue is debulked over the osseous aspect and completely excised from the dentine surface. The lamina is stored in autologous heparinized venous blood or temporarily replaced in the submuscular pocket to avoid drying during the preparation of the globe. The buccal membrane is partially reflected inferiorly to expose the cornea and sclera, leaving a large inferiorly attached base to preserve adequate blood supply. A Flieringa ring is sutured to the sclera. The central cornea is identified and trephined to match the posterior part of the optical cylinder.[86] Two relieving incisions are made in the cornea to allow either cryoextraction of the lens or removal of the IOL–capsule complex as per the Rome–Vienna protocol.[86] The iris is completely removed at its root and a core vitrectomy is performed. This amputation of all anterior segment structures is performed to prevent secondary glaucoma from angle closure, and the formation of severe inflammatory membranes behind the optic cylinder.[87] Watertight closure of the relieving incisions is performed. The prosthesis is placed with the dentine surface facing the cornea and anchored tightly with interrupted Vicryl sutures to the corneoscleral surface. Sterile air is injected via the pars plana by a 30-G needle to reform the globe. Indirect fundoscopy is performed to ascertain adequate centration of the optic cylinder. The Flieringa ring is removed. The buccal membrane is repositioned and sutured in place with multiple interrupted sutures. A central 3-mm trephination of the buccal membrane allows protrusion of the anterior optical cylinder.

A number of variations in surgical technique have been described between centers.[94] The Rome–Vienna protocol recommends an intracapsular cataract extraction,[87] whereas a number of centers favor an extracapsular approach.[94,95,96]

Proponents of the intracapsular procedure prefer this technique as it minimizes the risk of synechiae formation with lens capsule and avoids risk of incomplete removal of crystalline lens fragments owing to poor visualization.[84] Another difference is the size of the trephined cornea relative to the posterior portion of the optical cylinder. The Rome–Vienna protocol recommends equal sizing,[87] whereas other centers prefer to oversize the cornea by around 0.5 mm.[94,96,97]

7.5.4 Postoperative Management

Immediate Postoperative Period

Patients are admitted for 1 week after each stage and receive systemic and topical antibiotics, in addition to oral prednisone. Typically, oral antibiotic is administered for 1 week and oral prednisolone 20 mg in conjunction with a proton pump inhibitor is administered for 5 days.[88] Oral acetazolamide, in concert with pro re nata intravenous mannitol, is administered in anticipation of elevated IOP and is continued until IOP is normalized. After the first stage, meticulous oral hygiene is maintained with chlorhexidine and nystatin mouthwashes until the donor site has healed.[86] Following stage 2, topical broad-spectrum antibiotics are continued indefinitely once daily with a 3-month alternate cycling to reduce bacterial resistance. In dry eyes, the mucous membrane is lubricated with balanced salt solution. Eyes with lagophthalmos require ongoing nighttime lubricating ointment. The optical cylinder is cleaned with a sterile cotton-tipped applicator and protein deposits are removed with juice from a fresh-cut lemon.

Long-Term Follow-up

OOKP patients require lifelong follow-up. In the postoperative period, routine patients are seen at weekly intervals for 1 month, then monthly for 3 months, then every 2 months for 6 months, and quarterly thereafter. Important components of scheduled examinations include unaided and corrected vision, refraction, and digital estimation of IOP. The health of the mucous membrane graft is assessed for vascularization, dryness, and the presence of thinning or ulceration. The optical cylinder is examined for tilt, anterior protrusion, and the presence of a retroprosthetic membrane. Increased exposure of the anterior portion of the optical cylinder may indicate bone resorption and/or thinning of the overlying mucous membrane.[98] The lamina is evaluated for bone resorption by palpating the mass and dimensions of the lamina.[88] Baseline radiological volumetric analysis is performed with a multidetector CT scan; however, there is no consensus regarding the need for or the frequency of serial imaging to detect early bone resorption. Fundoscopy is performed at each visit to assess the optic nerve and macula, and exclude retinal detachment. B-scan ultrasonography can be used to detect early peripheral detachments.[88]

Glaucoma monitoring is essential to the long-term success of the prosthesis and is discussed in greater detail below.

7.5.5 Outcomes

The OOKP is reserved for the most desperate cases of bilateral ocular surface disease. The overall long-term anatomical survival in published OOKP series is 87.8% (range 67–100%) at 5 years and 81.0% (range 65–98%) at 20 years.[94] The encouraging success rate in this high-risk patient group compared with conventional keratoplasty is attributed to the replacement of an unstable ocular surface with durable biological constituents. More than half of patients (52%, range 46–72%) enjoy a vision better than 6/18 after OOKP.[94] Overall, around 80% of patients will experience an improvement in vision following OOKP[95,99] and failure to improve is mostly secondary to preoperative posterior pole damage and glaucoma.[86] However, the functional survival of the OOKP is finite in the majority of patients. In one large series, the 10-year functional survival was reported to be 49% in OOKP eyes and further reduced to 25% for tibial bone KPro.[100]

The OOKP is not a visual panacea and while the central visual acuity may be excellent, the visual field is severely constricted. Patients should understand preoperatively that the OOKP has the potential to restore reading and ambulatory vision, but driving vision will remain unattainable.[88] The view is analogous to looking through a tube as the cylinder is by necessity long and narrow.[88] The original optical cylinder design had a reported visual field of 40°[88] and subsequent modifications have improved the field of view, albeit to a still limited reported median 69°.[101] The visual field may be even further constricted in the high proportion of patients with concomitant glaucoma. Tilt and decentration of the optical cylinder will also diminish the visual field. Glare is another significant issue in OOKP eyes and patients also experience lower contrast sensitivity compared with age-matched controls.[101]

7.5.6 Complications

In common with other KPro designs, complications associated with the OOKP device include glaucoma, vitritis, endophthalmitis, and retinal detachment. Complications specific to OOKP implantation include injury to the maxillary sinus, facial, and jaw bone fractures, mucosal complications such as necrosis or overgrowth, and resorption of the osteodental lamina with the risk of extrusion. Mucous membrane necrosis, RPM formation, and bone resorption are more common in tibial bone OOKP than OOKP.[100] A list of complications reported in the literature is provided in ▶ Table 7.7.

Glaucoma

Glaucoma is a considerable challenge in OOKP eyes owing to a plethora of issues in diagnosis, monitoring, and management. Glaucoma may be primary to etiology, secondary to previous intraocular procedures and/or traumatic, inflammatory, or infectious events, or occur de novo after prosthesis implantation. The reported incidence of preoperative glaucoma ranges from 20 to 52%,[84,95,97,99,103] whereas the condition

Table 7.7 Complications of osteo-odonto-keratoprosthesis surgery

Complication	Study						
	Tan[94] (n = 35)	De La Paz[102] (n = 145)	Iyer[92] (n = 50)	Liu[95] (n = 36)	Hille[99] (n = 25)	Falcinelli[84] (n = 181)	Marchi[97] (n = 85)
Intraoperative							
Vitreous hemorrhage	48.6%	–	–	–	52.0%*	0.6%	–
Expulsive hemorrhage	–	–	–	2.8%	–	–	–
Subchoroidal hemorrhage	–	–	–	–	8%*	–	–
Choroidal detachment	–	–	–	–	20%*	0.6%	–
Mucous membrane defects	–	–	–	–	40%*	–	–
Postoperative							
Glaucoma	34.3%	11%	20%	47%	16%	6.6%	33%
Laminar resorption	2.9%	28.0%	4.0%	19.4%	8%	1.7%	2.3%
Mucous membrane ulceration	25.7%	–	18%**	27.8%	8%	7.7%	–
Mucous membrane overgrowth	22.9%	–	2%	33.3%	–	–	–
Vitreous hemorrhage	2.9%	3%	–	8.3%	–	3.3%	–
Sterile vitritis	8.6%	–	6%	–	–	–	–
Endophthalmitis	2.9%	–	2%	8.3%	0%	2.2%	–
Hypotonia	2.9%	–	2%	–	8%	–	–
Phthisis	–	–	–	2.8%	–	–	–
Retinal detachment	8.6%	16%	2%	8.3%	12%*	2.8%	3.5%
Retroprosthetic membrane	20.0%	5%	–	16.7%	8%	0.6%	3.5%
Fistula	–	–	6%	–	–	0.6%	–
Mandibular fracture	–	–	–	–	–	1.1%	–
Dental unit loss	–	–	–	–	–	0.6%	–

*Described as "perioperative."

**Described as lamina exposure in study (central 6%, peripheral 12%). Trophic alterations 8%.

has been reported to arise de novo in 0 to 33%.[84,95,97,103] The burden of postoperative glaucoma varies widely from 11 to 47%.[92,95,102] The wide range reflects disparate patient cohorts and also the constraints under which glaucoma is diagnosed in both the preoperative and postoperative periods. In some patients, disease progression has been observed despite aggressive treatment with medications, GDDs, and/or endo-laser photocoagulation.[55,99,103] Chemical injury eyes are particularly susceptible to glaucoma and this may be compounded by the toxic effect of the original chemical insult on the optic nerve.[104]

The pathogenesis of de novo glaucoma following OOKP is poorly understood. The procedure involves total iridectomy and intracapsular cataract extraction, which minimize the possibility of iridocorneal or iridocapsular adhesions.[93] Furthermore, anatomical distortion of the angle structures by peripheral corneal sutures does not occur. De novo glaucoma has been postulated to arise from extensive intraoperative manipulation and decompartmentalization of the anterior chamber.[50]

Glaucoma monitoring is encumbered by the absence of a reliable measure of IOP, which is effectively limited to estimation by digital palpation. Furthermore, the optics of the device result in a limited field of view for both patient and examiner. Therefore, assessment and diagnosis rely on stereo-biomicroscopic examination of the optic nerve head, serial visual field testing, and optic nerve tomographic imaging. The Goldmann visual field is superior to automated visual field testing, which is affected by the diameter of the PMMA cylinder.[105] All imaging devices are likely to encounter issues with reproducibility and quality relating to axial alignment along the small optical cylinder,[103] and all modalities will be altered compared with normal eyes.[106] Adjunctive tests of central visual field functioning may also be performed, including contrast sensitivity, pattern ERG, and VEPs, with the latter most accurate to detect glaucomatous change (sensitivity 75% and specificity 85%).[106]

Topical medications have questionable benefit due to a lack of absorption through the thick oral mucosal graft; however, they may be considered if areas of intact conjunctival epithelium are observed around the limits of the graft.[103] Systemic acetazolamide is the mainstay of medical therapy for glaucoma in OOKP eyes but should be used with caution particularly in SJS patients.[104] One series recommends its continued postoperative use for a period of 6 to 12 months in eyes with no pre-existing glaucoma.[93] Sublingual timolol may also be considered.

Drainage device implantation forms the backbone of surgical treatment and may be performed before or during stage 1, or at a later time after stage 2. Simultaneous drainage tube implantation during the stage 2 procedure is not recommended due to the risk of hypotony.[87] Early device insertion before the placement of the mucosal graft is preferable as the anatomy of the ocular surface has not yet been disturbed.[93] Furthermore, early tube placement could play a role in minimizing IOP spikes during subsequent procedures.[93] However, empiric GDD implantation is not warranted, considering the risk of complications and the absence of de novo glaucoma in some series.[93,103] The decision to place a drainage device should be continually reassessed as each stage of the procedure causes a varied response on IOP.[93]

In one series, the IOP stabilized in 73.3% of eyes with preexisting glaucoma following Ahmed GDD implantation in conjunction with systemic oral acetazolamide.[93] The success of drainage device surgery in OOKP eyes is complicated by unpredictable encapsulation and the obliteration of episcleral vessels.[86]

Endoscopic cyclophotocoagulation is another option but is associated with a high incidence of postoperative complications, in particular, vitreous hemorrhage.[107] Therefore, it should be considered as a last resort after alternatives have been exhausted.[107] Cyclocryocoagulation is not recommended because of the risk of inflammation and phthisis.

Bone Resorption

Bone resorption is an issue unique to the OOKP procedure and threatens the longevity of the lamina.[108] Loss of laminar volume and integrity is an important cause of anatomical failure, and in extreme cases, can result in extrusion of the cylinder or endophthalmitis.[86,109] Other sequelae include optic instability, RPM formation, vitreous hemorrhage, choroidal and retinal detachment, and aqueous leak.[110] Resorption may result in either focal or global thinning of the lamina.[86]

Clinically, significant resorption rates have been reported to range from 1.7 to 28%,[84,92,94,95,97,99,102] though a degree of resorption is thought to occur in all patients. Resorption is likely underreported since clinical detection is often a late manifestation.[86] Indeed, clinical examination alone fails to identify up to 60% of eyes with radiologic evidence of resorption.[98] The exact etiology of bone resorption is unknown but chronic subclinical inflammation, and ulceration and infection of the mucous membrane are implicated.[88,108,111] Increased rates of resorption have been observed in SJS, metabolically active young patients, tibial bone laminae, and tooth allografts.[95,110,112]

The diagnosis of resorption may be difficult as the process is insidious and the lamella is hidden beneath the oral mucosal membrane.[86] Clinical signs include a change in refraction, reduced vision, elongation or tilting of the optical cylinder, loss of bony resistance to palpation, and loss of lamina dimensions.[110] In more advanced cases, there may be aqueous leak with resultant hypotony.[88] Laminar resorption is commonly accompanied by a "sterile" vitritis[108] however, a high index of suspicion for endophthalmitis is necessary as these eyes are vulnerable to microbial ingress via external communication from a loosened cylinder.

Imaging of the lamina is typically performed with a multidetector CT scan. Baseline linear dimensions and volumetric data of the lamina are compared with subsequent serial measurements to estimate resorption. Currently, there is no consensus regarding the frequency of imaging, which must balance the advantage of early detection and intervention against the hazards of radiation.[98] The early detection of laminar resorption allows the use of prophylactic measures to preserve the lamina. One series describes augmentation of the bony lamina by mandibular bone graft, with encouraging results.[109] A technique to prolong the longevity of the lamina by reinforcing the same with bone morphogenic protein has been described.[108] Systemic bisphosphonates have been used to retard the bone and dentine resorption process, though the efficacy is indeterminate.[86] In cases of severe resorption, the lamina is exchanged to preserve the integrity and function of the eye.[86]

Buccal Mucous Membrane Complications

The buccal membrane graft is associated with a spectrum of complications ranging from mucous membrane overgrowth to ulceration and exposure of the lamina. The health of the mucous membrane may be compromised from the outset by the underlying inflammatory condition or poor orodental hygiene, smoking, chewing betel nuts, or heavy alcohol consumption.[113] A compromised mucosal membrane is particularly vulnerable to complications such as ulceration and necrosis. Patients with SJS are at an increased risk of mucosal complications.[114]

Mucous membrane ulceration arises secondary to ischemia, dryness, and infection. It requires prompt evaluation and treatment as it can lead to laminar erosion and intraocular infection. The rate has been reported in various studies to range from 8 to 27.8%.[84,92,94,95,99] In the event of mucous membrane ulceration, it is important to exclude and treat any underlying infection.[88] Mild ulcers can be treated with increased lubrication.[86] Large ulcers require mucosoplasty in the form of tarsal pedicle, mucosal rotation, bucket handle flaps, or free patch graft.[88] Advanced cases may require replacement with a new buccal membrane graft. Refractory ulceration may necessitate a modified tarsorrhaphy with an aperture for the optical cylinder to protrude.[88]

Buccal mucosal tissue overgrowth occluding the surface of the optical cylinder is a common and frequently recurrent condition that can cause visual obstruction. A stepladder approach to management is recommended.[86] Deliberate desiccation will retard membrane proliferation in the early postoperative period; however, lubrication should only be discontinued once vascularization is reestablished, a process which usually takes 3 weeks.[113] Recalcitrant mucosal overgrowth can be treated with trimming and cauterization. Recurrent cases are treated with repeat excision around the optic cylinder, followed by the off-label application of mitomycin C.[113]

Vitreoretinal Complications

Vitreoretinal complications have been reported to arise in 23 to 55.7% of OOKP eyes[91,115,116] and include sterile vitritis, retinal detachment, RPM formation, endophthalmitis, vitreous hemorrhage, serous choroidal detachment, hemorrhagic choroidal detachment, and leak related hypotony.[116]

Vitreous hemorrhage is commonly seen in the early postoperative period and arises from extensive anterior segment dissection and iatrogenic aniridia.[91] Most cases are mild, self-resolving, and therefore managed expectantly. RPM formation occurs in around 0.6 to 20.0% of OOKP eyes and occurs less frequently than with other forms of KPro owing to the surgical removal of the iris.[116] They are thought to occur secondary to chronic inflammation or due to an epithelial downgrowth after loss of the epithelial seal.[116] Medical management with a 1-week course of systemic steroids in combination with systemic antibiotics followed by a steroid taper has been described.[116] Visually significant membranes may be removed by YAG laser. In cases of dense RPM or recurrent RPM refractory to YAG laser, endoscopic membranectomy may be required.[88]

Retinal detachment has been reported in 2 to 16%[84,92,94,95,97,99,102] of OOKP eyes and is typically complex involving both tractional and rhegmatogenous components, further complicated by proliferative vitreoretinopathy.[91] Silicone oil is frequently required to achieve anatomical success, but this degrades optical quality, precludes ultrasonic visualization, and increases the already elevated risk of glaucoma.[91] Retinal detachment following OOKP has been associated with a poor visual outcome.[116,117]

Endophthalmitis can be a devastating complication of OOKP and may present with atypical signs and symptoms.[86] This behooves a high index of suspicion and any acute symptom of pain or decreased vision should be evaluated to exclude endophthalmitis.[86] The rate of endophthalmitis is reported at 0 to 8.3%,[84,92,94,95,99] and there is a strong association of endophthalmitis and laminar resorption.[116] According to the Rome–Vienna protocol, endophthalmitis necessitates immediate explantation of the OOKP, vitrectomy, intravitreal and systemic antibiotics, and tectonic closure with a corneal graft.[87]

Vitreoretinal surgery in OOKP eyes is beset with surgical difficulties. The OOKP obliterates anatomical landmarks and poses considerable challenges in the intraoperative visualization of the posterior segment.[91] Surgical tools to enable visualization include temporary KPro, wide-angle viewing systems, and endoscopic vitrectomy. In one series, one-third of patients required perioperative retinal surgery for either diagnosis or treatment complications.[91] Retinal surgery was indicated for the assessment of retina and optic nerve health prior to OOKP, endoscopic cyclophotocoagulation, endoscopic trimming of RPM, retinal detachment repair, and vitrectomy for endophthalmitis.[91]

7.5.7 Conclusion

The OOKP is a complex surgical technique that offers promising anatomical and functional results in patients with bilateral severe end-stage ocular surface disease. It is considered the most invasive and technically challenging keratoplasty technique and has the greatest cosmetic burden. Therefore, its applicability is restricted to the most challenging cases of ocular surface disease.

7.6 Keratoprosthesis Conclusion

The field of KPro is experiencing an exciting period of evolution. Innovations in design and surgical technique have broadened the clinical applicability and the number of

hitherto hopeless cases helped by KPro implantation continues to expand. Appropriate patient selection is vital to success and important considerations include etiology, visual potential, ocular surface status, and patient expectations.

The Boston KPro type I is the most commonly used device, though its applicability is limited to wet blinking eyes with adequate forniceal depth. The Boston KPro type II and the OOKP have both been deployed in the surgical treatment of eyes with severe end-stage ocular surface disease. To date, there is no formal study comparing the Boston KPro type II and the OOKP. Comparisons between the two devices are difficult because of differences in underlying patient populations and ongoing incremental improvements in device design and perioperative care.[79]

For many, the OOKP remains the gold standard for vision restoration in eyes with a severely dry keratinized or dermalized ocular surface.[2,78] The OOKP has more extensive published literature with longer follow-up periods and better-reported device retention.[2,86] The disadvantage of the OOKP is that it is a complicated, lengthy, multistage procedure, requiring experienced oral and ophthalmic subspecialists and can be done at only a few centers of excellence. The Boston KPro type II is comparatively more simple. Provided the facilities are available and there is suitable dentition, the OOKP is the procedure of choice.[78,90]

References

[1] Aravena C, Yu F, Aldave AJ. Long-term visual outcomes, complications, and retention of the Boston type I keratoprosthesis. Cornea 2018;37(1):3–10

[2] Lee R, Khoueir Z, Tsikata E, Chodosh J, Dohlman CH, Chen TC. Long-term visual outcomes and complications of Boston keratoprosthesis type II implantation. Ophthalmology 2017;124(1):27–35

[3] Salvador-, Culla B, Kolovou PE. Keratoprosthesis: A Review of Recent Advances in the Field. J Funct Biomater 2016;7(2):E13

[4] Akpek EK, Alkharashi M, Hwang FS, Ng SM, Lindsley K. Artificial corneas versus donor corneas for repeat corneal transplants. Cochrane Database Syst Rev 2014(11):CD009561

[5] Harissi-Dagher M, Khan BF, Schaumberg DA, Dohlman CH. Importance of nutrition to corneal grafts when used as a carrier of the Boston keratoprosthesis. Cornea 2007;26(5):564–568

[6] Khan BF, Harissi-Dagher M, Khan DM, Dohlman CH. Advances in Boston keratoprosthesis: enhancing retention and prevention of infection and inflammation. Int Ophthalmol Clin 2007;47(2):61–71

[7] Williamson SL, Cortina MS. Boston type 1 keratoprosthesis from patient selection through postoperative management: a review for the keratoprosthetic surgeon. Clin Ophthalmol 2016;10:437–443

[8] Belin MW, Güell JL, Grabner G. Suggested Guidelines for Reporting Keratoprosthesis Results: Consensus Opinion of the Cornea Society, Asia Cornea Society, EuCornea, PanCornea, and the KPRO Study Group. Cornea 2016;35(2):143–144

[9] Saeed HN, Shanbhag S, Chodosh J. The Boston keratoprosthesis. Curr Opin Ophthalmol 2017;28(4):390–396

[10] Yaghouti F, Nouri M, Abad JC, Power WJ, Doane MG, Dohlman CH. Keratoprosthesis: preoperative prognostic categories. Cornea 2001;20(1):19–23

[11] Ahmad S, Mathews PM, Srikumaran D, et al. Outcomes of Repeat Boston Type 1 Keratoprosthesis Implantation. Am J Ophthalmol 2016;161:181–7.e1

[12] Hager JL, Phillips DL, Goins KM, et al. Boston type 1 keratoprosthesis for failed keratoplasty. Int Ophthalmol 2016;36(1):73–78

[13] Ahmad S, Mathews PM, Lindsley K, et al. Boston Type 1 Keratoprosthesis versus Repeat Donor Keratoplasty for Corneal Graft Failure: A Systematic Review and Meta-analysis. Ophthalmology 2016;123(1):165–177

[14] Fadous R, Levallois-Gignac S, Vaillancourt L, Robert MC, Harissi-Dagher M. The Boston Keratoprosthesis type 1 as primary penetrating corneal procedure. Br J Ophthalmol 2015;99(12):1664–1668

[15] Kosker M, Suri K, Rapuano CJ, et al. Long-Term Results of the Boston Keratoprosthesis for Unilateral Corneal Disease. Cornea 2015;34(9):1057–1062

[16] Pineles SL, Ela-Dalman N, Rosenbaum AL, Aldave AJ, Velez FG. Binocular visual function in patients with Boston type I keratoprostheses. Cornea 2010;29(12):1397–1400

[17] Rahi JS, Cumberland PM, Peckham CS. Visual impairment and vision-related quality of life in working-age adults: findings in the 1958 British birth cohort. Ophthalmology 2009;116(2):270–274

[18] Mendes F, Schaumberg DA, Navon S, et al. Assessment of visual function after corneal transplantation: the quality of life and psychometric assessment after corneal transplantation (Q-PACT) study. Am J Ophthalmol 2003;135(6):785–793

[19] Williams KA, Ash JK, Pararajasegaram P, Harris S, Coster DJ. Long-term outcome after corneal transplantation. Visual result and patient perception of success. Ophthalmology 1991;98(5):651–657

[20] Fung SSM, Jabbour S, Harissi-Dagher M, et al. Visual Outcomes and Complications of Type I Boston Keratoprosthesis in Children: A Retrospective Multicenter Study and Literature Review. Ophthalmology 2017

[21] Ciolino JB, Belin MW, Todani A, Al-Arfaj K, Rudnisky CJ; Boston Keratoprosthesis Type 1 Study Group. Retention of the Boston keratoprosthesis type 1: multicenter study results. Ophthalmology 2013;120(6):1195–1200

[22] Kim KH, Mian SI. Diagnosis of corneal limbal stem cell deficiency. Curr Opin Ophthalmol 2017;28(4):355–362

[23] de Araujo AL, Charoenrook V, de la Paz MF, Temprano J, Barraquer RI, Michael R. The role of visual evoked potential and electroretinography in the preoperative assessment of osteo-keratoprosthesis or osteo-odonto-keratoprosthesis surgery. Acta Ophthalmol 2012;90(6):519–525

[24] Nguyen P, Chopra V. Glaucoma management in Boston keratoprosthesis type I recipients. Curr Opin Ophthalmol 2014;25(2):134–140

[25] Akpek EK, Aldave AJ, Aquavella JV. The use of precut, -irradiated corneal lenticules in Boston type 1 keratoprosthesis implantation. Am J Ophthalmol 2012;154(3):495–498.e1

[26] Harissi-Dagher M, Colby KA. Cataract extraction after implantation of a type I Boston keratoprosthesis. Cornea 2008;27(2):220–222

[27] Lim JI, Machen L, Arteaga A, et al. Comparison of Visual and Anatomical Outcomes of Eyes Undergoing Type I Boston Keratoprosthesis with Combination Pars Plana Vitrectomy with Eyes without Combination Vitrectomy. Retina 2018;38(Suppl 1):S125–S133

[28] Perez VL, Leung EH, Berrocal AM, et al. Impact of Total Pars Plana Vitrectomy on Postoperative Complications in Aphakic, Snap-On, Type 1 Boston Keratoprosthesis. Ophthalmology 2017;124(10):1504–1509

[29] Sayegh RR, Avena Diaz L, Vargas-Martín F, Webb RH, Dohlman CH, Peli E. Optical functional properties of the Boston Keratoprosthesis. Invest Ophthalmol Vis Sci 2010;51(2):857–863

[30] Sayegh RR, Dohlman CH. Wide-angle fundus imaging through the Boston keratoprosthesis. Retina 2013;33(6):1188–1192

[31] Behlau I, Martin KV, Martin JN, et al. Infectious endophthalmitis in Boston keratoprosthesis: incidence and prevention. Acta Ophthalmol 2014;92(7):e546–e555

[32] Kammerdiener LL, Speiser JL, Aquavella JV, et al. Protective effect of soft contact lenses after Boston keratoprosthesis. Br J Ophthalmol 2016;100(4):549–552

[33] Harissi-Dagher M, Beyer J, Dohlman CH. The role of soft contact lenses as an adjunct to the Boston keratoprosthesis. Int Ophthalmol Clin 2008;48(2):43–51

[34] Thomas M, Shorter E, Joslin CE, McMahon TJ, Cortina MS. Contact Lens Use in Patients With Boston Keratoprosthesis Type 1: Fitting, Management, and Complications. Eye Contact Lens 2015;41(6):334–340

[35] Wagoner MD, Welder JD, Goins KM, Greiner MA. Microbial Keratitis and Endophthalmitis After the Boston Type 1 Keratoprosthesis. Cornea 2016;35(4):486–493

[36] Lee WB, Shtein RM, Kaufman SC, Deng SX, Rosenblatt MI. Boston Keratoprosthesis: Outcomes and Complications: A Report by the American Academy of Ophthalmology. Ophthalmology 2015;122(7):1504–1511

[37] Zerbe BL, Belin MW, Ciolino JB; Boston Type 1 Keratoprosthesis Study Group. Results from the multicenter Boston Type 1 Keratoprosthesis Study. Ophthalmology 2006;113(10):1779.e1–1779.e7

[38] Greiner MA, Li JY, Mannis MJ. Longer-term vision outcomes and complications with the Boston type I keratoprosthesis at the University of California, Davis. Ophthalmology 2011;118(8):1543–1550

[39] Srikumaran D, Munoz B, Aldave AJ, et al. Long-term outcomes of Boston type 1 keratoprosthesis implantation: a retrospective multicenter cohort. Ophthalmology 2014;121(11):2159–2164

[40] Kamyar R, Weizer JS, de Paula FH, et al. Glaucoma associated with Boston type I keratoprosthesis. Cornea 2012;31(2):134–139

[41] Talajic JC, Agoumi Y, Gagné S, Moussally K, Harissi-Dagher M. Prevalence, progression, and impact of glaucoma on vision after Boston type 1 keratoprosthesis surgery. Am J Ophthalmol 2012;153(2):267–274.e1

[42] Crnej A, Paschalis EI, Salvador-, Culla B, et al. Glaucoma progression and role of glaucoma surgery in patients with Boston keratoprosthesis. Cornea 2014;33(4):349–354

[43] Aldave AJ, Sangwan VS, Basu S, et al. International results with the Boston type I keratoprosthesis. Ophthalmology 2012;119(8):1530–1538

[44] Goins KM, Kitzmann AS, Greiner MA, et al. Boston Type 1 Keratoprosthesis: Visual Outcomes, Device Retention, and Complications. Cornea 2016;35(9):1165–1174

[45] Aravena C, Bozkurt TK, Yu F, Aldave AJ. Long-Term Outcomes of the Boston Type I Keratoprosthesis in the Management of Corneal Limbal Stem Cell Deficiency. Cornea 2016;35(9):1156–1164

[46] Kang JJ, de la Cruz J, Cortina MS. Visual outcomes of Boston keratoprosthesis implantation as the primary penetrating corneal procedure. Cornea 2012;31(12):1436–1440

[47] Ali MH, Dikopf MS, Finder AG, et al. Assessment of Glaucomatous Damage After Boston Keratoprosthesis Implantation Based on Digital Planimetric Quantification of Visual Fields and Optic Nerve Head Imaging. Cornea 2018;37(5):602–608

[48] Magalhaes OA, Aldave AJ. Scleral Pneumatonometry in Penetrating Keratoplasty: A Clinical Study. Cornea 2017;36(10):1200–1205

[49] Lenis TL, Chiu SY, Law SK, Yu F, Aldave AJ. Safety of Concurrent Boston Type I Keratoprosthesis and Glaucoma Drainage Device Implantation. Ophthalmology 2017;124(1):12–19

[50] Baltaziak M, Chew HF, Podbielski DW, Ahmed IIK. Glaucoma after corneal replacement. Surv Ophthalmol 2018;63(2):135–148

[51] Patel V, Moster MR, Kishfy L, et al. Sequential versus concomitant surgery of glaucoma drainage implant and Boston keratoprosthesis type 1. Eur J Ophthalmol 2016;26(6):556–563

[52] Baratz KH, Goins KM. The Boston Keratoprosthesis: Highs and Lows of Intraocular Pressure and Outcomes. Ophthalmology 2017;124(1):9–11

[53] Li JY, Greiner MA, Brandt JD, Lim MC, Mannis MJ. Long-term complications associated with glaucoma drainage devices and Boston keratoprosthesis. Am J Ophthalmol 2011;152(2):209–218

[54] Chew HF, Ayres BD, Hammersmith KM, et al. Boston keratoprosthesis outcomes and complications. Cornea 2009;28(9):989–996

[55] Netland PA, Terada H, Dohlman CH. Glaucoma associated with keratoprosthesis. Ophthalmology 1998;105(4):751–757

[56] Robert MC, Dohlman CH. A review of corneal melting after Boston Keratoprosthesis. Semin Ophthalmol 2014;29(5–6):349–357

[57] Bouhout S, Robert MC, Deli S, Harissi-Dagher M. Corneal Melt after Boston Keratoprosthesis: Clinical Presentation, Management, Outcomes and Risk Factor Analysis. Ocul Immunol Inflamm 2017•:1–7

[58] Robert MC, Harissi-Dagher M. Boston type 1 keratoprosthesis: the CHUM experience. Can J Ophthalmol 2011;46(2):164–168

[59] Davies E, Chodosh J. Infections after keratoprosthesis. Curr Opin Ophthalmol 2016;27(4):373–377

[60] Durand ML, Dohlman CH. Successful prevention of bacterial endophthalmitis in eyes with the Boston keratoprosthesis. Cornea 2009;28(8):896–901

[61] Nouri M, Terada H, Alfonso EC, Foster CS, Durand ML, Dohlman CH. Endophthalmitis after keratoprosthesis: incidence, bacterial causes, and risk factors. Arch Ophthalmol 2001;119(4):484–489

[62] Barnes SD, Dohlman CH, Durand ML. Fungal colonization and infection in Boston keratoprosthesis. Cornea 2007;26(1):9–15

[63] Grassi CM, Crnej A, Paschalis EI, Colby KA, Dohlman CH, Chodosh J. Idiopathic vitritis in the setting of Boston keratoprosthesis. Cornea 2015;34(2):165–170

[64] Muzychuk AK, Durr GM, Shine JJ, Robert MC, Harissi-Dagher M. No Light Perception Outcomes Following Boston Keratoprosthesis Type 1 Surgery. Am J Ophthalmol 2017;181:46–54

[65] Rudnisky CJ, Belin MW, Todani A, et al; Boston Type 1 Keratoprosthesis Study Group. Risk factors for the development of retroprosthetic membranes with Boston keratoprosthesis type 1: multicenter study results. Ophthalmology 2012;119(5):951–955

[66] Bakhtiari P, Chan C, Welder JD, de la Cruz J, Holland EJ, Djalilian AR. Surgical and visual outcomes of the type I Boston Keratoprosthesis for the management of aniridic fibrosis syndrome in congenital aniridia. Am J Ophthalmol 2012;153(5):967–971.e2

[67] Tsai JH, Freeman JM, Chan CC, et al. A progressive anterior fibrosis syndrome in patients with postsurgical congenital aniridia. Am J Ophthalmol 2005;140(6):1075–1079

[68] Rudnisky CJ, Belin MW, Guo R, Ciolino JB; Boston Type 1 Keratoprosthesis Study Group. Visual Acuity Outcomes of the Boston Keratoprosthesis Type 1: Multicenter Study Results. Am J Ophthalmol 2016;162:89–98.e1

[69] Gibbons A, Leung EH, Haddock LJ, et al. Long-term outcomes of the aphakic snap-on Boston type I keratoprosthesis at the Bascom Palmer Eye Institute. Clin Ophthalmol 2018;12:331–337

[70] Samarawickrama C, Strouthidis N, Wilkins MR. Boston keratoprosthesis type 1: outcomes of the first 38 cases performed at Moorfields Eye Hospital. Eye (Lond) 2018;32(6):1087–1092

[71] Dunlap K, Chak G, Aquavella JV, Myrowitz E, Utine CA, Akpek E. Short-term visual outcomes of Boston type 1 keratoprosthesis implantation. Ophthalmology 2010;117(4):687–692

[72] Duignan ES, Ní Dhubhghaill S, Malone C, Power W. Long-term visual acuity, retention and complications observed with the type-I and type-II Boston keratoprostheses in an Irish population. Br J Ophthalmol 2016;100(8):1093–1097

[73] Aquavella JV, Qian Y, McCormick GJ, Palakuru JR. Keratoprosthesis: current techniques. Cornea 2006;25(6):656–662

[74] Goldman DR, Hubschman JP, Aldave AJ, et al. Postoperative posterior segment complications in eyes treated with the Boston type I keratoprosthesis. Retina 2013;33(3):532–541

[75] Bradley JC, Hernandez EG, Schwab IR, Mannis MJ. Boston type 1 keratoprosthesis: the University of California Davis experience. Cornea 2009;28(3):321–327

[76] Sejpal K, Yu F, Aldave AJ. The Boston keratoprosthesis in the management of corneal limbal stem cell deficiency. Cornea 2011;30(11):1187–1194

[77] Noel CW, Isenberg J, Goldich Y, et al. Type 1 Boston keratoprosthesis: outcomes at two Canadian centres. Can J Ophthalmol 2016;51(2):76–82

[78] Zarei-Ghanavati M, Shalaby Bardan A, Liu C. 'On the capability and nomenclature of the Boston Keratoprosthesis type II'. Eye (Lond) 2018;32(1):9–10

[79] Pujari S, Siddique SS, Dohlman CH, Chodosh J. The Boston keratoprosthesis type II: the Massachusetts Eye and Ear Infirmary experience. Cornea 2011;30(12):1298–1303

[80] Sivaraman KR, Aakalu VK, Sajja K, Cortina MS, de la Cruz J, Setabutr P. Use of a porous polyethylene lid spacer for management of eyelid retraction in patients with Boston type II keratoprosthesis. Orbit 2013;32(4):247–249

[81] Nanavaty MA, Avisar I, Lake DB, Daya SM, Malhotra R. Management of skin retraction associated with Boston type II keratoprosthesis. Eye (Lond) 2012;26(10):1384–1386

[82] Poon LY, Chodosh J, Vavvas DG, Dohlman CH, Chen TC. Endoscopic Cyclophotocoagulation for the Treatment of Glaucoma in Boston Keratoprosthesis Type II Patient. J Glaucoma 2017;26(4):e146–e149

[83] Ament JD, Stryjewski TP, Pujari S, et al. Cost-effectiveness of the type II Boston keratoprosthesis. Eye (Lond) 2011;25(3):342–349

[84] Falcinelli G, Falsini B, Taloni M, Colliardo P, Falcinelli G. Modified osteo-odonto-keratoprosthesis for treatment of corneal blindness: long-term anatomical and functional outcomes in 181 cases. Arch Ophthalmol 2005;123(10):1319–1329

[85] Avadhanam VS, Liu CS. A brief review of Boston type-1 and osteo-odonto keratoprostheses. Br J Ophthalmol 2015;99(7):878–887

[86] Zarei-Ghanavati M, Avadhanam V, Vasquez Perez A, Liu C. The osteo-odonto-keratoprosthesis. Curr Opin Ophthalmol 2017;28(4):397–402

[87] Hille K, Grabner G, Liu C, et al. Standards for modified osteo-odonto-keratoprosthesis (OOKP) surgery according to Strampelli and Falcinelli: the Rome-Vienna Protocol. Cornea 2005;24(8):895–908

[88] Liu C, Paul B, Tandon R, et al. The osteo-odonto-keratoprosthesis (OOKP). Semin Ophthalmol 2005;20(2):113–128

[89] De Leo D, Hickey PA, Meneghel G, Cantor CH. Blindness, fear of sight loss, and suicide. Psychosomatics 1999;40(4):339–344

[90] Vazirani J, Mariappan I, Ramamurthy S, Fatima S, Basu S, Sangwan VS. Surgical Management of Bilateral Limbal Stem Cell Deficiency. Ocul Surf 2016;14(3):350–364

[91] Lim LS, Ang CL, Wong E, Wong DW, Tan DT. Vitreoretinal complications and vitreoretinal surgery in osteo-odonto-keratoprosthesis surgery. Am J Ophthalmol 2014;157(2):349–354

[92] Iyer G, Pillai VS, Srinivasan B, et al. Modified osteo-odonto keratoprosthesis--the Indian experience--results of the first 50 cases. Cornea 2010;29(7):771–776

[93] Iyer G, Srinivasan B, Agarwal S, et al. Glaucoma in modified osteo-odonto-keratoprosthesis eyes: role of additional stage 1A and Ahmed glaucoma drainage device-technique and timing. Am J Ophthalmol 2015;159(3):482–9.e2

[94] Tan A, Tan DT, Tan XW, Mehta JS. Osteo-odonto keratoprosthesis: systematic review of surgical outcomes and complication rates. Ocul Surf 2012;10(1):15–25

[95] Liu C, Okera S, Tandon R, Herold J, Hull C, Thorp S. Visual rehabilitation in end-stage inflammatory ocular surface disease with the osteo-odonto-keratoprosthesis: results from the UK. Br J Ophthalmol 2008;92(9):1211–1217

[96] Fukuda M, Hamada S, Liu C, Shimomura Y. Osteo-odonto-keratoprosthesis in Japan. Cornea 2008;27(Suppl 1):S56–S61

[97] Marchi V, Ricci R, Pecorella I, Ciardi A, Di Tondo U. Osteo-odonto-keratoprosthesis. Description of surgical technique with results in 85 patients. Cornea 1994;13(2):125–130

[98] Sipkova Z, Lam FC, Francis I, Herold J, Liu C. Serial 3-dimensional computed tomography and a novel method of volumetric analysis for the evaluation of the osteo-odonto-keratoprosthesis. Cornea 2013;32(4):401–406

[99] Hille K, Hille A, Ruprecht KW. Medium term results in keratoprostheses with biocompatible and biological haptic. Graefes Arch Clin Exp Ophthalmol 2006;244(6):696–704

[100] Charoenrook V, Michael R, de la Paz MF, Temprano J, Barraquer RI. Comparison of long-term results between osteo-odonto-keratoprosthesis and tibial bone keratoprosthesis. Ocul Surf 2018;16(2):259–264

[101] Lee RM, Ong GL, Lam FC, et al. Optical functional performance of the osteo-odonto-keratoprosthesis. Cornea 2014;33(10):1038–1045

[102] De La Paz MF, De Toledo JA, Charoenrook V, et al. Impact of clinical factors on the long-term functional and anatomic outcomes of osteo-odonto-keratoprosthesis and tibial bone keratoprosthesis. Am J Ophthalmol 2011;151(5):829–839.e1

[103] Kumar RS, Tan DT, Por YM, et al. Glaucoma management in patients with osteo-odonto-keratoprosthesis (OOKP): the Singapore OOKP Study. J Glaucoma 2009;18(5):354–360

[104] Iyer G, Srinivasan B. Glaucoma with modified osteo-odonto keratoprosthesis. Cornea 2012;31(9):1092

[105] Parthasarathy A, Aung T, Oen FT, Tan DT. Endoscopic cyclophotocoagulation for the management of advanced glaucoma after osteo-odonto-keratoprosthesis surgery. Clin Exp Ophthalmol 2008;36(1):93–94

[106] Falcinelli GC, Falsini B, Taloni M, Piccardi M, Falcinelli G. Detection of glaucomatous damage in patients with osteo-odontokeratoprosthesis. Br J Ophthalmol 1995;79(2):129–134

[107] Lee RM, Al Raqqad N, Gomaa A, Steel DH, Bloom PA, Liu CS. Endoscopic cyclophotocoagulation in osteo-odonto-keratoprosthesis (OOKP) eyes. J Glaucoma 2011;20(1):68–69, author reply 69

[108] Iyer G, Srinivasan B, Agarwal S, Shanmugasundaram S, Rajan G. Structural and functional rehabilitation in eyes with lamina resorption following MOOKP—can the lamina be salvaged? Graefes Arch Clin Exp Ophthalmol 2014;252(5):781–790

[109] Iyer G, Srinivasan B, Agarwal S, et al. Bone augmentation of the osteo-odonto alveolar lamina in MOOKP—will it delay laminar resorption? Graefes Arch Clin Exp Ophthalmol 2015;253(7):1137–1141

[110] Norris JM, Kishikova L, Avadhanam VS, Koumellis P, Francis IS, Liu CS. Comparison of 640-Slice Multidetector Computed Tomography Versus 32-Slice MDCT for Imaging of the Osteo-odonto-keratoprosthesis Lamina. Cornea 2015;34(8):888–894

[111] Avadhanam V, Liu C. Managing laminar resorption in osteo-odonto-keratoprosthesis. Am J Ophthalmol 2014;158(2):213–214.e2

[112] Iyer G, Srinivasan B, Agarwal S, Rachapalle SR. Laminar resorption in modified osteo-odonto-keratoprosthesis procedure: a cause for concern. Am J Ophthalmol 2014;158(2):263–269.e2

[113] Avadhanam VS, Herold J, Thorp S, Liu CS. Mitomycin-C for mucous membrane overgrowth in OOKP eyes. Cornea 2014;33(9):981–984

[114] Basu S, Pillai VS, Sangwan VS. Mucosal complications of modified osteo-odonto keratoprosthesis in chronic Stevens-Johnson syndrome. Am J Ophthalmol 2013;156(5):867–873.e2

[115] Hughes EH, Mokete B, Ainsworth G, et al. Vitreoretinal complications of osteoodontokeratoprosthesis surgery. Retina 2008;28(8):1138–1145

[116] Rishi P, Rishi E, Agarwal V, et al. Vitreoretinal Complications and Outcomes in 92 Eyes Undergoing Surgery for Modified Osteo-Odonto-Keratoprosthesis: A 10-Year Review. Ophthalmology 2018;125(6):832–841

[117] Vilaplana F, Nadal J, Temprano J, Julio G, Barraquer RI. Results of Retinal Detachment Surgery in Eyes with Osteo-Keratoprosthesis. Retina 2017

8 Patch Grafts

Sonal Tuli

Summary

Patch grafts are usually indicated for localized corneal defects and perforations. The most common indications are infectious keratitis or autoimmune peripheral ulcerative keratitis. Corneal tissue, conjunctival grafts, or amniotic membranes are most commonly used as patches. Often, these are used as temporary emergency treatment until a more definitive surgery can be performed under more controlled circumstances, although, for peripheral defects, no further management may be required. The advantage of patch grafts over conventional penetrating corneal transplants is that as they are usually small, rejection is not as much of an issue.

Keywords: Patch graft, crescent graft, conjunctival pedicle graft, amniotic membrane patch

8.1 Introduction

Patch grafts are usually needed in localized corneal problems for either tectonic or therapeutic reasons. In these cases, full penetrating keratoplasties may be unnecessary or not appropriate. Patch grafts may also be used temporarily in urgent situations where good quality corneal tissue for a penetrating keratoplasty is not immediately available. The most common indications are localized loss of tissue and infectious keratitis. Peripheral pathology is particularly suitable for patch grafts as the pathology often resolves without needing any further definitive treatment. Some of the common indications for patch grafts are seen in ▸ Table 8.1. Patch grafts may be constructed from corneal tissue, conjunctival tissue, amniotic membranes, or even synthetic materials.[1]

8.2 Mini Patch Grafts

Localized peripheral infectious keratitis, especially deep keratomycosis, and localized traumatic tissue loss are good indications for small corneal grafts. In these cases, as the central cornea is unaffected, patching the peripheral area alone can decrease the long-term complications of traditional corneal transplantation. Lamellar or full-thickness patches may be performed, depending on the depth of the pathology. As the area covered by these grafts is very small and peripheral, graft rejection or endothelial failure is usually not significant even in full-thickness grafts as the host endothelium can replace this limited area easily. Another advantage is that corneal tissue that would not typically be useful for traditional keratoplasty can be used for patch grafting. Therefore, tissue with low endothelial cell counts or stromal opacities may be used. Irradiated and glycerol-preserved tissues, which have long shelf lives, can be kept on hand and used emergently in this manner. Tissue left over from small incision lenticule extraction surgery or Descemet's stripping endothelial keratoplasty stromal caps may be used, and one cornea can be used for multiple grafts.

A dermal punch of appropriate diameter (usually 3.0, 3.5, or 4.0 mm) is selected and used to cut the host and donor cornea (▸ Fig. 8.1). The same size can be used for both corneas. In case of a lamellar transplant, dissection is performed of the host cornea to remove the necrotic tissue. Alternatively, the punch is used to punch out a full-thickness button of the host cornea encompassing the entire pathology. The donor corneal button is then sutured into position using 6 to 8 sutures (▸ Fig. 8.2). Sutures close to the pupil are usually placed more obliquely to avoid distorting the visual axis (▸ Fig. 8.3). It is

Table 8.1 Indications for patch grafts

Infectious keratitis

Neurotrophic ulcers

Autoimmune peripheral ulcerative keratitis

Degenerative conditions:

- Pellucid marginal degeneration
- Terrien marginal degeneration

Traumatic tissue loss

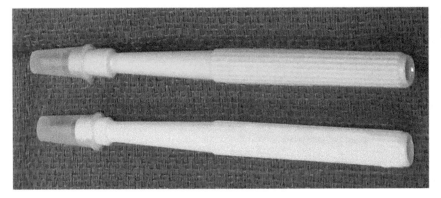

Fig. 8.1 Dermal punches used for mini-grafts.

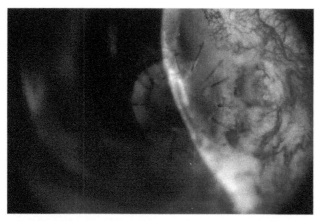

Fig. 8.2 Mini-graft measuring 4 mm in diameter performed for a fungal ulcer with severe thinning.

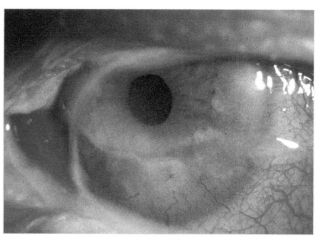

Fig. 8.4 Peripheral corneal melt from peripheral ulcerative keratitis.

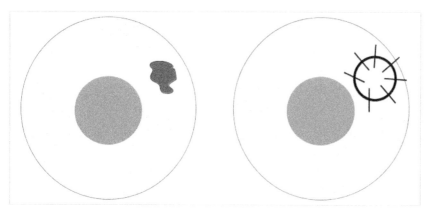

Fig. 8.3 Suture the graft, to avoid the visual axis if possible, to minimize the effect on the vision.

seldom necessary to redo these transplants for the above reasons and they usually incorporate well into the host cornea, obviating the need for further procedures.[2]

8.3 Crescent Grafts

These require a little more skill to construct but are particularly good for pathologies that result in peripheral melts in a crescentic fashion like peripheral ulcerative keratitis from autoimmune diseases such as rheumatoid arthritis or granulomatosis with angiitis (formerly called Wegener's granulomatosis) (▶ Fig. 8.4). Degenerative conditions, such as Terrien marginal degeneration or Pellucid degeneration, also result in severe peripheral thinning in a crescent fashion. All these conditions can perforate either spontaneously or with minimal trauma. Performing a traditional penetrating keratoplasty in these situations would require a very large transplant, and its proximity to the limbus would increase the risk of rejection. Rejection of a crescentic graft, however, is not as significant as a mini-graft, and the endothelial surface area is much smaller and can be replaced by host endothelium. Crescent transplants can be full-thickness or, if the corneal endothelium is intact and the melt or defect is localized to the stroma and endothelium, a lamellar graft can be performed in a similar manner.[3]

The graft is constructed first by marking the host corneal pathology with two trephines. The first trephine is approximately the diameter of the cornea and is placed

peripheral to the pathology. The second trephine is 2 to 3 mm larger, based on the size of the pathology. It is placed just central to the innermost aspect of the pathology (▶ Fig. 8.5). The cornea is then cut out with scissors along the marks created by the two trephines. The same trephines are then used to punch the donor cornea in a similar fashion. The crescent graft is then sutured into place using interrupted or running sutures (▶ Fig. 8.6). Similar to the mini-graft, multiple crescent grafts can be fashioned from one donor cornea and corneal tissue not suitable for traditional transplantation may be used.

8.4 Conjunctival Pedicle Patches

Conjunctival tissue is a good option for peripheral ulcers, especially neurotrophic ulcers that occur due to a lack of growth factors and sensation. The conjunctival tissue and its associated lymphatic and blood vessels recruit vital growth factors and nutrients while allowing removal of proinflammatory proteases. Once adequate healing has occurred with corresponding vascularization and scarring after several months, the conjunctival flap may be removed. However, in peripheral ulcers, it is usually left permanently to maintain healthy tissue in the affected area, preventing recurrence of the ulceration.

The surgical technique consists of debulking of necrotic tissue and de-epithelializing the area immediately around the affected area. A peritomy is performed, and the conjunctiva with or without Tenon capsule (depending on the thickness of

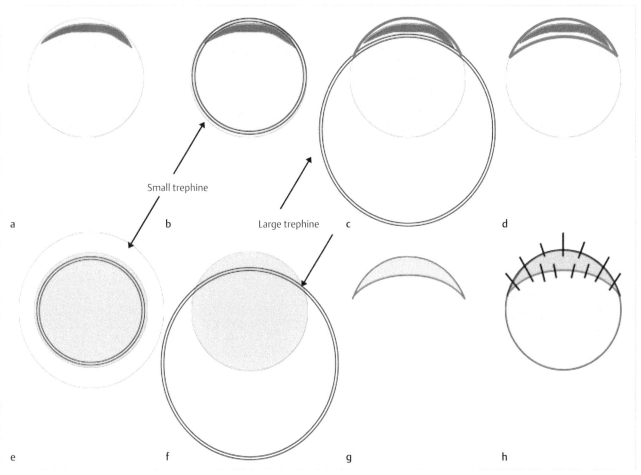

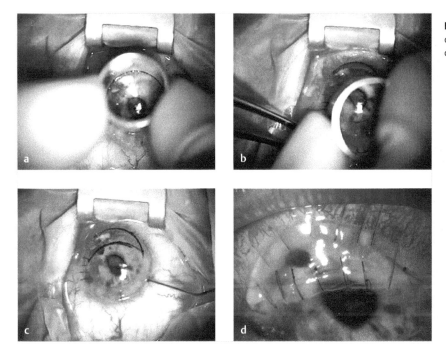

Fig. 8.5 **(a–h)** Preparation of a crescent graft using two trephines. The host cornea is marked with two trephines and cut freehand. The donor cornea is then punched with the same two trephines.

Fig. 8.6 **(a–d)** Steps in the preparation of crescent graft for a patient with a perforated cornea due to Terrien marginal degeneration.

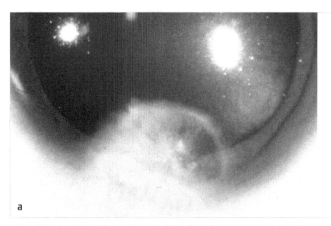
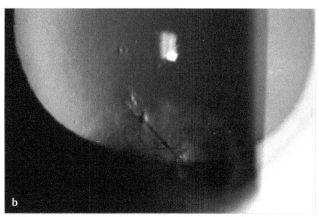

Fig. 8.7 (a, b) Pedicle conjunctival flap for inferior neurotrophic ulcer.

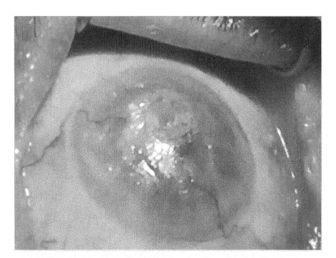

Fig. 8.8 Circular piece of sterile drape used as patch graft for a perforated corneal ulcer.

tissue required) is mobilized over the peripheral corneal defect and sutured into place using nonabsorbable sutures, which are subsequently removed (▶ Fig. 8.7). Care is taken to limit traction on the flap.

An alternative technique is a superior forniceal conjunctival advancement pedicle technique, which incorporates Tenon fascia and a prominent blood vessel into a pedicle that is created by two parallel superior conjunctival incisions 4 to 5 mm apart in the forniceal recess and attaching it to the diseased cornea.[4] Thicker flaps are used with deep corneal ulcers or perforations and thinner ones are used for more superficial ulceration. A further modification involves using just a small patch of Tenon's membrane to plug the perforation.[5]

8.5 Amniotic Membrane Patches

Amniotic membrane transplantation (AMT) is frequently used in ocular surface diseases. Human amniotic membrane is available in various configurations, including cryopreserved, glycerol-preserved, and dehydrated, among others. It provides structural support as well as a variety of growth factors, which help facilitate epithelial cell migration and adhesion. In addition, it has anti-inflammatory and antiangiogenic effects.[6]

Ulcerations lacking depth or significant stromal thinning respond well to a single-layered AMT approach. It can be secured with sutures or glued to the defect using tissue glue. However, deeper defects require a multilayered approach.[7] Here, several layers of AMT are stacked within the defect to build the stromal thickness. Then, a large overlay membrane is placed over the entire corneal–limbal surface and secured with Vicryl or nylon sutures or glued in place.[8] The amniotic membrane usually integrates into the cornea, resulting in restoration of the corneal structure by thicking the corneal stroma.[9] For corneal perforations, the dehydrated AMT can be placed in the wound and allowed to rehydrate. Fibrin glue may be used to assist the adhesion of the AMT to the corneal stroma.[10]

Another innovative method to adhere to the amniotic membrane to the cornea without sutures or fibrin glue while adding tensile strength uses light-activated bonding. The amniotic membrane is soaked in rose bengal and applied to the corneal defect. It is then activated using green light, which bonds the amniotic membrane to the cornea.[11] Rose bengal bonding may be used with corneal tissue alone to close corneal lacerations using a similar technique but applying rose bengal to the edges of the corneal laceration before green light application. These bonds are able to tolerate considerable intraocular pressure elevations.[12]

8.6 Other Techniques and Materials

In emergent conditions, where corneal or other biological tissue is not available for patching the cornea, temporarily, other materials may be used. Large perforations that are not directly amenable to cyanoacrylate glue application may be candidates for the drape method where a piece of sterile drape material is cut to slightly larger than the corneal defect. A small drop of glue is placed on the drape and, after drying the ulcer bed, it is everted over the defect so that the edges of the drape get glued to the edges of the ulcer (▶ Fig. 8.8). This seals off the ulcer until a more definitive procedure can be performed.[13] A double-drape modification of this technique prevents the glue from entering the anterior chamber by using a drape patch to cover the perforation, followed by glue and a larger drape patch over the glue, followed by a bandage contact lens.[14]

Another useful device for corneal melts and perforations is a contact lens; both rigid and soft varieties may be used. Tight soft contact lenses may be adequate by themselves to seal corneal defects and impending perforations, acting like a bandage. However, another option is to glue the contact lens to the edges of the ulcerated area to protect the area as well as act as a temporary patch until more definitive treatment can be performed.[15]

8.7 Conclusion

There are a number of patch grafts that can be used either temporarily or permanently to provide tectonic or therapeutic support to the cornea. The most appropriate technique depends on the condition being treated, whether it is a temporary fix or a permanent procedure, and the location of the pathology. Small, peripheral ulcerations and defects can be definitively treated with mini-grafts, cyanoacrylate glue, or conjunctival flaps. Autoimmune peripheral melts are best treated with lamellar or full-thickness crescentic corneal grafts. If corneal tissue is not available, amniotic membranes, conjunctiva, or even plastic drapes and contact lenses can be used as patches. While synthetic grafts have only structural support, biologic patches have the additional advantage of recruiting growth factors and other beneficial proteins to the corneal pathology.

References

[1] Tuli S, Gray M. Surgical management of corneal infections. Curr Opin Ophthalmol 2016;27(4):340–347

[2] Mannis M, Holland E. Cornea. 4th ed. Elsevier; 2016. Amsterdam, The Netherlands

[3] Jabbarvand M, Hashemian H, Khodaparast M, Hassanpour N, Mohebbi M. Intrastromal lamellar keratoplasty in patients with pellucid marginal degeneration. J Cataract Refract Surg 2015;41(1):2–8

[4] Sandinha T, Zaher SS, Roberts F, Devlin HC, Dhillon B, Ramaesh K. Superior forniceal conjunctival advancement pedicles (SFCAP) in the management of acute and impending corneal perforations. Eye (Lond) 2006;20(1):84–89

[5] Korah S, Selvin SS, Pradhan ZS, Jacob P, Kuriakose T. Tenons Patch Graft in the Management of Large Corneal Perforations. Cornea 2016;35(5):696–699

[6] Tseng SC, Espana EM, Kawakita T, et al. How does amniotic membrane work? Ocul Surf 2004;2(3):177–187

[7] Prabhasawat P, Tesavibul N, Komolsuradej W. Single and multilayer amniotic membrane transplantation for persistent corneal epithelial defect with and without stromal thinning and perforation. Br J Ophthalmol 2001;85(12):1455–1463

[8] Kruse FE, Rohrschneider K, Völcker HE. Multilayer amniotic membrane transplantation for reconstruction of deep corneal ulcers. Ophthalmology 1999;106(8):1504–1510, discussion 1511

[9] Berguiga M, Mameletzi E, Nicolas M, Rivier D, Majo F. Long-term follow-up of multilayer amniotic membrane transplantation (MLAMT) for non-traumatic corneal perforations or deep ulcers with descemetocele. Klin Monatsbl Augenheilkd 2013;230(4):413–418

[10] Kara S, Arikan S, Ersan I, Taskiran Comez A. Simplified technique for sealing corneal perforations using a fibrin glue-assisted amniotic membrane transplant-plug. Case Rep Ophthalmol Med 2014;2014:351534

[11] Soeken TA, Zhu H, DeMartelaere S, et al. Sealing of Corneal Lacerations Using Photoactivated Rose Bengal Dye and Amniotic Membrane. Cornea 2018;37(2):211–217

[12] Wang T, Zhu L, Peng Y, et al. Photochemical Cross-Linking for Penetrating Corneal Wound Closure in Enucleated Porcine Eyes. Curr Eye Res 2017;42(11):1413–1419

[13] Vote BJ, Elder MJ. Cyanoacrylate glue for corneal perforations: a description of a surgical technique and a review of the literature. Clin Exp Ophthalmol 2000;28(6):437–442

[14] Gandhewar J, Savant V, Prydal J, Dua H. Double drape tectonic patch with cyanoacrylate glue in the management of corneal perforation with iris incarceration. Cornea 2013;32(5):e137–e138

[15] Kobayashi A, Shirao Y, Segawa Y, et al. Temporary use of a customized, glued-on hard contact lens before penetrating keratoplasty for descemetocele or corneal perforation. Ophthalmic Surg Lasers Imaging 2003;34(3):226–229

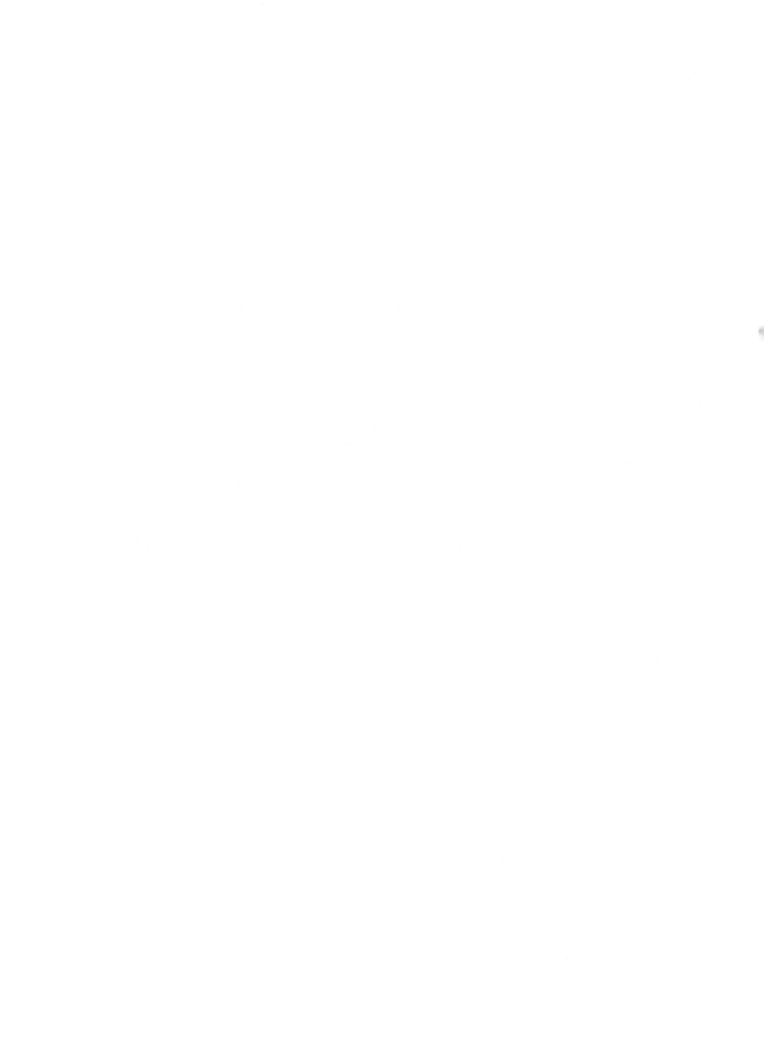

Section II

Reconstructing the Iris

9 Single-Pass Four-Throw Pupilloplasty

Priya Narang, Amar Agarwal

Summary

Single-pass four-throw pupilloplasty is a surgical technique that involves passage of the 10–0 suture needle only once through the anterior chamber (AC) and involves taking of four throws through the loop withdrawn from the AC. The technique creates an approximation of loop that has a self-retaining and a self-locking mechanism.

Keywords: Pupilloplasty, single-pass four-throw, Siepser's technique, modified Siepser's

9.1 Introduction

Pupilloplasty procedures are aimed at restoring the configuration of the iris contour, thereby preventing any hindrance to its functionality and cosmetic aspect. Iris defects may be congenital, traumatic, or may be induced iatrogenically during the intraocular maneuvers. Irrespective of the etiology of iris defect, it needs to be surgically corrected as conformation of the shape and size of the pupil to the normal configuration is extremely essential to avoid unpleasant outcomes like glare and photophobia.

In 1976, McCannel introduced the concept of iris suturing within the confines of the anterior chamber (AC) by creating corneal paracentesis incisions.[1] The flaw with the procedure was that the iris tissue was often overstretched and it was a bit inconvenient to perform. Modified McCannel technique overcame this aspect although it also required intraocular manipulation of suture thread to tie the knot.[2] Siepser's introduced the slipknot technique[3] that was further modified by Osher et al and was known as modified Siepser's knot.[4] Single-pass four-throw (SFT) technique[5] is the newer variant in the arena of pupilloplasty procedures and is also a modification of the modified Siepser's slipknot technique, wherein only one pass is made into the AC with four throws taken around the loop of the suture.

9.2 Surgical Technique

9.2.1 Principle

A surgical knot comprises an approximation loop initially followed by a securing knot. The SFT technique comprises only the approximation loop and a second pass to take the securing knot is not taken. In the creation of the initial approximation loop, four throws are taken and a helical configuration is created that frames a secured knot that is self-locking and self-retaining (▶ Video 9.1).

Under peribulbar anesthesia, two paracentesis incisions are created and a 10–0 suture attached to the long arm of the needle is introduced into the AC. An end-opening forceps is introduced through the paracentesis incision and the proximal iris leaflet is held. The 10–0 needle is passed through the proximal iris tissue (▶ Fig. 9.1a, b). A 26-G needle is introduced from the paracentesis incision from the opposite quadrant and is passed through the distal iris leaflet after being held with an end-opening forceps. The tip of the 10–0 needle is then passed through the barrel of the 26-G needle that is then pulled out from the paracentesis incision (▶ Fig. 9.1c–e). This also pulls the 10–0 needle out of the AC along with the 26-G needle.

A Sinskey's hook is passed through the paracentesis incision and a loop of suture is withdrawn from the eye (▶ Fig. 9.1f, ▶ Fig. 9.2a). The suture end is passed through the loop four times, that is, in a way, four throws are taken through the loop taking care to pass the suture through the loop in the same direction (▶ Fig. 9.2b, c). Both the suture ends are pulled and the loop slides inside the eye approximating the iris tissue edges (▶ Fig. 9.2d, e). The suture ends are then cut with a microscissors (▶ Fig. 9.2f). The procedure is then repeated in the second half quadrant to achieve a pupil of the desired configuration.

9.3 Discussion

The surgical repair of iris is of substantial benefit to the patient as it filters the amount of light entering inside the eye and helps to eliminate glare and photophobia (▶ Video 9.2).

SFT is a simplified procedure of surgical repair that works on the principle of approximation of loops creating a helical structure that does not open up even though a securing knot is not taken. The approximated loop has a self-retaining and a self-locking mechanism. The procedure has been tried with three throws that tend to loosen and eventually open up, whereas with five throws, no extra benefit was noted. Therefore,

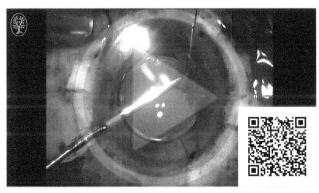

Video 9.1 Single-pass four-throw pupilloplasty. https://www.thieme.de/de/q.htm?p=opn/tp/311890101/9781684200979_video_09_01&t=video

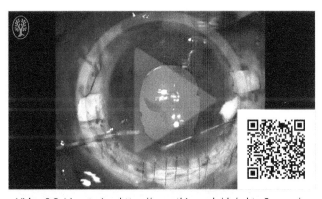

Video 9.2 Iris suturing. https://www.thieme.de/de/q.htm?p=opn/tp/311890101/9781684200979_video_09_02&t=video

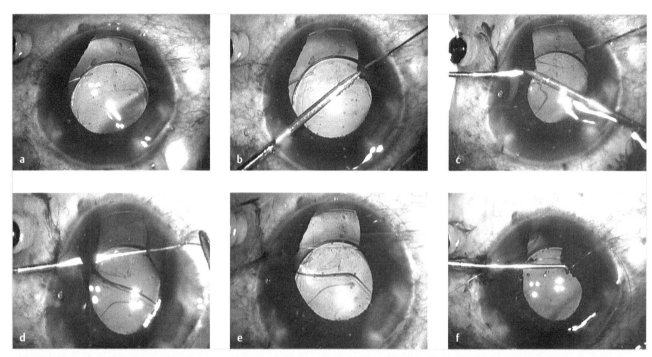

Fig. 9.1 Technique of single-pass four-throw pupilloplasty. **(a)** A case of iris coloboma that needs pupilloplasty to prevent glare induced from the edges of the intraocular lens placed in the eye. **(b)** Paracentesis incisions are framed. The proximal end of the iris tissue is held with an end-opening forceps. A 10–0 suture attached to the long-arm needle is passed through it. **(c)** A 26-G needle is introduced from the opposite paracentesis incision and the distal iris tissue is also held with an end-opening forceps to facilitate the passage of the needle. **(d)** The 10–0 needle is docked into the barrel of the 26-G needle. **(e)** The 26-G needle is pulled and the suture can be seen passing through the iris edges from the anterior chamber. **(f)** A Sinskey's hook is passed and the suture loop is pulled into the anterior chamber.

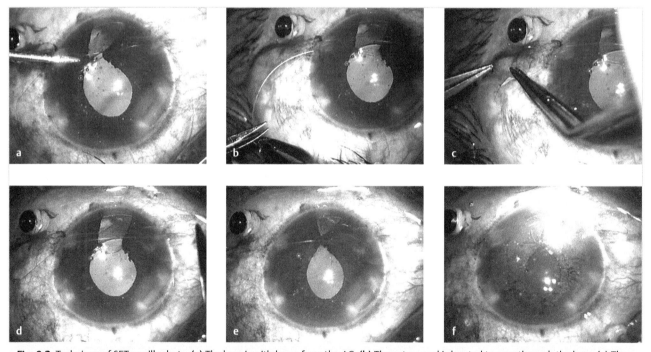

Fig. 9.2 Technique of SFT pupilloplasty. **(a)** The loop is withdrawn from the AC. **(b)** The suture end is located to pass through the loop. **(c)** The suture end is passed through the loop four times. **(d)** Both the suture ends are pulled. **(e)** The iris tissue is approximated. **(f)** The suture ends are cut with microscissors. AC, anterior chamber; SFT, single-pass four-throw.

four throws were considered to be optimal with good apposition of the iris tissue.

The applications of SFT technique are numerous and it has been clinically proven in various situations. SFT is considered to be safe for an endothelial keratoplasty procedure as there is no knot formation that does not hinder with the graft unrolling and also does not rub against the graft endothelium.[6] The knot lies almost parallel to the surface of the iris and it has been verified on anterior segment optical coherence tomography (AS-OCT) where the AS-OCT image taken at the level of iris demonstrated an elevation of the iris about 145 µm (longitudinal meridian; range from 136 to 160 µm) and 165 µm (cross section meridian; range from 160 to 175 µm) from the adjoining iris plane. The end on view of the suture end was observed above the iris plane for about 47 µm (range from 40 to 65).

In select cases of angle-closure glaucoma (ACG) with plateau iris syndrome, Urrets-Zavalia syndrome, and in cases of chronic, ACG with peripheral anterior synechiae, the SFT technique is considered as a procedure of choice where it has been documented on gonioscopy and on AS-OCT to lead to the breakage of PAS due to mechanical pull created due to the pupilloplasty procedure (▶Fig. 9.3).[7] SFT has also been documented to be effective in cases with secondary ACG post-silicon oil tamponade.[8] Thus, in summary, this technique (▶Fig. 9.4, ▶Fig. 9.5, ▶Fig. 9.6, ▶Fig. 9.7 and ▶Fig. 9.8) has tremendous applications with benefits in varied clinical scenarios.

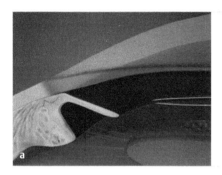
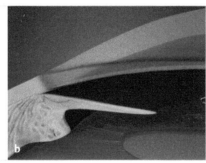

Fig. 9.3 (a, b) Animation describing the pull on the peripheral iris induced by the pupilloplasty that leads to breakage of the peripheral anterior synechiae and opens up the anterior chamber angle structures.

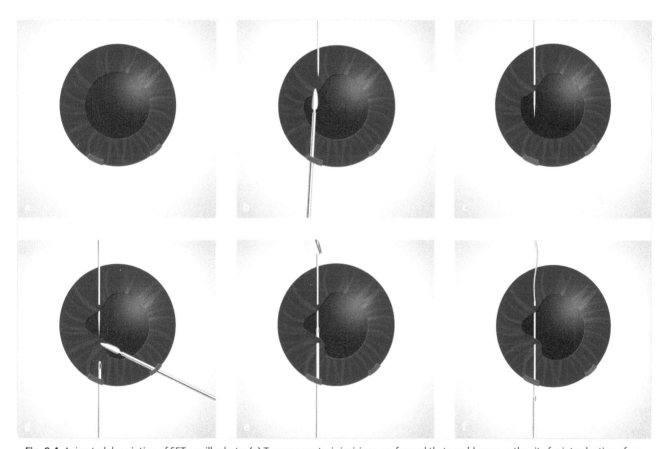

Fig. 9.4 Animated description of SFT pupilloplasty. (a) Two paracentesis incisions are framed that would serve as the site for introduction of an end-opening forceps and the 26-G needle for performing pupilloplasty (paracentesis sites as marked in red). (b) A 10–0 suture attached to the long arm of the needle is passed through the clear cornea. An end-opening forceps is introduced from the opposite end and the proximal part of the iris tissue that is to be repaired is held with the forceps. This makes the iris taut and facilitates its passage through the iris. (c) The 10–0 needle is passed through the proximal iris tissue. (d) A 26-G needle is introduced from the opposite side through the paracentesis incision and the iris edge is grasped by an end-opening forceps introduced from the adjacent paracentesis incision. (e) The 10–0 needle is docked into the barrel of the 26-G needle. (f) The 10–0 needle is pulled and withdrawn from the AC through the paracentesis incision. AC, anterior chamber; SFT, single-pass four-throw.

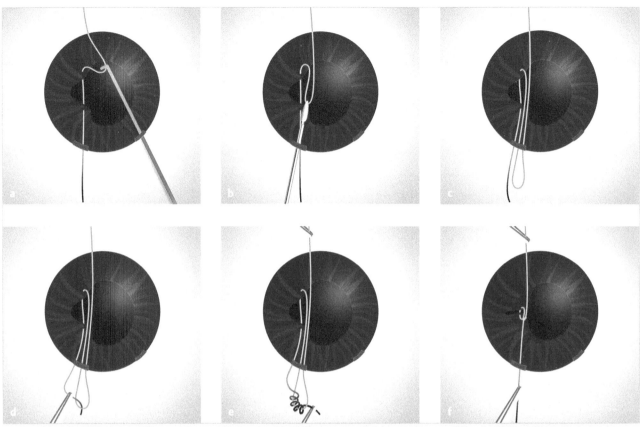

Fig. 9.5 Animated description of SFT pupilloplasty. **(a)** Using a dialer, form a loop of the distal suture end intraocularly. **(b)** Using micrograspers/intraocular end-opening forceps, externalize the loop via the paracentesis. **(c)** Distal suture loop externalized through the paracentesis and maintained immediately outside the paracentesis. **(d)** Leading end of the suture is passed through the loop. **(e)** Four throws of the leading end are passed through the loop with care being taken to pass the suture through the loop in the same direction. **(f)** Pull both the distal and proximal end of the suture, internalizing the helical knot. SFT, single-pass four-throw.

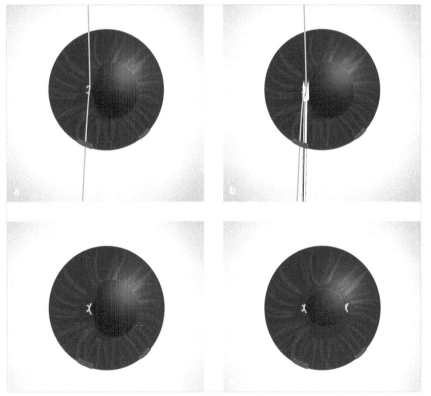

Fig. 9.6 Animated description of single-pass four-throw pupilloplasty. **(a)** Helical knot is formed. **(b)** Microscissors are used to cut the ends of the knot. **(c)** Pupilloplasty complete on one side. **(d)** Pupilloplasty complete on the other side with the resultant desired pupil.

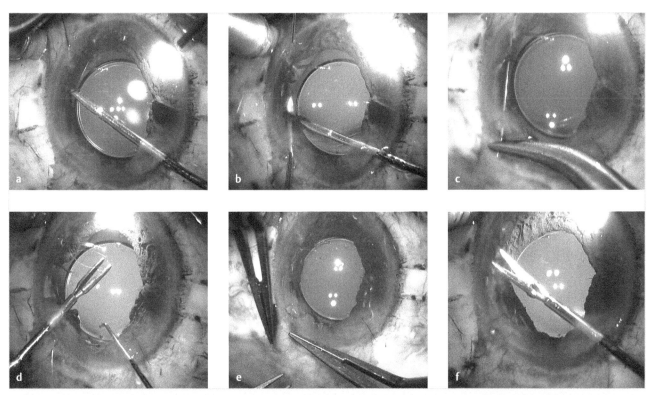

Fig. 9.7 SFT pupilloplasty—surgical technique. **(a)** The proximal end of the iris leaflet is held with an end-opening forceps and a 10–0 long-arm needle is passed through it from the side-port incision. **(b)** A 26-G needle is passed through the opposite side and it passes from the distal edge of the iris tissue. **(c)** The long-arm needle is passed into the barrel of the 26-G needle and is pulled out of the eye. **(d)** A Sinskey's hook is passed and it engages the suture that is pulled inside the AC, creating a loop. **(e)** The loop is pulled out and the suture end is passed four times through the loop. **(f)** Both the ends of the suture are pulled and this leads to the sliding of the loops inside the AC. After the loops are secured, the suture is cut in a way that it leaves 1 mm of end on either side. AC, anterior chamber; SFT, single-pass four-throw.

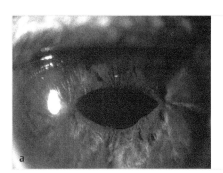
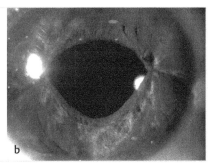

Fig. 9.8 **(a, b)** Dilatation of the pupil after SFT. Predilation pupil after SFT and the post-dilation with tropicacyl plus at 40 minutes. SFT, single-pass four-throw.

References

[1] McCannel MA. A retrievable suture idea for anterior uveal problems. Ophthalmic Surg 1976;7(2):98–103

[2] Alpar JJ. The use of Healon in McCannel suturing procedures. Trans Ophthalmol Soc U K 1985;104(Pt 5):558–562

[3] Siepser SB. The closed chamber slipping suture technique for iris repair. Ann Ophthalmol 1994;26(3):71–72

[4] Osher RH, Snyder ME, Cionni RJ. Modification of the Siepser slip-knot technique. J Cataract Refract Surg 2005;31(6):1098–1100

[5] Narang P, Agarwal A. Single-pass four-throw technique for pupilloplasty. Eur J Ophthalmol 2017;27(4):506–508

[6] Narang P, Agarwal A, Kumar DA. Single-pass 4-throw pupilloplasty for pre-Descemet endothelial keratoplasty. Cornea 2017;36(12):1580–1583

[7] Narang P, Agarwal A, Kumar DA. Single-pass four-throw pupilloplasty for angle-closure glaucoma. Indian J Ophthalmol 2018;66(1):120–124

[8] Narang P, Agarwal A, Agarwal A. Single-pass four-throw pupilloplasty for secondary angle-closure glaucoma associated with silicon oil tamponade. Eur J Ophthalmol 2018:1120672118780809; [Epub ahead of print]

10 Iridodialysis Repair

Priya Narang, Amar Agarwal

Summary

The correction of iridodialysis is crucial to prevent glare and photophobia. Following iridodialysis repair, corectopia is often observed that leads to potential problems on the functional as well as cosmetic aspect. The chapter deals with methods and techniques to repair the iris disinsertion as well as achieve a satisfactory outcome from the patient's perspective. The chapter also describes the twofold technique to deal with iridodialysis of varying severity.

Keywords: Iridodialysis, single-pass four-throw, twofold technique, nonappositional iris repair, pupilloplasty

10.1 Introduction

The term *iridodialysis* implies the disinsertion of iris root from the ciliary body that can be traumatic, iatrogenic, or rarely congenital in origin. Numerous techniques have been described in peer literature for the management of this clinical scenario.[1,2,3,4,5,6,7,8,9,10] It is extremely important to treat this entity as it leads to glare, photophobia, and monocular diplopia. Corectopia is often observed following an iridodialysis repair that often needs to be corrected with iris repair techniques to achieve the proper pupil shape and contour. For iridodialysis repair, one of the most commonly employed techniques is the nonappositional or hangback iris repair technique.[11]

10.2 The Essentials and Basics of Iridodialysis Repair

The procedure is performed under peribulbar anesthesia. Conjunctival peritomy is done throughout the extent of the area of iridodialysis and the area is cauterized. A scleral groove is made about 1.5 mm away from the limbus along the entire extent.

10.3 Nonappositional Iridodialysis Repair

This technique comprises the application of the passage of a 10–0 double-arm polypropylene suture attached to the curved long-arm needle. One arm of the needle is passed through the torn peripheral iris tissue and the needle is then passed and pulled out through the scleral groove. The second arm of the needle is passed through the adjacent iris tissue that is to be apposed and the needle is similarly pulled out from the adjacent corresponding scleral portion of the groove. Both the sutures are pulled and this apposes the iris tissue to its base. Both the sutures are then tied and the knot is buried in the scleral groove. The procedure is repeated until the entire iris tissue is reapposed to its base.

10.4 Twofold Technique (TFT) for Iridodialysis Repair

This technique[12] comprises the combination of nonappositional repair and single-pass four-throw (SFT) pupilloplasty.[13] TFT is applicable in all cases of iridodialysis with varied degree of severity (▶ Video 10.1). To describe the clinical line of management, iridodialysis has been clinically classified into:
- Massive iridodialysis (>120°).
- Moderate iridodialysis (45–120°).
- Minimal iridodialysis (<45°).

10.4.1 Massive Iridodialysis

This type is encountered in cases with massive trauma and it is often associated with either an absence of iris tissue or sectoral avulsion of the iris to the extent that it is difficult to reattach it to the iris base on the sclera. Under such circumstances, TFT is applied and the amount of iris that can be reapposed to the sclera is done with nonappositional technique. Following this, SFT is performed to cover up the missing iris tissue. This helps to restore the continuity of the iris structure and also helps to achieve a functional pupil (▶ Fig. 10.1, ▶ Fig. 10.2, ▶ Fig. 10.3, and ▶ Fig. 10.4).

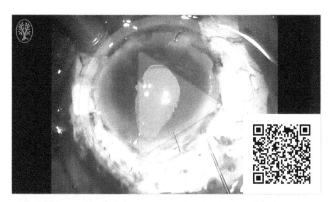

Video 10.1 Iridodialysis. https://www.thieme.de/de/q.htm?p=opn/tp/311890101/9781684200979_video_10_01&t=video

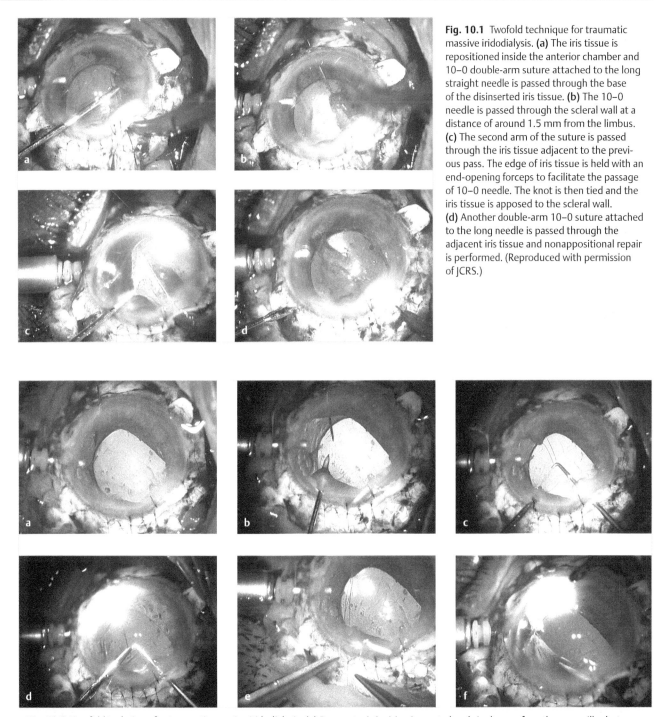

Fig. 10.1 Twofold technique for traumatic massive iridodialysis. **(a)** The iris tissue is repositioned inside the anterior chamber and 10–0 double-arm suture attached to the long straight needle is passed through the base of the disinserted iris tissue. **(b)** The 10–0 needle is passed through the scleral wall at a distance of around 1.5 mm from the limbus. **(c)** The second arm of the suture is passed through the iris tissue adjacent to the previous pass. The edge of iris tissue is held with an end-opening forceps to facilitate the passage of 10–0 needle. The knot is then tied and the iris tissue is apposed to the scleral wall. **(d)** Another double-arm 10–0 suture attached to the long needle is passed through the adjacent iris tissue and nonappositional repair is performed. (Reproduced with permission of JCRS.)

Fig. 10.2 Twofold technique for traumatic massive iridodialysis. **(a)** Paracentesis incision is created and single-pass four-throw pupilloplasty procedure where a 10–0 single-arm suture attached to the long needle is passed through the proximal iris tissue. **(b)** A 26-G needle is introduced from the paracentesis incision from the opposite side that is passed through the distal iris tissue. **(c)** The 10–0 needle is threaded into the barrel of 26-G needle and it is then withdrawn. A Sinskey's hook is passed and a loop of the suture is withdrawn into the anterior chamber. **(d)** The loop is held with an end-opening forceps and is withdrawn outside the anterior chamber. **(e)** The suture end is passed through the loop and four throws are taken. **(f)** Both the suture ends are pulled and the iris tissue is approximated. The suture ends are cut with microscissors. (Reproduced with permission of JCRS.)

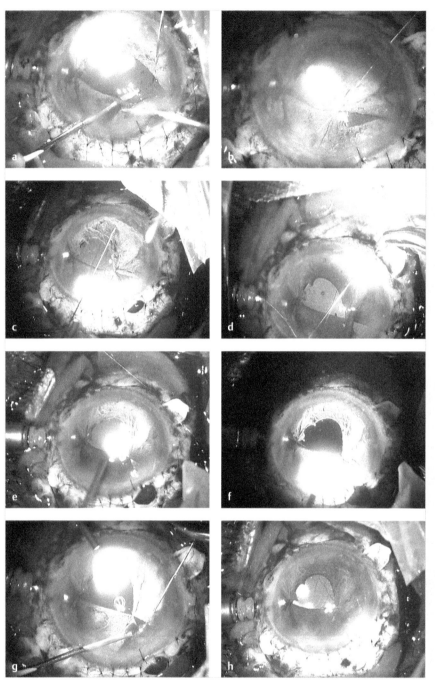

Fig. 10.3 Twofold technique for traumatic massive iridodialysis. **(a)** SFT is being performed in the opposite quadrant. **(b)** Iris tissue is apposed and central pupillary contour is achieved. **(c)** Nonappositional repair is being performed in the remaining area of iridodialysis. **(d)** The second arm of 10–0 suture is passed through the adjacent iris tissue. **(e)** The knot is tied and is buried in the scleral groove. **(f)** Effective functional pupil contour is achieved. **(g)** SFT pupilloplasty is being performed to close the peripheral iris tissue gap. **(h)** Complete iris repair is achieved. SFT, single-pass four-throw. (Reproduced with permission of JCRS.)

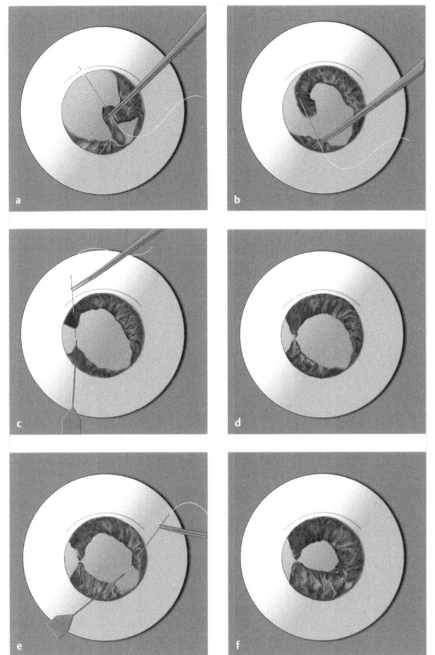

Fig. 10.4 Animated illustration of twofold technique for massive iridodialysis. **(a)** Long-arm needle is passed through the edge of the peripheral iris tear tissue and the needle is exteriorized through the corresponding scleral area. **(b)** The adjacent iris tissue is also fixed to the scleral wall with nonappositional technique. **(c)** Sectorial iris tissue defect is observed. SFT is performed by engaging the adjoining iris tissue. **(d)** The gap is closed or minimized with SFT procedure and pupil contour is achieved in one quadrant. **(e)** SFT is performed in other quadrant. **(f)** Functional iris configuration is achieved in a case of massive iridodialysis. SFT, single-pass four-throw. (Reproduced with permission of JCRS.)

10.4.2 Moderate Iridodialysis

In this type of clinical situation, SFT is performed initially along the edges of the base of the disinserted iris tissue, taking care to appose the approximating iris tissue so as to narrow down the defect of iridodialysis. Nonappositional repair is then performed and the remaining iris base is attached to the scleral wall (►Fig. 10.5, ►Fig. 10.6, and ►Fig. 10.7).

The advantage in doing so is that the iridodialysis gap is shortened by performing SFT initially following which minimal passes are needed to fix the iris tissue to its base.

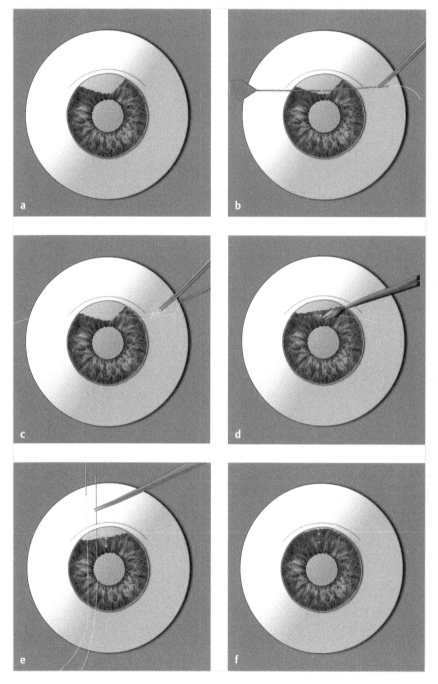

Fig. 10.5 Animated illustration of twofold technique for moderate iridodialysis. **(a)** The image depicts a moderate amount of iridodialysis. **(b)** SFT procedure is being performed along the edge of the base of the iris tissue. A 10–0 suture on long-arm needle is passed from one side and a 26-G needle is passed from the corresponding iris tissue on the other side. **(c)** The 10–0 needle is threaded into the 26-G needle and is withdrawn from the AC. A loop of the suture is withdrawn from the AC and the suture end is passed from the loop taking four throws. **(d)** Both the suture ends are pulled and the iris tissue is approximated. The suture ends are cut with microscissors. Note the narrowing of the iridodialysis defect. **(e)** A 10–0 double-arm suture on long needle is passed to reappose the peripheral iris defect with hangback technique. **(f)** The peripheral iris defect is sealed. AC, anterior chamber; SFT, single-pass four-throw. (Reproduced with permission of JCRS.)

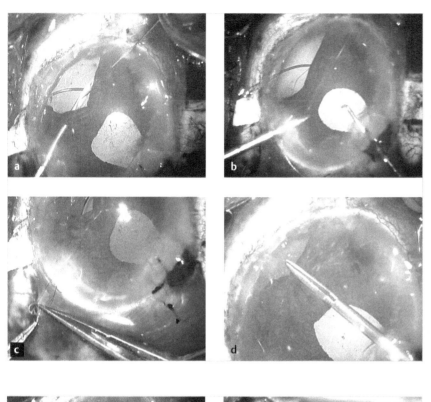

Fig. 10.6 Twofold technique for moderate iridodialysis. **(a)** A 10–0 suture attached to the long-arm needle is passed from the proximal iris tissue defect and the needle is threaded into the barrel of 26-G needle introduced from the opposite side that engages the distal iris tissue that is to be apposed. **(b)** The suture loop is withdrawn from anterior chamber. **(c)** Four throws are taken through the loop. **(d)** Both the suture ends are pulled and the iris defect is narrowed down to a great extent. The suture ends are then cut with microscissors. (Reproduced with permission of JCRS.)

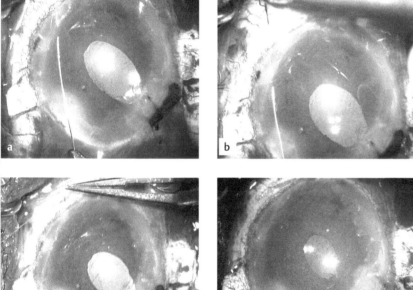

Fig. 10.7 Twofold technique for moderate iridodialysis. **(a)** Nonappositional repair is being performed and a 10–0 long-arm needle is passed from the paracentesis incision in a way that it engages the peripheral iris tissue that needs to be apposed. **(b)** The needle is withdrawn from the scleral side. **(c)** The second arm of suture is passed through the adjacent iris tissue and the needle exits the eye on the scleral side. Both suture ends are tied. **(d)** The knot is formed that is then buried in the scleral wall. (Reproduced with permission of JCRS.)

10.4.3 Minimal Iridodialysis

A minimal iris base defect can be easily covered with nonappositional repair. Corectopia is often noticed following an iridodialysis repair due to either retraction of iris tissue or fibrosis or due to engagement of a greater amount of iris tissue in the needle to fix it to the base. Performing SFT procedure helps to achieve optimal pupil shape and size, following an iris base repair (▶ Fig. 10.8 and ▶ Fig. 10.9).

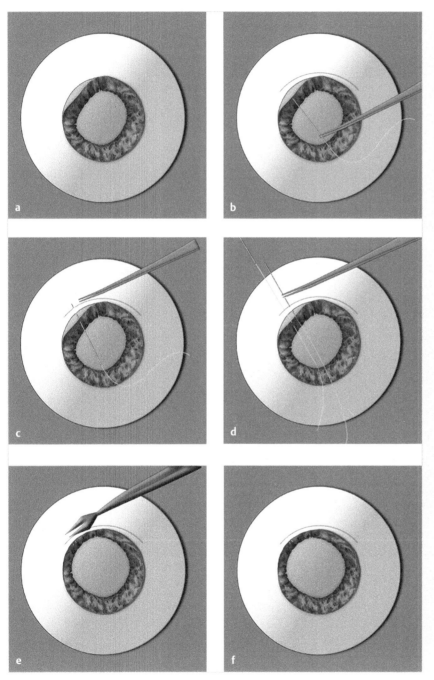

Fig. 10.8 Animated illustration of twofold technique for minimal iridodialysis. **(a)** A case of minimal iridodialysis. **(b)** A 10–0 suture attached to long-arm needle is being passed through the iris defect. **(c)** The needle is passed through the iris defect and is exteriorized from the corresponding scleral side. **(d)** The second arm of suture is passed corresponding through the previous path and the needle is exteriorized. **(e)** Both the suture threads are pulled and the knot is tied. **(f)** Suture ends are cut. The iris base gets approximated. Note the retraction of pupil in the iris repair area. (Reproduced with permission of JCRS.)

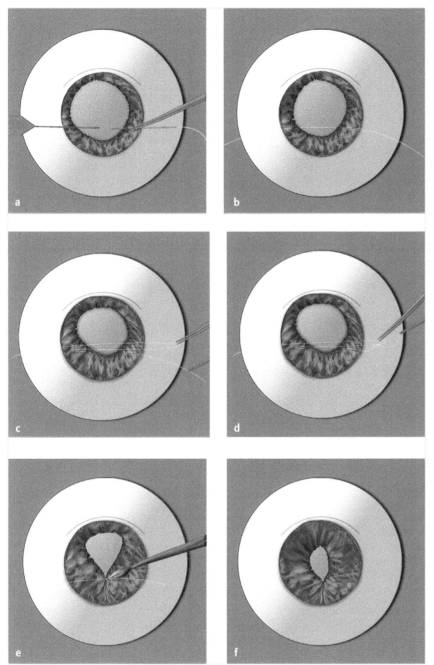

Fig. 10.9 Animated illustration of twofold technique for minimal iridodialysis. **(a)** There is the retraction of pupil following iridodialysis repair. SFT is performed to overcome corectopia. The 10–0 suture attached to the long-arm needle is passed through the proximal iris tissue and the needle tip is threaded into the barrel of 26-G needle introduced from the opposite side that engages the distal iris tissue. **(b)** The needle is withdrawn from the AC. **(c)** A Sinskey's hook is passed through the paracentesis and the loop of the suture is withdrawn from the AC. **(d)** The suture end is passed through the loop four times. **(e)** Both the suture ends are pulled and this leads to sliding of the knot internally. **(f)** SFT is performed again in the opposite quadrant and appropriate pupil shape and size are achieved. AC, anterior chamber; SFT, single-pass four-throw. (Reproduced with permission of JCRS.)

10.5 Discussion

Kaufman et al[4] first reported the technique to repair iridodialysis with straight needle double-arm suture wherein the iris tissue was reapposed with mattress suture without making any scleral flaps.[4] This was a closed globe technique that helped to reappose the iris tissue. Various techniques like *sewing machine*,[10] *single-knot sewing machine*,[9] have been described that are technically demanding and require multiple knots for larger iridodialysis. Snyder et al described the *nonappositional technique* that is comparatively easier to perform and offers excellent visual, functional, and cosmetic result. It also has an added advantage of not compromising the trabecular meshwork during reapposition of the iris.

Siepser's[14] described the sliding suture closed chamber technique to perform pupilloplasty that Osher et al further modified and was known as modified Siepser's slipknot technique.[15] Both these techniques comprise creating a locking knot by taking more than two passes from the anterior chamber (AC). Performing an SFT has an advantage of passing the needle only once from the AC and this indirectly translates into lesser AC inflammation in an already inflamed eye. In addition to this, SFT has been shown to allow adequate pupil dilation postoperatively, thus facilitating retinal examination without any hindrance.[16]

Thus, performing a TFT is beneficial as it encompasses the advantages of both the nonappositional and SFT technique. In addition to this, it gives optimal results (▶ Fig. 10.10) as it helps to refix the iris tissue to its base and also guides to keep in check the element of corectopia (▶ Fig. 10.11, ▶ Fig. 10.12, and ▶ Fig. 10.13).

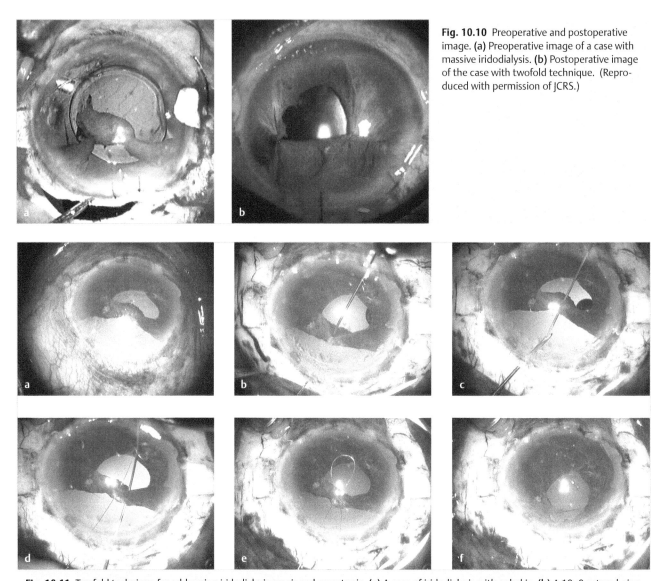

Fig. 10.10 Preoperative and postoperative image. **(a)** Preoperative image of a case with massive iridodialysis. **(b)** Postoperative image of the case with twofold technique. (Reproduced with permission of JCRS.)

Fig. 10.11 Twofold technique for addressing iridodialysis repair and corectopia. **(a)** A case of iridodialysis with aphakia. **(b)** A 10–0 suture being passed from the iris tissue as in a non-appositional repair. **(c)** The 10–0 needle is threaded in to the 26 G needle that is passed from the scleral groove form the base of the iris tissue. **(d)**The second arm of 10–0 needle is passed from the adjacent iris tissue. **(e)** A loop of 10–0 suture is created along the iris base. **(f)** Both the suture ends are pulled and are tied to the scleral base.

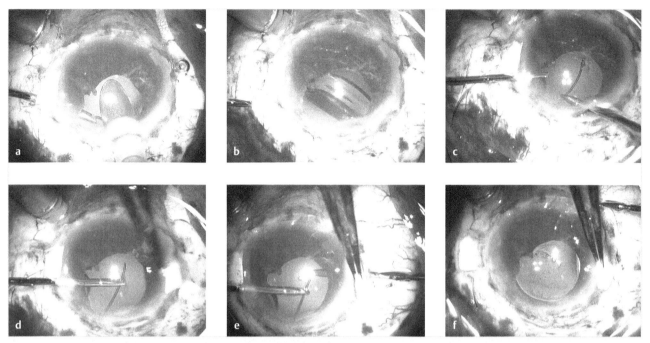

Fig. 10.12 Twofold technique for addressing iridodialysis repair and corectopia. **(a)** A 3-piece foldable intraocular lens is injected inside the anterior chamber and the tip of the haptic is held with an end opening forceps introduced from the left sclerotomy site. **(b)** The tip of the leading haptic is pulled and externalized. **(c)** The trailing haptic is flexed inside and a no-assistant technique is performed. **(d, e)** Handshake technique is performed and the tip of trailing haptic is held. **(f)** The trailing haptic is pulled and externalized.

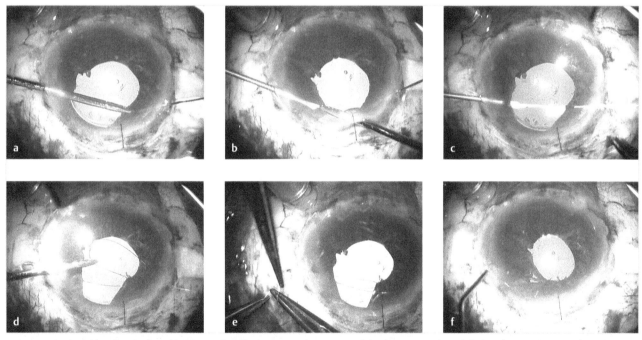

Fig. 10.13 Twofold technique for addressing iridodialysis repair and corectopia. **(a)** Corectopia is observed. Therefore single-pass four-throw technique is being performed where the 10–0 suture needle is passed from the proximal iris tissue. **(b, c)** A 26 G needle is passed from the distal iris tissue and the 10–0 needle is threaded in to the barrel of 26 G needle. **(d)** The suture loop is withdrawn from anterior chamber. **(e)** The suture end is passed from the loop 4 times. **(f)** Both the suture ends are pulled and the loop slides inside the anterior chamber approximating the iris tissue.

References

[1] Viestenz A, Küchle M. Ocular contusion caused by elastic cords: a retrospective analysis using the Erlangen Ocular Contusion Registry. Clin Exp Ophthalmol 2002;30(4):266–269

[2] McCannel MA. A retrievable suture idea for anterior uveal problems. Ophthalmic Surg 1976;7(2):98–103

[3] Brown SM. A technique for repair of iridodialysis in children. J AAPOS 1998;2(6):380–382

[4] Kaufman SC, Insler MS. Surgical repair of a traumatic iridodialysis. Ophthalmic Surg Lasers 1996;27(11):963–966

[5] Bardak Y, Ozerturk Y, Durmus M, Mensiz E, Aytuluner E. Closed chamber iridodialysis repair using a needle with a distal hole. J Cataract Refract Surg 2000;26(2):173–176

[6] Zeiter JH, Shin DH, Shi DX. A closed chamber technique for repair of iridodialysis. Ophthalmic Surg 1993;24(7):476–480

[7] Nunziata BR. Repair of iridodialysis using a 17-millimeter straight needle. Ophthalmic Surg 1993;24(9):627–629

[8] Richards JC, Kennedy CJ. Sutureless technique for repair of traumatic iridodialysis. Ophthalmic Surg Lasers Imaging 2006;37(6):508–510

[9] Silva JL, Póvoa J, Lobo C, Murta J. New technique for iridodialysis correction: Single-knot sewing-machine suture. J Cataract Refract Surg 2016;42(4):520–523

[10] Ravi Kumar KV. Sewing Machine Technique for Iridodialysis Repair. DJO. 2014;24:248–51. Presented at the 26th annual meeting of the Asia-Pacific Association of Cataract & Refractive Surgeons. Singapore. July 2013. [Last accessed on 2018 May 09]. Available from: http://www.apacrs.org/filmfestival.asp?info=6

[11] Snyder ME, Lindsell LB. Nonappositional repair of iridodialysis. J Cataract Refract Surg 2011;37(4):625–628

[12] Narang P, Agarwal A, Agarwal A, Agarwal A. Twofold technique of non-appositional repair with single pass four throw pupilloplasty for iridodialysis. J Cataract Refract Surg 2018:2018 Dec;44(12):1413-1420

[13] Narang P, Agarwal A. Single-pass four-throw technique for pupilloplasty. Eur J Ophthalmol 2017;27(4):506–508

[14] Siepser SB. The closed chamber slipping suture technique for iris repair. Ann Ophthalmol 1994;26(3):71–72

[15] Osher RH, Snyder ME, Cionni RJ. Modification of the Siepser slip-knot technique. J Cataract Refract Surg 2005;31(6):1098–1100

[16] Kumar DA, Agarwal A, Srinivasan M, Narendrakumar J, Mohanavelu A, Krishnakumar K. Single-pass four-throw pupilloplasty: Postoperative mydriasis and fundus visibility in pseudophakic eyes. J Cataract Refract Surg 2017;43(10):1307–1312

11 Iris Cerclage: 360 Degree Running Pupil Margin Suture

Gregory S. H. Ogawa, Michael E. Snyder

Summary

A pupillary cerclage procedure is an elegant and effective method to wind a 10-0 polypropylene suture around a dysfunctional, mydriatic pupil margin, effectuating a more physiologic aperture to reduce undesired photic symptoms and restore a more normal body image.

Keywords: Mydriasis, pupil, cerclage, iris

11.1 Introduction

Permanent mydriasis creates significant disability both during the day with photophobia and at night with glare from lights. When the mydriasis is due to focal areas of iris sphincter dysfunction, the condition may be treated with localized suturing. When the sphincter dysfunction is diffuse with no areas of meaningful contraction, then a 360° suturing solution becomes more beneficial. The most commonly used iris cerclage technique today utilizes a curved needle and a finishing knot tied inside the eye. It was first presented and then published in the peer review literature in the late 1990s.[1,2,3,4,5,6,7,8]

11.2 Preoperative Assessment

The preoperative evaluation in the office usually provides all the information needed to determine if the symptomatic mydriasis is due to nonfunctional iris sphincter. In the nonpharmacologically dilated state, if the pupil is large when examining it through the slit lamp with very little light, and there are no areas of the sphincter that appreciably constrict when widely opening the light diaphragm on the slit lamp, then the sphincter dysfunction is very likely diffuse and rather complete. One can further confirm the lack of iris sphincter activity if instillation of an iris sphincter relaxing drop, such as tropicamide, does not make the pupil larger, or instillation of a sphincter constricting drop, such as pilocarpine, does not make it smaller.

In contrast, if there is something like a 180° of pupillary sphincter that constricts well, then the mydriasis might be reparable with interrupted (two-bite, or multibite) sutures in the dysfunctional area. The pupil activity assessment may be confirmed intraoperatively by injecting acetylcholine (Miochol) into the anterior chamber and observing the pupil response. When making an intraoperative assessment, one should avoid using epinephrine or phenylephrine in the infusion bottle for any concomitant procedures as this tends to significantly blunt the constricting effect of acetylcholine. In fact, if the pupil is large enough, then no preoperative dilation drops are even needed for a concomitant procedure, which further decreases the chance of confounding the assessment. If one is not efficient at performing an iris cerclage suture, then strong consideration should be given to using a corneal light shield to protect the macula. Although we standardly perform iris cerclage at the same time as cataract surgery in eyes that have need for both procedures, one may wish to consider staging the cerclage 1.5 months or more after a primary cataract/intraocular lens (IOL) surgery to allow time for the capsule to seal around the IOL or to decrease the amount of surgical time per session that the patient experiences.

11.3 Surgical Technique

For the procedure, the globe needs to be kept pressurized using either a limbal infusion cannula with relatively normotensive infusion pressure (if the lens capsule diaphragm is disrupted) or ophthalmic viscosurgical device (OVD) in the anterior chamber (if the lens capsule diaphragm is intact). Rectus bridle sutures can be helpful for stabilizing and elevating the globe during surgery, which may make performing the procedure easier for some surgeons.

The surgeon creates three to five paracentesis openings at the limbus with the inside of the paracentesis wider than the outside to facilitate exiting the eye at the paracenteses as well as passing the needle in through the paracentesis on its way to the iris. If a concomitant procedure was performed with an incision, then that incision can be utilized as one of the paracenteses. Generally, a cerclage for very large pupils needs more paracenteses than for moderately large pupils because of the geometry involved in accessing the pupil margin when it is far in the periphery.

It is important to realize that the central most part of the mydriatic pupil is not always the actual pupillary margin. As the iris dilator muscles are in the back of the iris, they can cause the pupil margin to roll posteriorly when the pupillary sphincter activity is lost. Hence, using an IOL manipulator with a knob to hook the underside of the pupil to unfurl the iris may be needed in some cases to retrieve and expose the pupil margin. In other situations, intraocular forceps may be able to grasp the pupil margin and pull it centrally to prestretch the iris before suturing (▶Fig. 11.1).

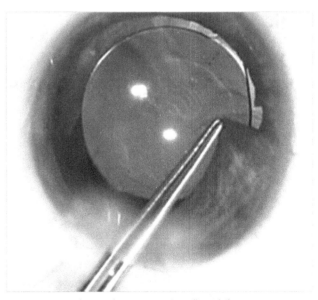

Fig. 11.1 Gently stretching iris centripetally with forceps to decrease iris tension and better position the iris tissue for passing the cerclage needle.

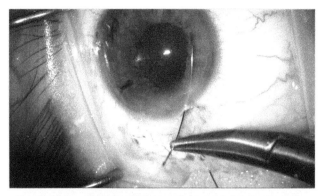

Fig. 11.17 In preparation for tying a Siepser-style intraocular knot, the needle is redirected back through the phaco incision (without catching corneal tissue) and passed out through the limbus in a location selected for Siepser-style knot tying.

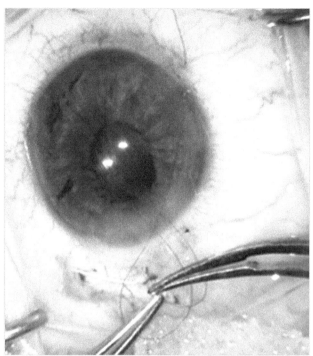

Fig. 11.18 Performing suture wraps for the first throw of a Siepser-style intraocular sliding knot.

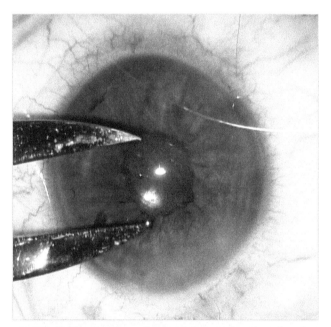

Fig. 11.19 The entrance pupil measured externally with a caliper at roughly 4 mm.

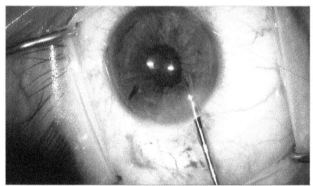

Fig. 11.20 A 23-G intraocular scissors trimming the suture tails at approximately 1.5-mm length after finalization of the knot.

tightened, the new size of the pupil is determined. Approximately, a 4-mm pupil (as measured externally) is generally large enough for retinal examination yet small enough to control photophobia (▶ Fig. 11.19). The pupil can be made larger or smaller than that depending on the individual patient needs. If with the first throw of the knot, the pupil becomes smaller than desired, a pair of IOL manipulators with rounded knobs may be used opposite each other inside the pupil to pull outward, causing the first throw to slide and the pupil size to become larger. This same maneuver

may be performed if, as the second throw is tightened, the knot does not cinch and both throws start sliding, making a smaller pupil. Once the knot is finalized, then coaxial intraocular scissor works well for trimming the suture tails, leaving them about 1.5-mm long (▶ Fig. 11.20). The procedure is completed with gentle removal of any OVD and sealing of incisions as well as any other surgeon-preferred case completion steps, such as verification of IOL position and/ or pupil centration by inspecting Purkinje image alignment (▶ Fig. 11.21) (▶ Video 11.1).[10]

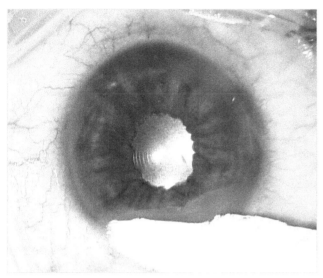

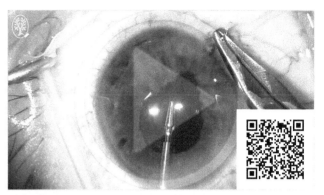

Video 11.1 Iris Cerclage: 360 degrees running pupil margin suture. https://www.thieme.de/de/q.htm?p=opn/tp/311890101/9781684200979_video_11_01&t=video

Fig. 11.21 Note the pupil aligned with the Purkinje images 1, 3, and 4 indicating good intraocular lens and pupil position.

References

[1] Ogawa GSH. Iris cerclage suture: a running suture technique for permanent/traumatic mydriasis. New Techniques Category of the Film Festival at the American Society of Cataract and Refractive Surgery's Annual Symposium on Cataract, IOL and Refractive Surgery. Boston, MA. April 26 & 28, 1997

[2] Ogawa GSH. The iris cerclage suture for permanent mydriasis: a running suture technique. Ophthalmic Surg Lasers 1998;29(12):1001–1009

[3] Bucher P. Iris cerclage. Audiovisual J Cataract Implant Surg 1991;7(3)

[4] Behndig A. Small incision single-suture-loop pupilloplasty for postoperative atonic pupil. J Cataract Refract Surg 1998;24(11):1429–1431

[5] Ogawa GSH, O'Gawa GM. Single wound, in situ tying technique for iris repair. Ophthalmic Surg Lasers 1998;29(11):943–948

[6] Siepser SB. The closed chamber slipping suture technique for iris repair. Ann Ophthalmol 1994;26(3):71–72

[7] Osher RH, Snyder ME, Cionni RJ. Modification of the siepser slip-knot technique. J Cataract Refract Surg 2005;31(6):1098–1100

[8] Ahmed IK. The Siepser sliding knot for iris repair. https://www.youtube.com/watch?v=4QipgGl1HTk. Accessed August 7, 2018

[9] Snyder M. Cerclage gone wrong. Video Journal of Cataract and Refractive Surgery 2016;XXXII(2)

[10] Ogawa G. Cerclage in America. Video Journal of Cataract and Refractive Surgery 2016;XXXII(2)

13 Iris Prosthesis Implantation

Walter T. Parker, David R. Hardten, Michael E. Snyder

Summary

This chapter reviews the various iris prosthesis options currently available worldwide, including surgical tips for their application for afflicted patients.

Keywords: Iris defect, iris prosthesis, custom iris, intraocular implant, aniridia, albinism

13.1 Introduction

Iris defects are a significant ophthalmic challenge, yet these can be associated with rewarding clinical and surgical outcomes. The iris serves many functions for the eye and is quite dynamic. Understanding the anatomy of the iris helps us comprehend the different functions. One obvious role to the patient is the cosmetic appearance caused by pigment or lack of pigment in the stromal layer, but the iris also serves as a modulator of light by reducing glare and photophobia. The muscle layers located within the posterior stromal layer act as a sphincter by constricting with parasympathetic innervation and dilating with sympathetic innervation. These muscles lie just anterior to the posterior pigment epithelial layer, which reduces light transmission. The iris sphincter also helps provide better visual quality for the patient by accommodative miosis and by reducing aberrations.[1]

It is important to assess the individual patient and identify the cause of the particular complaints, as the details of the iris defect may dictate a unique solution. The size of the particular defect, for example, does not necessarily correlate directly to the patient's severity of symptoms. Surgeons are urged to abstain from inadvertently focusing attention on what seems like an obvious abnormality to the examiner, yet may not be the problem that is bothering the patient. Additionally, comorbidities such as retinal, glaucomatous, or corneal diseases may exacerbate an already existing problem. This should be taken into account when assessing the patient and planning for repair or treatment. Some patients with iris defects experience such severe light sensitivity that it prevents them from venturing outdoors or even in intensely lighted indoor locations. These patients can experience such decreased visual quality and noxious glare that they will sometimes request that the eye be fogged, covered, or completely removed. Other times, in pseudophakic patients, the pupil can be extremely dilated—leaving the edges of the usually 6-mm optic exposed to ambient light. This causes the image to appear washed out from light entering around the intraocular lens (IOL) optic or can induce edge glare from light striking the optic margin. Patients with polycoria from their iris defects have to constantly endure multiple images. Often, underappreciated psychosocial side effects of these iris defects include insecurity, anxiety, and depression, resulting from the abnormal cosmesis of the eyes and the altered body image that this confers.[2]

13.2 Alternative Management Options for Iris Defects

13.2.1 Contact Lens

The artificial iris is incredibly useful in patients because it can be effective even when there is no residual native iris tissue. However, sometimes we can use a nonsurgical or alternative surgical approaches to these iris abnormalities. One solution is the use of an opaque periphery contact lens that acts to block out the incoming light with an outer diaphragm, coined "aniridic contacts." (▶Fig. 13.1) In many cases, however, patients report so much discomfort from the lenses due to the thickness and lesser oxygen transmission of these contacts that they would rather deal with their previous symptoms than wear them. Additionally, these lenses are not ideal in patients with coexisting corneal abnormalities, many times, presenting hand in hand with iris defects. The incoming light is blocked more anteriorly relative to the nodal point of the eye in these cases, at the corneal plane, which can still cause persisting photic symptoms in pseudophakic patients and can induce a visual field limitation in other patients.

13.2.2 Corneal Tattoos

In other cases, corneal tattoos have been performed on select patients. The femtosecond laser has even been used to help create a pocket for the pigmentation. However, this treatment is not reversible and may inhibit examination of the other parts of the eye, particularly the fundus. Studies have reported successful treatments of patients with minimal adverse effects. However, Alio et al, in a more recent study, reviewed 234 eyes that underwent treatment, and up to 49% of those patients experienced some level of light sensitivity. Others experienced visual

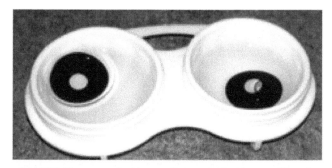

Fig. 13.1 Opaque contact lenses. Opaque contact lenses, although useful for glare and light sensitivity and are often thicker than typical contact lenses, can block peripheral vision, and when move with blink, they can cover the central visual axis, leading to frustration with the vision and comfort.

field defects and difficulty with magnetic resonance imaging. The learning curve is steep for this procedure and severe complications can result.[3,4,5,6]

13.2.3 Direct Suturing

When there is enough residual iris tissue to adequately resolve the defect, a suture iridoplasty may be helpful. In patients with a localized iris defect of minimal clock hours or sectors, either a Siepser knot or one of its variants[7,8] can be used. For more peripheral defects, a direct closure with a McCannel suture can be employed.[9] In cases of large pupillary dilation, an iris cerclage technique can be performed to decrease the size of the pupil. However, in lighter irides or subtle translucencies, the patient can still experience photic discomfort even if the pupil appears cosmetically improved.[10] Other patients with symptomatic iridodialysis can be repaired by utilizing a 9–0 or 10–0 prolene suture on a double-armed needle and suturing it to the scleral wall. However, many times, this can distort the pupil, even if a hang back technique is used to help prevent this distortion. While all the above techniques can be employed in the right patients, many times, an artificial iris prosthesis accomplishes many of the goals of repair that most of the other alternatives lack.

13.3 Iris Prosthesis: Indications

One of the many advantages of artificial iris is its versatility in treating iris defects. A useful way to think about potential candidates is to go back to the basic anatomy and functions of the iris. Is a deficiency in one of these areas causing symptoms severe enough to warrant surgery? We can break down the deficiencies into different categories based on a simplified view of the iris as a whole. Many of the categories can be broken into congenital/genetic causes versus acquired/traumatic causes.

13.3.1 Complete or Near-Complete Iris Deficiency

This type of deficit can be broken down into congenital, acquired, or traumatic causes. Congenital aniridia is a panophthalmic disorder that's most notable feature is a hypoplastic iris. The severity of hypoplasia ranges from total absence (at least rudimentary stump is present in all cases) to only a mild deficit of iris tissue. The condition is either spontaneous or familial in the form of an autosomal dominant inheritance of a defect in the PAX6 gene on band 11p13. The familial condition has complete penetrance but variable expressivity. The sporadic form is associated with Wilms tumor, aniridia, genitourinary anomalies, and mental retardation syndrome, specifically Wilms tumor. As discussed previously, many iris defects are associated with concomitant ocular conditions. In the case of congenital aniridia, the effects can range from isolated iris deficiency to abnormalities of the lens, optic nerve, fovea, and cornea; just to name a few. The mild iris hypoplasia variant could be confused with Axenfeld–Rieger syndrome; therefore, careful examination of these patients is the most prudent way to prepare for possible challenges during surgery.[11,12]

Performing surgery on aniridia patients can be quite challenging due to inherent zonular instability and thin capsules.[13] Additionally, a small percentage of these patients can experience a phenomenon called aniridia fibrosis syndrome that can be devastating and sight-threatening. This progressive fibrosis can occur in around 5% of patients with aniridia with no particular preference towards the type of intraocular surgery as the inciting factor.[14,15] Though no exact cause is known at this time and no specific type of surgery is known to cause the progression, we recommend placement of the artificial iris within the capsular bag, when possible, versus the sulcus. If possible, this could be performed at the time of cataract surgery, obviating a sulcus device and potential irritation of the residual native iris tissue and/or the ciliary body.

Although it is somewhat uncommon to see a complete or near-complete iris deficiency from trauma, a large iridodialysis from blunt trauma can cause functional aniridia. Contusion or penetrating injuries in rare cases could be severe enough to leave a patient functionally aniridic as well. Even iatrogenic injuries during cataract surgery in a patient with intraoperative floppy iris syndrome (IFIS) or from a complication from insertion or removal of an intraocular device could potentially leave a patient with a large defect. These patients should be carefully managed for coexisting medical and surgical problems caused by the trauma itself.

13.3.2 Partial Iris Deficiency

This category encompasses a large variety of potential iris defects that, like the previous category, can be broken into congenital/acquired versus traumatic/iatrogenic causes. Axenfeld–Rieger syndrome is one of the most common causes of stromal hypoplasia. It is inherited in an autosomal dominant fashion by mutations in the PITX2 gene on band 4q25. The iris anomalies can vary from mild transillumination defects to such severe hypoplasia that can be confused with congenital aniridia. Notably, these patients experience polycoria that renders functional vision almost entirely impossible. In many cases, there will not be enough iris tissue to repair directly; therefore, an iris prosthesis would be more effective. The importance of concomitant disease is again stressed because up to 50% of these patients can have glaucoma that should be coordinated with their glaucoma provider should you choose to take on the task.

Patients with more sectoral defects like in iris coloboma, typically located in the inferonasal quadrant and associated with posterior uveal colobomas, might be able to be repaired without a prosthesis utilizing a suture iridoplasty approach if small and enough iris tissue is present. Individual analysis of the iris parameters can help predict whether this approach will be successful.[11] Other partial iris deficiencies like iridocorneal endothelial (ICE) syndrome are characterized by epithelial-like metaplasia and abnormal proliferation of the corneal endothelium, resulting in the spread of the "ICE" cells to other parts of the anterior segment, including the iris.[16,17] These membranes can cause an iris that would not stretch with the previously described suturing techniques; therefore, likely an iris prosthesis is the best choice in these patients.

Iatrogenic iris damage from IFIS can occur during cataract surgery, which can vary in severity. Additionally, penetrating trauma can result in varying iris deficiencies. In some cases, a tumor excision will leave a small enough sectoral defect that can be repaired directly, but this is heterogeneous as well.

13.3.3 Pigment Deficiency

These particular patients can range from congenital absence of melanin like in ocular albinism to conditions acquired from surgical complications, intraocular infections, or chronic inflammation. Ocular albinism has an X-linked inheritance and results in patients with normal iris anatomy but a lack of melanin in the posterior pigment epithelial layer. These patients can experience severe photoaversion that tends to be the main complaint. Normally, incident light exits only through the pupil, but in these patients, the light penetrates directly through the iris. It can be made even worse by implantation of an IOL as the light penetrates and reflects directly off the haptics.[18]

This similar lack of pigment can also be found in systemic diseases like Chediak–Higashi syndrome and Hermansky–Pudlak syndrome, both of which have serious associated systemic health issues. IFIS also leads to a surgical cause of pigment deficiency without full-thickness defects that can be symptomatic in some patients. Many of these types of syndromes and causes would be excellent candidates for an iris prosthesis.

13.3.4 Constriction Deficiency

Most of these types of patients are a result of trauma, increased intraocular pressure (IOP), Adie's tonic pupil, or inflammatory disease. As discussed earlier in the chapter, an iris cerclage might be an adequate option in some cases, but light transmission could still be an issue. A discussion with the patient about the possible options, risks, and benefits might yield an iris prosthesis as the most satisfying solution.

13.4 A Brief History: From Pioneers to Food and Drug Administration (FDA) Approval

Surgeons have been developing different variations of iris prosthetic devices for over 50 years. As of today, there is only one US FDA approved iris prosthesis device: the CustomFlex Artificial Iris (HumanOptics AG).[19] Before the first phacoemulsification surgery was ever performed, Peter Choyce had already implanted the first prosthetic iris in the 1960s. These polymethyl methacrylate (PMMA) lenses were implanted directly in the angle and tended to cause glaucoma or corneal failure; therefore, they were eventually abandoned. However, this started the quest for a solution that has led us to where we are today.[20,21]

The next generation of devices came along in 1991 with the addition of a PMMA optic with a black outer PMMA diaphragm created by Sundmacher et al along with Morcher GMBH. As one could imagine, this very large diameter device required

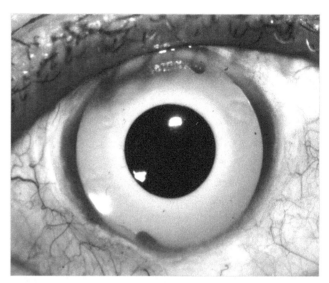

Fig. 13.2 Ophtec 311. Ophtec 311 green device with the incorporated optic in situ in an eye.

an extremely large incision.[22,23] This was the case until Volker Rasch and Morcher created a new injectable multiple piece iris prosthesis (also PMMA and black in color) that was a capsular tension ring-type device implanted in the capsular bag. Kenneth Rosenthal first implanted this and then later Robert Osher in 1996.[10,24] These types of fins, either partial or total, have evolved over the years since that time.

Later, Ophtec began creating small incision iris prosthetic devices that could also be implanted into the capsular bag and came in colors other than black (blue, light green, and brown). However, these colors still did not appear as natural compared to the fellow eye. Ophtec also provides a larger single-piece model, the Ophtec 311, that comes with or without an optic (▶ Fig. 13.2). Heino Hermeking created the multipiece models that can be inserted into the capsular bag and then lock the optic into place without any movement. However, placing the optic into the locking ring can prove quite difficult.

Morcher continued to develop iris prosthetic devices with an IrisMatch (30B) series that gave the patient and surgeon a large variety of color palette of up to 45 choices. This was a combination of iris and optic created by a PMMA main piece with a white diaphragm that could be colored to match the fellow eye. This device required a very large incision, and although much improved in cosmesis compared to older generation devices, still did not match exactly the fellow eye. There are scattered anecdotal reports of optic opacification in these 30B devices. They are no longer available.

HumanOptics along with Hans Reinhard Koch began designing a silicone-based custom iris prosthetic device in the early 2000s. The iris prosthesis is foldable and can be placed in the capsular bag or in the sulcus. It can be sutured into place with or without an optic as well or left without fixation passively in the sulcus (▶ Fig. 13.3). This device has been used for many years internationally and by compassionate-use and clinical trials in the United States. Just recently, the device was FDA approved based on the results of its clinical trial (ClinicalTrials.gov Identifier: NCT01860612).

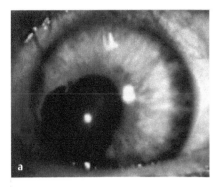
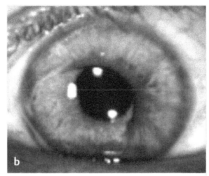
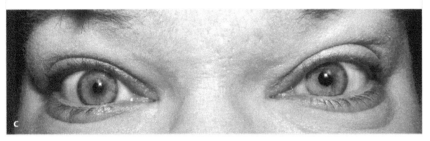

Fig. 13.3 HumanOptics. Eye with significant iris loss from iris melanoma resection **(a)**. The patient experienced a significant level of glare from the large loss of iris. The iris prosthesis significantly reduced glare and improved the cosmetic appearance in this eye **(b)**. The balance of the two eyes is excellent **(c)**.

13.5 Model Designs: Reviewing the Current Choices

There are many different designs currently available to surgeons, but they can be divided into several different categories that we will review below. The importance of preoperatively planning and counseling with the patient cannot be stressed enough because a "perfect" surgical outcome from a patient's perspective can differ greatly from the surgeon's perspective. Many patients feel strongly about the symmetric appearance between both eyes. For example, if a patient had a previous model with an unnatural appearance placed in one eye, many of these patients will strongly desire a matched color and model in the other eye even if a newer model comes on the market with a more natural appearance. In other patients who might have had asymmetrical eye color before their accident, it might be just as important for them to receive an implant that matched their previous appearance.

13.5.1 Iris–Lens Diaphragm Models

Ever since the first implantation of this type of model by Sundmacher, there have been a few updated designs over the years. The major advantage of this type of design is that it solves a problem of aniridia and aphakia all in one device and surgery. As we reviewed earlier, of the currently available designs, this model type has been around the longest compared to the other designs. Its long history lends us years of experience with its advantages and disadvantages.[25,26,27] The design has reasonable outcomes despite some disadvantages. First, the material of PMMA is rigid and the models are large, requiring an incision up to 10 mm to implant the device safely without breakage. Because the current models only come in a few select colors (mostly black), these can appear unnatural to patients and aesthetically artificial. Additionally, in the smaller optic models, some patients can experience dysphotopsias.

Two companies currently distribute this type of model, Ophtec BV and Morcher, with updates and variations. Ideally, these models are implanted into the capsular bag. However, since that can prove difficult in many cases, they can also be implanted into the sulcus passively or with scleral fixation. Morcher offers variable designs based on the patient's needs, all available in the color black. Some of the models come in smaller sizes that are asymmetric for the use in patients with only sectoral loss. This reduces the need for a larger incision for implantation. The optics range in size from 3 to 6.5 mm and from 10 to 30 D, and the overall diameter of the models ranges from 12.5 to 13.75 mm. The pseudopupillary apertures range in size as well. The process that is used to make the black PMMA opaque results in a more brittle material that can be prone to breakage during maneuvering.

The Ophtec 311 models give the advantage of a few different color choices (light blue, light green, or brown). The pseudopupil diameter is 4 mm and the overall diameter is 13.75 mm. The optic comes in a range of 1 to 30 D in 0.5-D increments as well as a plano lens. This material reflects ambient light and can appear unnatural compared to the fellow eye. However, the haptics are a bit more resistant to flex; therefore, breakage is less common than the Morcher models. Like the Morcher model, the overall large diameter makes placement in the capsular bag more difficult due to the possibility of capsular tear or zonular stress. The optic has a rounded edge to help reduce glare and is inset with a bevel into the iris complex. Both Morcher and Ophtec offer designs with or without optics. Ophtec also offers an Artisan iris-fixated lens with an optic as well. However, these types of lenses require enough iris tissue to safely fixate the lens; therefore, they are used less often.

Reper, a relative newcomer to space, is a Russian firm, which manufactures a similar combined IOL–iris diaphragm device made from hydrophobic acrylic with a variety of colors of embedded pigment. The Russian unit comes in a number of geometries for different anatomic placement or configuration. This device has been used sporadically inter-

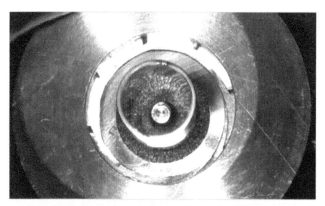

Fig. 13.10 Trephination of the iris prosthesis when a smaller diameter is desired. In cases that require trephination, careful centering of the central aperture can be improved through a device that allows centering of the device with careful precision.

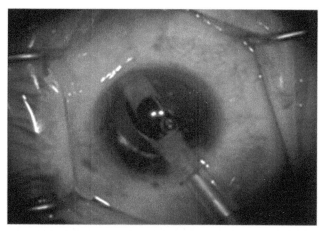

Fig. 13.11 Injecting a device into the capsular bag using an injector. After injection, because the iris is larger than the capsular bag, using two microtyers, using an overfold technique reduces the circumference of the iris and allows it to be placed into the capsular bag more easily.

sular support for the previous techniques. This requires at least a 7.0-mm scleral incision, first for insertion of a PMMA IOL and then for implantation of the iris prosthesis. The lens and the iris prosthesis should be sutured either through the same sclerotomies or at separate sclerotomies a few clock hours apart. The device with embedded fiber meshwork will allow for more secure use for sutures.

Scleral Fixation of Iris Prosthesis and Lens as a Complex in Aphakia

This option allows for insertion of the iris prosthesis and IOL at the same time, using just two fixation sites to the sclera instead of four sites as described in the previous technique. If a foldable IOL is used, then the haptics should be directly secured to the iris prosthesis. There are several methods that have been described for fixing the IOL to the iris, either with direct suturing the haptics to the mid-periphery of the device or placing the haptics through two sleeve-like pseudoiridectomies 180° apart.[45] The implant/iris combination can be folded and inserted through a 5.5- to 6.0-mm scleral incision with suture fixation. Others advocate using a PMMA IOL like the CZ70BD with haptic loops directly sutured to the iris prosthesis. This, however, will require a slightly larger 8- to 9-mm incision. One of the authors prefers to perform a cow-hitch with Gore-Tex suture on a PMMA IOL and then pass the suture through the peripheral iris and then fixate this through sclerotomies as one piece, while another of us prefers to fixate the devices separately, highlighting that there are multiple viable solutions. Utilizing 23-G trocars can provide scleral rigidity for passing the sutures during the surgical procedure (▶Fig. 13.12).

Open Sky During Penetrating Keratoplasty

This technique allows for easier insertion of the iris prosthesis, while the large opening from the penetrating keratoplasty is made after it is appropriately sized by trephination. Any of the above techniques for fixating the iris to the IOL can be used

in the open sky technique, though this obviously increases the open sky time somewhat.

13.7 Concomitant Ocular Abnormalities and Surgical Planning

Many eyes that require an iris prosthesis have comorbidities like corneal, glaucoma, strabismus, and retinal disease. These other diseases may have warranted placement of hardware like a tube shunt or silicone oil that can make surgical planning even more important. In other patients with systemic diseases, the impact of surgery and anesthesia during the procedure requires careful coordination with other specialists taking care of the patient.

An important consideration should be the crystalline lens and the timing of removal if other procedures are needed. In a traumatic aniridia patient with glaucoma in need of a tube shunt but also with associated visually significant corneal scar, it would be prudent to remove the cataract lens first to make room for the tube shunt. If there is associated proliferative vitreoretinopathy from the trauma, then this could be combined with a pars plana vitrectomy with membrane peel, cataract surgery, and pars plana tube placement in anticipation of a possible future corneal transplant or corneal stem cell transplant. The timing of the iris prosthesis and penetrating keratoplasty could be performed at the same time as the previously mentioned surgeries or at a later date when the other complicating factors have stabilized. The status of the zonular stability will also impact the decision of where and how to place the lens and artificial iris. Many of these eyes with multiple comorbid pathologies may require a team approach to management and not uncommonly combined multispecialty surgical procedures.

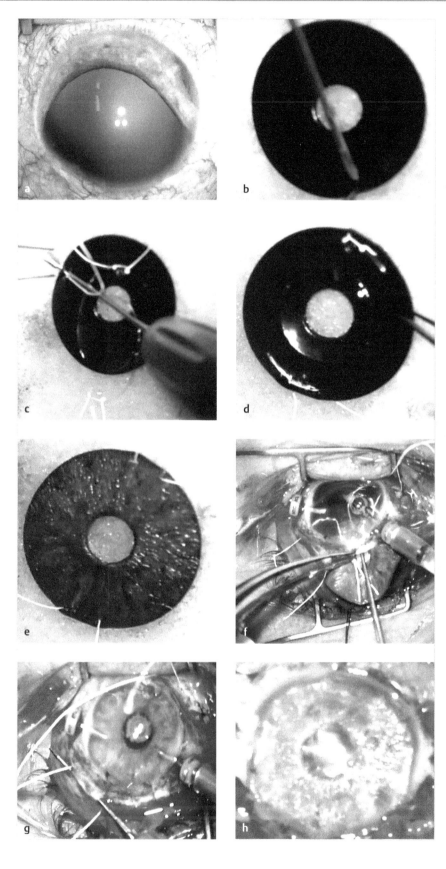

Fig. 13.12 Scleral incision traumatic aniridia case. **(a)** Preoperatively with a large traumatic iris defect and aphakia. **(b)** Vitrectomy has been done and Gore-Tex has been attached to an Alcon CZ70BD IOL with a cow-hitch suture technique. A 23-G MVR blade is used to make a small slit in the iris prosthesis 0.5 mm from the edge of the iris. Two slits are made in one meridian of the iris 2 mm apart. Another two slits are made 180° from the initial slits. **(c)** The IOL is oriented in a manner that is upside down compared to the usual insertion into the eye. The Gore-Tex from each tail is passed through the slits. **(d)** The IOL–iris complex from the posterior view. The IOL should be centered on the iris opening centrally. **(e)** The IOL–iris complex from the anterior view. **(f)** The IOL–iris complex is inserted through the scleral incision after the Gore-Tex is retrieved from sclerotomies 2.5 mm posterior to the limbus, 4 mm apart, and 180° apart. **(g)** Once the IOL is in place, the Gore-Tex is threaded through a previously created shallow tunnel between the sclerotomies. The end where the suture will be tied is on the counterclockwise end of the IOL haptic so that the knot can be rotated once it is tied. Differential amounts of burying the suture can help center the IOL–iris complex on the limbus. It is critical to have the sclerotomies the same distance from the limbus and 180° apart to achieve good centration. **(h)** After the incision and the conjunctiva are closed, the IOL/iris complex is well centered. IOL, intraocular lens; MVR, microvitreoretinal.

14 Cosmetic Iris Implant Complication and Management

Priya Narang, Amar Agarwal

Summary

Cosmetic color implants are employed for eye color change by individuals who are often not cognizant of the potential complications associated with the procedure and its after-effects in an otherwise normal eye. The chapter highlights and discusses in detail all the associated complications and the management strategy for these cases that can be salvaged with proper preoperative counseling and with adoption of appropriate surgical procedures.

Keywords: Cosmetic implants, eye color change, cosmetic lenses, endothelial decompensation, cataract, IOP, inflammation

14.1 Introduction

Cosmetic color implants are employed for iris color change by individuals who are unsatisfied with the current color of their iris and aim to go for a change for purely cosmetic reasons often being unaware of the hazardous complications associated with the procedure. Cosmetic iris implants are anterior chamber (AC) implants that are placed on to the anterior surface of the iris. They are made of silicon-graded material and are available in a single size with 15-mm diameter.

Since the implantation of cosmetic iris implants, significant complications have been reported in the postoperative period that range from corneal degeneration to AC angle structure involvement with raised intraocular pressure (IOP), inflammation, uveitis, and cataract formation.[1,2,3] Significant complications have also been reported even during the explantation of these cosmetic iris implants with the requirement of secondary procedures for the correction of these defects.[1,2]

Theories have been formulated that cite the possible cause for the damage caused by these implants to be the peripheral edges of the implants mounted in the AC angle that lead to constant friction and mechanical trauma to the corneal endothelium and the angle structures.[4] This leads to pigment dispersion and development of peripheral anterior synechiae that eventually leads to raised IOP and development of glaucoma. The hazardous effects of these implants often cause irreversible changes in the eye with the depletion of endothelial cell counts, cataract formation, raised IOP, uveitis-glaucoma-hyphema syndrome, and neovascular glaucoma.[1,2,3,4,5,6,7,8,9,10,11,12,13,14,15,16,17,18,19,20,21]

Surgical procedures such as cataract removal, Descemet's stripping endothelial keratoplasty,[4] Descemet's stripping automated endothelial keratoplasty (DSAEK),[1,2] penetrating keratoplasty,[1] trabeculectomy[1,8] and shunt operations[1] have been described to rectify the complications. It is essential to remove the iris implants atraumatically and it is also essential to perform additional surgical procedures to optimize the potential visual outcomes.

14.2 Surgical Procedure

After the explantation of the implants, the surgical procedure involves the performance of surgical techniques that are necessary as per the type of complications that manifest. These eyes are typically associated with cataract formation, iris deformation, and endothelial decompensation. For such a clinical scenario, the most common surgical procedure performed is a compilation of phacoemulsification (▶Fig. 14.1) with single-pass four-throw (SFT) pupilloplasty (▶Fig. 14.2)[22,23] and pre-Descemet's endothelial keratoplasty (PDEK) (▶Fig. 14.3).[24]

The surgical technique of SFT and PDEK has been discussed, respectively, in Chapters 9 and 6 of this book.

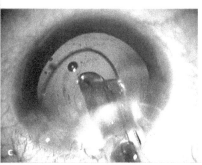
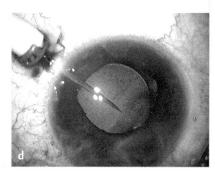
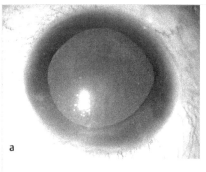
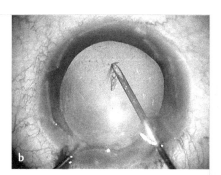

Fig. 14.1 Cosmetic iris implant. **(a)** Cataract with endothelial decompensation and atrophic iris after explantation of iris implant. **(b)** Capsulorhexis initiated. **(c)** A three-piece foldable IOL is inserted inside the bag. **(d)** Trocar anterior chamber maintainer placed in position for fluid and air infusion. IOL, intraocular lens.

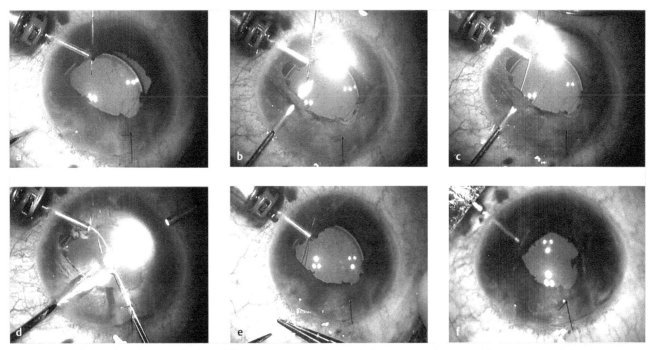

Fig. 14.2 Single-pass four-throw pupilloplasty. **(a)** A 10–0 suture attached to the long-arm needle is passed from the proximal iris tissue. **(b)** A 26-G needle is introduced from the opposite end through the paracentesis incision and it engages the distal iris tissue. **(c)** The 10–0 needle is docked into the barrel of 26-G needle. **(d)** A Sinskey's hook is passed and the loop of suture is withdrawn. **(e)** The suture end is passed through the loop four times. **(f)** Both the suture ends are pulled and this leads to sliding of the knot inside the anterior chamber, thereby approximating the iris defect. The suture ends are cut with microscissors.

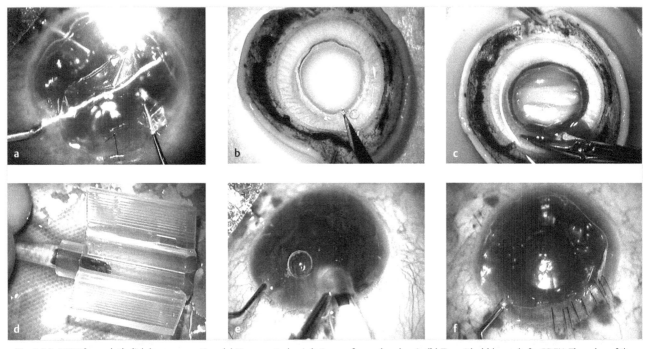

Fig. 14.3 PDEK for endothelial decompensation. **(a)** Descemetorhexis being performed under air. **(b)** Type 1 bubble made for PDEK. The edge of the bubble is punctured with a stab knife. **(c)** Trypan blue is injected inside the bubble and the graft is obtained by cutting it around the edge of the bubble with corneoscleral scissors. **(d)** The graft is loaded on to the cartridge of a foldable IOL. **(e)** The graft is injected inside the AC. **(f)** The donor graft is unfolded using air and fluidics. Air is injected inside the AC and the graft is attached to the recipient bed. Corneal sutures are taken to prevent the escape of air and maintain effective air tamponade. AC, anterior chamber; IOL, intraocular lens; PDEK, pre-Descemet's endothelial keratoplasty.

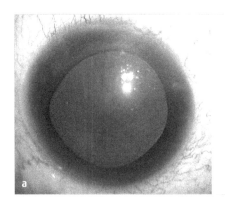
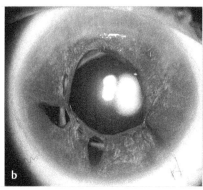

Fig. 14.4 Preoperative and postoperative image. **(a)** Preoperative image after explantation of the cosmetic iris implant. **(b)** Postoperative image at 3 weeks follow-up.

14.3 Discussion

Studies state under-reporting of the complications with these devices in peer literature and that the explantation of these devices should be considered at the earliest sign of inflammation. Apart from the techniques described for the removal of the cosmetic iris implant,[4] various surgical procedures such as trabeculectomy, goniosynechiolysis, DSAEK, and cataract extraction are advised in cases that are complicated with the placement of cosmetic iris implants.

Management of these cases with phacoemulsification, SFT, and PDEK helps to restore the sanctity of the eye, although surgical difficulties are encountered while performing the procedure. As the iris tissue is friable, difficulty is observed in performing SFT. The second attempt is often needed to perform SFT due to the cut through the suture in the iris. Gentle handling of the iris tissue along with a second attempt at the procedure often facilitates the completion of the procedure. In reported cases, the most common cause of low vision was the development of glaucoma that led to glaucomatous visual field defects. Nevertheless, the triple procedure can be performed with considerable ease and is feasible with potentially good visual outcomes in cases with earlyintervention.

The triple procedure can be performed as a single-stage or a two-stage procedure. The advantage of performing a single-stage procedure is that unnecessary exposure to surgery for the second time is averted and the patient has to undergo lesser postoperative follow-ups. The outcome with the triple procedure for handling the complications of cosmetic iris implants is a feasible procedure with potentially good visual outcomes (▶Fig. 14.4).

References

[1] Hoguet A, Ritterband D, Koplin R, et al. Serious ocular complications of cosmetic iris implants in 14 eyes. J Cataract Refract Surg 2012;38(3):387–393

[2] Hull S, Jayaram H, Mearza AA. Complications and management of cosmetic anterior chamber iris implants. Cont Lens Anterior Eye 2010;33(5):235–238

[3] Sikder S, Davis SW, Holz H, Moshirfar M. Complications of NewColorIris implantation in phakic eyes: a review. Clin Ophthalmol 2011;5:435–438

[4] Arjmand P, Gooi P, Ahmed II. Surgical technique for explantation of cosmetic anterior chamber iris implants. J Cataract Refract Surg 2015;41(1):18–22

[5] Shweikh Y, Ameen S, Mearza A. Complications secondary to cosmetic artificial iris anterior chamber implants: a case report. BMC Ophthalmol 2015;15:97

[6] Thiagalingam S, Tarongoy P, Hamrah P, et al. Complications of cosmetic iris implants. J Cataract Refract Surg 2008;34(7):1222–1224

[7] Mamalis N. Cosmetic iris implants. J Cataract Refract Surg 2012;38(3):383

[8] Arthur SN, Wright MM, Kramarevsky N, Kaufman SC, Grajewski AL. Uveitis-glaucoma-hyphema syndrome and corneal decompensation in association with cosmetic iris implants. Am J Ophthalmol 2009;148(5): 790–793

[9] Anderson JE, Grippo TM, Sbeity Z, Ritch R. Serious complications of cosmetic NewColorIris implantation. Acta Ophthalmol 2010;88(6):700–704

[10] Chaurasia S. Devastating complication of cosmetic iris implants. Indian J Ophthalmol 2017;65(8):771–772

[11] Galvis V, Tello A, Corrales MI. Postoperative results of cosmetic iris implants. J Cataract Refract Surg 2016;42(10):1518–1526

[12] Li S, Noble J, Lloyd JC. Risks of cosmetic iris implantation. Can J Ophthalmol 2012;47(6):e50–e51

[13] Luk S, Spiteri A, Muthusamy K, Mearza AA. Cosmetic iris implantation complicated by secondary angle closure. Cont Lens Anterior Eye 2015;38(2): 142–143

[14] Kelly A, Kaufman SC. Corneal endothelial cell loss and iritis associated with a new cosmetic iris implant JAMA Ophthalmol 2015;133(6):723–724

[15] Mansour AM, Ahmed II, Eadie B, et al. Iritis, glaucoma and corneal decompensation associated with BrightOcular cosmetic iris implant. Br J Ophthalmol 2016;100(8):1098–1101

[16] Morales-Fernandez L, Martinez-de-la-Casa JM, Borrego L, et al. Glaucoma and corneal decompensation following cosmetic iris prosthesis implantation: a case report. JSM Ophthalmol 2015;3:1031

[17] Jonsson NJ, Sahlmüller MC, Ruokonen PC, Torun N, Rieck P. Komplikationen nach kosmetischer Irisimplantation. [Complications after cosmetic iris implantation]. Ophthalmologe 2011;108(5):455–458

[18] Garcia-Pous M, Udaondo P, Garcia-Delpech S, Salom D, Díaz-Llopis M. Acute endothelial failure after cosmetic iris implants (NewIris®). Clin Ophthalmol 2011;5:721–723

[19] McCall D, Hamilton A, Grigg J, Chau-Vo S. Severe glaucoma and vision loss due to cosmetic iris implants. [Letter]. Med J Aust 2015;202(4):182

[20] Veldman PB, Behlau I, Soriano E, Starling JC, Pineda R. Two cases of cosmetic iris implant explantation secondary to uveitis, glaucoma, and corneal decompensation. Arch Ophthalmol 2012;130(6):787–789

[21] Shah RD, Randleman JB. New color iris implants. Ophthalmology 2012;119(7):1495–1495.e2

[22] Narang P, Agarwal A. Single-pass four-throw technique for pupilloplasty. Eur J Ophthalmol 2017;27(4):506–508

[23] Narang P, Agarwal A. Single pass four throw (SFT) pupilloplasty for angle closure glaucoma. Indian J Ophthalmol 2018;66(1):120–124

[24] Agarwal A, Dua HS, Narang P, et al. Pre-Descemet's endothelial keratoplasty (PDEK). Br J Ophthalmol 2014;98(9):1181–1185

15 Pinhole Pupilloplasty

Priya Narang, Amar Agarwal

Summary

The chapter explains the concept and applicability of performing pinhole pupilloplasty in cases with higher order irregular corneal astigmatism. The pinhole effect channelizes the incident light through the narrow aperture and blocks the peripheral stray light induced from peripheral irregular cornea.

Keywords: Pinhole, pupilloplasty, PPP, single-pass four-throw, irregular astigmatism, corneal irregularity, aberrations

15.1 Introduction

Corneal astigmatism may be of the regular or irregular variant. With regular variant, good visual acuity can be attained either by correction with glasses or surgically by performing astigmatic keratotomy. The irregular variant is difficult to correct with spectacles due to induced aberrations. Therefore, for such cases, other interventions like placing the corneal inlays and pinhole intraocular lenses (IOLs) have been suggested. The concept of pinhole or small aperture optics has established a definite value in the field of ophthalmology.[1,2,3,4,5,6,7,8,9,10]

Pupilloplasty[11,12,13,14,15] is usually performed to achieve adequate pupil shape and size, following any disruption in the pupil architecture. Pinhole pupilloplasty (PPP) is a concept put forward to narrow down the pupillary aperture and achieve a pinhole kind of functionality, thereby benefitting patients suffering from higher order irregular corneal astigmatism. David Chang suggested the terminology of PPP (▶ Video 15.1).

15.2 Principle

By creating a pinhole or a small aperture (▶ Fig. 15.1), the impact of higher order aberrations caused by irregular corneal astigmatism can be minimized. The pinhole allows passage of rays of light from the central aperture and blocks the rays emanating from the peripheral irregular cornea.

Another possible mechanism could be "the Stiles–Crawford effect"[16,17] of the first kind (▶ Fig. 15.2). In this phenomenon, the light entering the eye near the edge of the pupil produces a lower photoreceptor response compared to the light of equal intensity entering near the center of the pupil. Therefore, it is conceptualized that the photoreceptor response is significantly lower than expected by the reduction in the photoreceptor

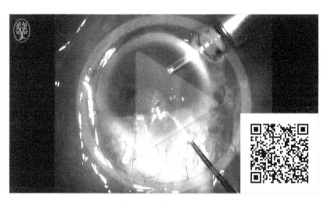

Video 15.1 Pinhole pupilloplasty. https://www.thieme.de/de/q.htm?p=opn/tp/311890101/9781684200979_video_15_01&t=video

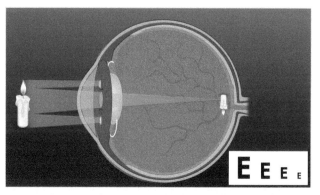

Fig. 15.1 Animated image depicting the principle of pinhole pupilloplasty. A clear focused image is obtained when the rays from the central cornea are focused on the retina.

Fig. 15.2 Stiles–Crawford effect.

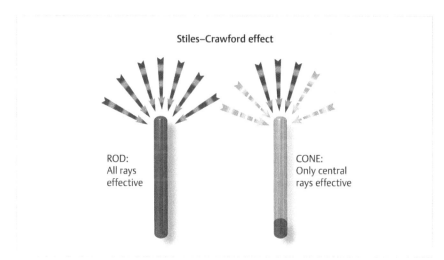

Stiles–Crawford effect

ROD:
All rays
effective

CONE:
Only central
rays effective

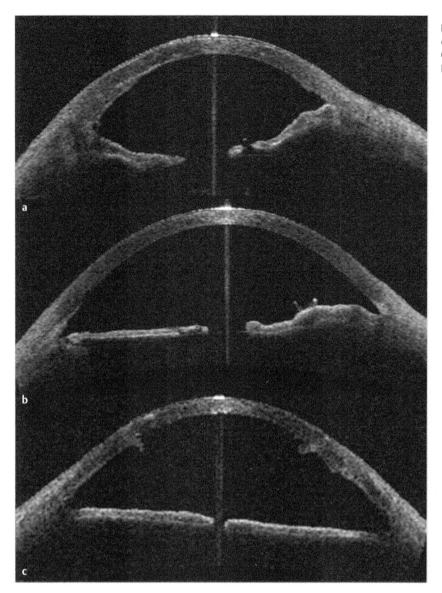

Fig. 15.6 (a–c) Anterior segment OCT of cases 1, 2, and 3 showing the PPP. OCT, optical coherence tomography; PPP, pinhole pupilloplasty.

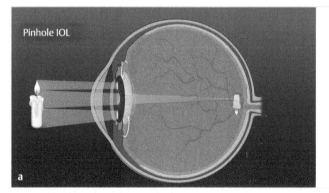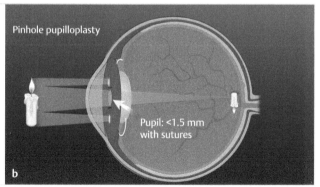

Fig. 15.7 (a, b) Pinhole IOL in comparison with PPP. Both work on the same principle. IOL, intraocular lens; PPP, pinhole pupilloplasty.

To determine whether a patient is a good candidate for PPP, a pinhole acuity test should be done preoperatively. The patient can be apprised of the vision that will follow the PPP procedure. This may also help to increase patient compliance and confidence in the surgical procedure.

References

[1] Trindade CLC, Trindade LC. Novel pinhole intraocular implant for the treatment of irregular corneal astigmatism and severe light sensitivity after penetrating keratoplasty. J Cataract Refract Surg 2015;3:4–7

[2] Trindade CC, Trindade BC, Trindade FC, Werner L, Osher R, Santhiago MR. New pinhole sulcus implant for the correction of irregular corneal astigmatism. J Cataract Refract Surg 2017;43(10):1297–1306

[3] Dick HB, Piovella M, Vukich J, Vilupuru S, Lin L; Clinical Investigators. Prospective multicenter trial of a small-aperture intraocular lens in cataract surgery. J Cataract Refract Surg 2017;43(7):956–968

[4] Schultz T, Dick HB. Small-aperture intraocular lens implantation in a patient with an irregular cornea. J Refract Surg 2016;32(10):706–708

[5] Trindade BLC, Trindade FC, Trindade CLC, Santhiago MR. Phacoemulsification with intraocular pinhole implantation associated with Descemet membrane endothelial keratoplasty to treat failed full-thickness graft with dense cataract. J Cataract Refract Surg 2018;44(10):1280–1283

[6] Srinivasan S. Small aperture intraocular lenses: The new kids on the block. J Cataract Refract Surg 2018;44(8):927–928

[7] Barnett V, Barsam A, Than J, Srinivasan S. Small-aperture intraocular lens combined with secondary piggyback intraocular lens during cataract surgery after previous radial keratotomy. J Cataract Refract Surg 2018;44(8):1042–1045

[8] Waring GO IV. Correction of presbyopia with a small aperture corneal inlay. J Refract Surg 2011;27(11):842–845

[9] Seyeddain O, Hohensinn M, Riha W, et al. Small-aperture corneal inlay for the correction of presbyopia: 3-year follow-up. J Cataract Refract Surg 2012;38(1):35–45

[10] Dexl AK, Seyeddain O, Riha W, Hohensinn M, Hitzl W, Grabner G. Reading performance after implantation of a small-aperture corneal inlay for the surgical correction of presbyopia: two-year follow-up. J Cataract Refract Surg 2011;37(3):525–531

[11] Siepser SB. The closed chamber slipping suture technique for iris repair. Ann Ophthalmol 1994;26(3):71–72

[12] Osher RH, Snyder ME, Cionni RJ. Modification of the Siepser slip-knot technique. J Cataract Refract Surg 2005;31(6):1098–1100

[13] McCannel MA. A retrievable suture idea for anterior uveal problems. Ophthalmic Surg 1976;7(2):98–103

[14] Schoenberg ED, Price FW Jr. Modification of Siepser sliding suture technique for iris repair and endothelial keratoplasty. J Cataract Refract Surg 2014;40(5):705–708

[15] Narang P, Agarwal A. Single-pass four-throw technique for pupilloplasty. Eur J Ophthalmol 2017;27(4):506–508

[16] Westheimer G. Directional sensitivity of the retina: 75 years of Stiles-Crawford effect. Proc Biol Sci 2008;275(1653):2777–2786

[17] Stiles WS, Crawford BH. The luminous efficiency of rays entering the eye pupil at different points. Proc R Soc Lond, B 1933;112(778):428–450

16 Minimally Invasive Glaucoma Surgery and Valves

Priya Narang, Amar Agarwal

Summary

The chapter describes various types of minimally invasive glaucoma surgery and the different devices used for the minimally invasive glaucoma surgery (MIGS) procedure along with the mechanism of the pathway of function.

Keywords: MIGS, iStent, Hydrus implant, XEN Gel, Trabectome, Schlemm's canal, GATT, glaucoma, primary open-angle glaucoma, open-angle glaucoma

16.1 Minimally Invasive Glaucoma Surgery

MIGS is an abbreviation that stands for minimally invasive glaucoma surgery. Traditionally, the treatment of primary open-angle glaucoma[1,2,3,4,5,6,7] comprises a medical line of management followed by trabeculectomy for advanced cases and shunt surgeries for refractory cases of glaucoma. While they are very often effective at lowering eye pressure and preventing the progression of glaucoma, they have a long list of potential complications due to the invasive nature of the procedure.

MIGS has been introduced that potentially helps in mild to moderate cases of glaucoma. These procedures have a higher safety profile with fewer complications and more rapid recovery time than other invasive techniques (▶Video 16.1).

MIGS procedures work by using microscopic-sized equipment and tiny incisions (▶Video 16.2).

There are four main approaches by which MIGS works.

16.1.1 Enhancing Trabecular Meshwork Outflow

Trabecular meshwork forms an important component of the aqueous humor drainage pathway. The trabecular meshwork can either be destroyed (Trabectome) or bypassed using a tiny snorkel-like device (the iStent). These procedures are Food and Drug Administration (FDA) approved but generally do not get the eye pressure very low and therefore are most useful in

early to moderate stages of glaucoma. Currently, three devices (iStent, iStent inject [Glaukos Inc., Laguna Hills, CA, USA], and Hydrus [Ivantis Inc., Irvine, CA, USA]) target the juxtacanalicular part of the trabecular meshwork, which is believed to represent the greatest resistance to aqueous humor outflow in patients with open-angle glaucoma. One limitation of all of these procedures is that the postoperative intraocular pressure (IOP) cannot fall below the episcleral venous pressure, which is difficult to evaluate but is reported in different studies in a range of 7.6 to 9.1 mm Hg.

iStent

iStent is the first-generation device, whereas iStent inject is the second-generation device that is FDA approved. iStent measures 0.3 mm in height and 1 mm in length. It is a heparin-coated, nonferromagnetic titanium stent with a snorkel shape to facilitate implantation. The device is placed using a single-use, sterile inserter through a 1.5-mm corneal incision. The applicator is inserted into the anterior chamber (AC) and across the nasal angle. The pointed tip allows penetration of the trabecular meshwork and insertion into Schlemm's canal and three retention arches ensure that the device will be held in place.

iStent inject is a much smaller device with a length of 360 µm and a diameter of 230 µm. The iStent inject stents are delivered in an injector system, which injects the stents automatically into Schlemm's canal through a stainless steel insertion tube. The injector is released by the surgeon by pressing a button. Usually, two iStent inject stents are implanted nasally into the trabecular meshwork and Schlemm's canal with a distance of 30 to 60°.

Trabectome

Trabectome (NeoMedix, CA) allows a trabeculotomy to be performed via an internal approach. In this procedure, a strip of trabecular meshwork is removed along with the inner wall of Schlemm's canal to create a path for the drainage of aqueous humor. It is a single-use disposable device that allows *electrocautery, irrigation, and aspiration.* It has a three-stage foot pedal

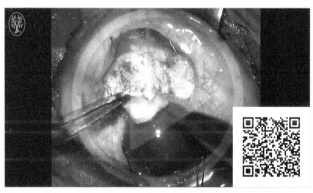

Video 16.1 Ahmed glaucoma valve tube tribulations. https://www.thieme.de/de/q.htm?p=opn/tp/311890101/9781684200979_video_16_01&t=video

Video 16.2 Leaking blebs: grafts, patches, and rotational flaps. https://www.thieme.de/de/q.htm?p=opn/tp/311890101/9781684200979_video_16_02&t=video

control that initiates irrigation, aspiration, and electrocautery in sequence. Continuous irrigation and aspiration allow for removal of debris and regulation of temperature. Ablation of 60 to 120° is recommended for re-establishment of the drainage pathway.

Hydrus Microstent

The Hydrus Microstent (Ivantis Inc.) is made from super-elastic, biocompatible, nickel–titanium alloy (nitinol) and is 8 mm in size. The "intracanalicular scaffold" is inserted into Schlemm's canal to maintain patency and establish outflow. The procedure can be performed in conjunction with cataract surgery and uses the same corneal incision. The microstent is implanted ab interno with a preloaded injector through a clear corneal incision into Schlemm's canal. The beveled tip of the injector is used to perforate the trabecular meshwork and to position the microstent in Schlemm's canal. After implantation, the Hydrus Microstent dilates Schlemm's canal in the complete nasal quadrant, allowing aqueous humor to bypass the trabecular meshwork through multiple collector channels.

Gonioscopy-Assisted Transluminal Trabeculotomy (GATT)

GATT is a type of ab interno trabeculotomy where in under the guidance of a gonioscopy lens, a goniotomy is made in the nasal trabecular meshwork, which serves as the entry point for the iTrack microcatheter (iScience Interventional Corp, Menlo Park, CA). Alternatively, a 4–0 nylon suture can also be employed instead of the microcatheter. Microsurgical forceps are used to advance the microcatheter into Schlemm's canal circumferentially 360°, tracking its progress with its illuminated distal tip. Once it has been passed through the entire canal, the catheter is externalized to create a 360° trabeculotomy.

16.1.2 Subconjunctival Filtration

This subset comprises performing *microtrabeculectomies* where tiny, microscopic-sized tubes are inserted to drain the aqueous fluid from the AC to underneath the conjunctiva.

Two new devices fall into this category: the XEN Gel Stent and InnFocus MicroShunt have shown excellent pressure lowering with improved safety over trabeculectomy in studies. The XEN Gel implant is inserted and placed into position with the help of an inserter introduced from the corneal incision.

16.1.3 Decreasing Aqueous Production

Endocyclophotocoagulation

This comprises performing an endocyclodiode wherein ablation of ciliary processes is performed under endoscopic control to reduce aqueous production.

Valves

Glaucoma drainage devices are generally used to lower IOP in refractory glaucomas. They act by allowing aqueous humor to drain into an extrascleral reservoir through a small-caliber tube. Of the many glaucoma drainage devices available, the Ahmed glaucoma valve (AGV) has gained popularity because of its valved, unidirectional mechanism of action.

This was introduced in 1993 and is now available in many different models.

The AGV acts by utilizing a specially designed, tapered trapezoidal chamber to create a Venturi effect to help aqueous flow through the device. This reduces internal friction within the valve system. As demonstrated by Bernoulli's equation of hydrodynamic principle, the inlet velocity of aqueous entering the larger port of the Venturi chamber increases significantly as it exits the smaller outlet port of the tapered chamber. The increased exit velocity helps in evacuating aqueous from the valve, thereby helping to reduce valve friction. The AGV also has a nonobstructive, self-regulating mechanism for fluid flow and elastic membranes help to regulate fluid flow at all times, consistently by changing their shape. The tension on these membranes is responsible for reducing hypotony.

16.1.4 Suprachoroidal Drainage

CyPass

CyPass is a polyamide, supraciliary device for ab interno implantation. The goal of the device is to create a controlled cyclodialysis with stented outflow to the supraciliary space. The stent is 6.35 mm long with an outer diameter of 0.51 mm. During surgery, the implant is loaded onto a retractable guide wire, inserted through the initial phacoemulsification incision, and advanced toward the sclera spur. The guide wire is used to perform blunt dissection of the ciliary body in order to allow passage into the supraciliary space where the stent can be placed.

On August 29, 2018, Alcon announced an immediate, voluntary market withdrawal of the CyPass Microstent from the global market and advised surgeons to immediately cease further implantation with the CyPass Microstent. The decision was based on an analysis of five-year post-surgery data from the COMPASS-XT long-term safety study. At five years, the CyPass Microstent group experienced statistically significant endothelial cell loss compared to the group who underwent cataract surgery alone.

16.2 Surgical Technique

The Ahmed valve comes in various models of which we prefer the FP7 for adults. It is made of medical-grade silicone and has a 13 × 16 mm plate and a tube. Our technique of insertion consists of making a conjunctival peritomy and creating space under the Tenon's. The valve is primed using balanced salt solution and a 27-G cannula (►Fig. 16.1) and inserted under the Tenon's in between the recti till it is about 8 to 10 mm from the limbus. Any impingement on the recti should be carefully avoided to prevent postoperative diplopia. Once sutured, the position of the flap is marked and a superficial scleral flap is dissected. Too thin flaps are avoided to prevent tube erosion. A 23-G needle is then used to enter the AC under the flap making an oblique passage through the sclera. The tube is cut to its desired length with a 30° bevel. It is then inserted into the AC and its position verified. Once satisfied, the flap is sutured over the tube making sure that the tube cannot move under the flap. Fibrin glue, if available, seals the flap completely around the tube. A stay suture is also applied around the tube and anchored to the sclera. We believe these three simple steps prevent tube migration (►Fig. 16.2). The peritomy is then closed. The conjunctiva may also be closed using fibrin glue

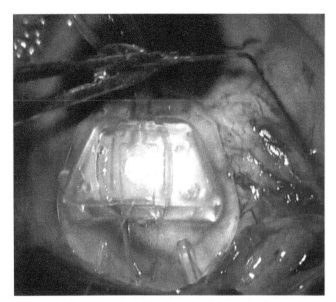

Fig. 16.1 An adult model Ahmed valve being primed prior to insertion.

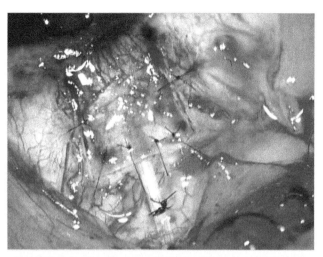

Fig. 16.2 Tube migration is avoided by an oblique passage through the sclera, an anchoring scleral stay suture, and a tight flap.

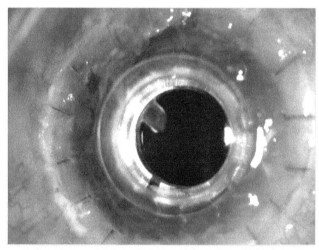

Fig. 16.3 An Ahmed valve is often combined with a Boston keratoprosthesis.

making sure that the glue is not applied posteriorly but only at the anterior edge at the limbus. The glue should not seal off the posterior conjunctival space.

16.3 Complex Situations

A pre-existing trabeculectomy or a previous Ahmed valve implantation might preclude implantation in the superotemporal quadrant, which is generally the preferred site for AGV implantation. In this case, one can implant the valve superonasally to lie in between the superior and medial recti. The rest of the steps remain the same. It may also be implanted inferotemporally to lie in between the inferior and lateral recti.

Tube corneal endothelial touch can cause corneal decompensation and should be avoided at all costs. For this reason, in pseudophakic eyes, we prefer tube implantation in the posterior chamber in between the iris and the IOL. This is accomplished in the same way except that the needle is directed towards the posterior chamber parallel to the posterior iris surface. This keeps a safe distance between the tube and corneal endothelium and avoids long-term corneal decompensation. In phakic eyes, the tube is placed in the AC. However, it should be avoided in quadrants with peripheral anterior synechiae as they might result in anteroplacement of the tube with a resultant corneal touch. In such cases, a different quadrant may be selected or it may be placed in the posterior chamber after performing a cataract extraction.

Regardless of AC or posterior chamber implantation, the tube needs to remain parallel to the iris so as to avoid iris pigment dispersion as well as iris plugging. A large flaccid iris may require an iridoplasty. Careful insertion should be done to avoid damage to the iris root or the ciliary body and hyphema.

We also utilize intravitreal placement of the AGV tube in selected cases. This includes patients with an absent posterior capsule, secondarily scleral-fixated IOL, and so forth. In this case, it is essential to perform a thorough anterior vitrectomy to prevent vitreous strands from occluding the tube. We particularly perform additional vitrectomy near the tube tip. We

avoid tube migration by an oblique passage through the sclera, the anchoring stay suture, and a tight flap.

We use the pediatric FP8 model for refractory glaucomas in children and have found encouraging results. We also use the AGV in cases with post-penetrating keratoplasty glaucoma. Such eyes generally have deformed ACs and large areas of peripheral anterior synechiae. Trabeculectomy with or without antimetabolites may fail in such eyes. The AGV by acting as a drainage device can be combined with other anterior segment reconstructive procedures such as secondary IOL fixation, pupilloplasty, and so forth to get good postoperative results. We fix the tube tip behind the iris, in front of the IOL in such cases, or in the anterior vitreous after a thorough vitrectomy in eyes with no posterior capsule.

Another group of patients requiring special consideration are those undergoing Boston keratoprosthesis (BKPro) implantation. These patients sometimes develop increased IOP in the postoperative period and especially so if they also have deformed, complex anterior segments to start with. Measuring the IOP in the presence of a BKPro is difficult and often the surgeon only relies on digital estimation. We prefer to have a low threshold for implanting an Ahmed valve in such patients and very often combine the two procedures (▶ Fig. 16.3). The

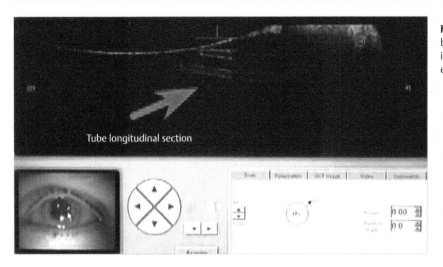

Fig. 16.4 The anterior segment OCT may be used to visualize the tube tip in eyes with inadequate media clarity. OCT, optical coherence tomography.

Tube longitudinal section

tube is placed in front of the IOL in case of a pseudophakic BKPro with intact posterior capsule. In case of a monocameral eye or in an eye with an aphakic BKPro and absent posterior capsule, a thorough vitrectomy is done to prevent vitreous from clogging the tube tip. We do not routinely use the pars plana clip for pars plana placement of the AGV but rather use a more oblique entry through the scleral wall as well as a stay suture on the tube.

16.4 Complications

Careful attention should be paid to the tube. Any inflammation within the eye needs to be treated aggressively before it causes a block in the tube tip. Vitreous blocking the tube tip might need a vitrectomy. A too long tube may remain in the visual axis and cause symptoms. A tube that is too long may require to be removed from the AC, shortened, and replaced back. Other tube-related complications can include tube migration, tube erosion, tube cornea touch, tube lenticular touch, tube iris touch, and so forth.

The tube tip is sometimes difficult to see and may require an anterior segment optical coherence tomography (AS-OCT) to visualize (▶ Fig. 16.4). The AS-OCT can also visualize the tube tract under the sclera and conjunctiva as well as the plate of the AGV. It may also be used to visualize the tip of the tube and the presence of any block.

Though we routinely elevate a lamellar scleral flap for tube coverage, a donor scleral patch graft or a scleral autograft or preserved dura might also be used to cover the tube primarily or secondarily in an exposed tube. This has the disadvantage of requiring donor tissue or of additional site surgery.

Early postoperative hypotony can be avoided by using a Vicryl suture for temporarily ligating the tube. This helps avoid attendant complications such as choroidal effusion and suprachoroidal hemorrhage. Late hypertensive phase, if it occurs, may be managed medically. Bleb encapsulation and fibrosis leading to increased IOP and failure may be managed by a second AGV implantation or by needling the bleb.

16.5 Conclusion

To conclude, we have found encouraging results with the AGV even in eyes with refractory glaucomas and complex ACs. Nevertheless, its use does require greater surgical skill, meticulousness, and close attention to surgical details.

References

[1] Wilson MR, Martone J. Epidemiology of chronic open-angle glaucoma. In: Ritch R, Shields MB, Krupin T, eds. The glaucomas – clinical science. 2nd ed. St. Louis: Mosby; 1996:729–738

[2] Jonas JB, Budde WM, Panda-Jonas S. Ophthalmoscopic evaluation of the optic nerve head. Surv Ophthalmol 1999;43(4):293–320

[3] Ramrattan RS, Wolfs RCW, Jonas JB, Hofman A, de Jong PT. Determinants of optic disc characteristics in a general population: the Rotterdam study. Ophthalmology 1999;106(8):1588–1596

[4] Weinreb RN. Assessment of optic disc topography for diagnosing and monitoring glaucoma. Arch Ophthalmol 1998;116(9):1229–1231

[5] Fitzke FW, McNaught AI. The diagnosis of visual field progression in glaucoma. Curr Opin Ophthalmol 1994;5(2):110–115

[6] Lütjen-Drecoll E. Functional morphology of the trabecular meshwork in primate eyes. Prog Retin Eye Res 1999;18(1):91–119

[7] Polansky JR. HTM cell culture model for steroid effects on intraocular pressure. In: Lutjen-Drecoll E, Rohen JW, eds. Basic aspects of glaucoma research III. Stuttgart: Schattaeur Press; 1993:307–318

17 Single-Pass Four-Throw Pupilloplasty for Angle-Closure Glaucoma

Priya Narang, Amar Agarwal

Summary

Secondary angle-closure glaucoma (ACG) often develops due to the fall back of iris tissue in the anterior chamber (AC) angle, thereby inadvertently blocking the trabecular outflow. Performing surgical pupilloplasty in the initial stages helps to prevent the formation of peripheral anterior synechiae (PAS) as well as break the newly formed PAS. This chapter deals with the aspect of preventing the further progression of AC angle changes in selected cases of secondary ACG and treating them with surgical pupilloplasty. Single-pass four-throw pupilloplasty helps to pull the peripheral iris, thereby preventing the trabecular meshwork from being blocked mechanically in cases with plateau iris syndrome, Urrets-Zavalia syndrome, and select cases of secondary angle closure.

Keywords: Angle-closure glaucoma, surgical pupilloplasty, single-pass four-throw, peripheral anterior synechiae, gonioscopy, iris traction, Urrets-Zavalia syndrome, intraocular pressure, silicone oil glaucoma

17.1 Introduction

Glaucoma is one of the leading causes of blindness worldwide. It is further categorized as open-angle or angle-closure glaucoma (ACG). ACG may be primary or secondary in nature and it may also be either acute or chronic in nature. Laser peripheral iridotomy (LPI) is the modality of treatment for ACG in cases with suspected pupillary block. However, in cases with plateau iris, Urrets-Zavalia syndrome (UZS),[1,2,3,4] and secondary angle closure due to development of peripheral anterior synechiae (PAS), LPI works seldom. The creeping of the iris tissue on the trabecular meshwork followed by the development of PAS over a long-standing period leads to raised intraocular pressure (IOP).

Surgical pupilloplasty with single-pass four-throw (SFT) technique[5,6,7] has been found helpful in resolving the raised IOP with breakage of PAS and opening of the angle structures in cases with plateau iris, UZS, and silicone oil-induced secondary angle closure (▶ Fig. 17.1 and ▶ Fig. 17.2).

17.2 Surgical Technique

In cases with UZS and in secondary angle closure due to the formation of PAS, the initial step is performed a bit differently (▶ Video 17.1). With an end-opening forceps introduced inside the AC, the peripheral edge of the iris tissue is held and is pulled slightly in a controlled way towards the center of the pupil. This helps to assess the amount of peripheral iris tissue available for the pupilloplasty procedure, and secondly, it also helps to relieve and break the PAS that are formed.

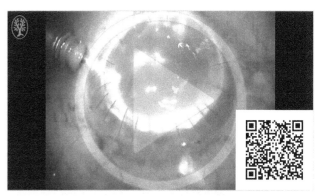

Video 17.1 Urrets–Zavalia syndrome. https://www.thieme.de/de/q.htm?p=opn/tp/311890101/9781684200979_video_17_01&t=video

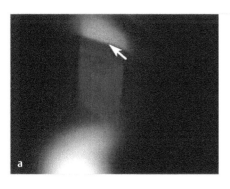
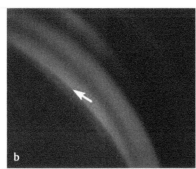

Fig. 17.1 Anterior chamber angle images following surgical pupilloplasty. **(a)** Bunching of the iris tissue in AC angle leading to angle closure. **(b)** The AC angle opens up following surgical pupilloplasty with SFT technique. AC, anterior chamber; SFT, single-pass four-throw.

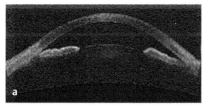
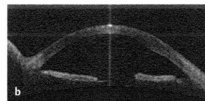

Fig. 17.2 Anterior segment optical coherence tomography (AS-OCT) imaging for AC angles. **(a)** Narrowing of the AC angles following an attack of secondary angle closure. **(b)** Opening of the angle structures post surgical pupilloplasty.

18 Jacob Paper Clip Capsule Stabilizer

Vinanti Kangale, Soosan Jacob

Summary

Subluxated cataracts are managed depending on the degree of zonular dialysis. For a subluxation of up to one quadrant, a capsular tension ring may be used. However, for larger subluxations, scleral fixation with sutures is necessary to avoid a decentered or subluxated bag in the postoperative period. To avoid suture related difficulties and complications, Dr. Jacob has designed a new device called the "paper clip capsule stabiliser" that is aimed at fixating the capsular bag in a sutureless manner to the scleral wall. It is made of blue polymethyl methacrylate and is a single-piece device, which has a fixation element and a haptic. The fixation element fixes onto the rhexis rim and thus engages the rhexis. The haptic is 13-mm long with indentations and it passes trans-sclerally through a sclerotomy made under a scleral flap and is then tucked into an intrascleral Scharioth tunnel. The fixation element is 2.5-mm wide and can be easily passed into the anterior chamber (AC) through the phaco incision. This device has its own advantages that it allows easier, faster, and safer surgery. The surgery requires less manoeuvring than sutured segments to be able to anchor the capsular bag to the scleral wall. The lack of sutures also removes all postoperative suture-related complications. Intraoperative centration of the intraocular lens (IOL) may be done easily by adjusting the degree of tuck of the haptic. For larger degrees of subluxation, two capsule stabilizers may be used. Subluxated in-the-bag IOLs may also be refixated easily using the Jacob capsule stabilizer.

Keywords: Subluxated cataract, sutureless fixation, Jacob paper clip capsule stabiliser, subluxated IOL, glued capsular hook, zonular dialysis, subluxation, dislocation

18.1 Introduction

Subluxated cataracts[1,2] are managed depending on the degree of zonular dialysis. For a subluxation of up to one quadrant, a capsular tension ring may be used.[3,4,5] However, for larger subluxations, some form of scleral fixation is necessary to avoid a decentered or subluxated bag in the postoperative period. The currently available devices for scleral fixation are all sutured and include the Ahmed segment,[6] the Cionni single- and double-hook rings,[5] the Assia segment,[7] and so forth. All these devices, once implanted, are sutured onto the sclera wall using either 9–0 Prolene suture or Gore-Tex suture. The disadvantages of having to suture these devices to the scleral wall are many. It involves the manipulations required to pass long and thin needles across the AC, which can involve complicated maneuvering. This makes surgery more difficult and also takes a longer time. In addition, the tension with which the suture knot is tied down determines the degree of centration of the IOL. If the knot happens to be tied either too loose or too tight, the IOL remains decentered. This situation would necessitate cutting the suture and performing the entire complicated maneuvering of sutured scleral fixation again. One of the authors (Jacob) had described the glued endocapsular ring[8,9] and the glued capsular hook[10] technique for sutureless capsular bag stabilization. In addition, Jacob also designed the Jacob capsule stabilizer (Morcher GmbH, Germany), which makes this a simple procedure to perform. It is a new device that is aimed at fixating the capsular bag in a sutureless manner to the scleral wall.[11,12,13,14]

18.2 Design of the Device

The paper clip capsule stabilizer is made of blue polymethyl methacrylate and is a single-piece device, which has a fixation element and a haptic. The fixation element has two flanges on either side and a central extension that together forms a paper clip component (▶Video 18.1). This paper clip component fixes onto the rhexis rim and thus engages the rhexis. The haptic passes trans-sclerally through a sclerotomy that has been made under a scleral flap and is then tucked into an intrascleral Scharioth tunnel. The haptic is 13-mm long and has indentations, which help to obtain a firm grip within the Scharioth tunnel. The fixation element is 2.5-mm wide and can be easily passed into the AC through the phaco incision (▶Fig. 18.1).

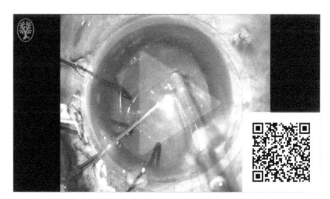

Video 18.1 Why suture: glued capsular hook. https://www.thieme.de/de/q.htm?p=opn/tp/311890101/9781684200979_video_18_01&t=video

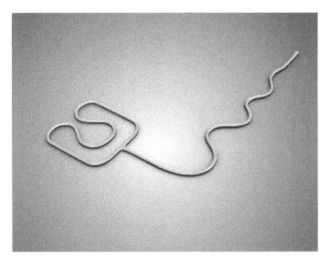

Fig. 18.1 Design of the device: The Jacob paper clip capsule (Morcher GmbH) stabilizer consists of 2 parts. **(1)** A fixation element that is 2.5-mm wide. It has two flanges on either side and a central extension that together forms a paper clip component. **(2)** The haptic is 13-mm long and has indentations.

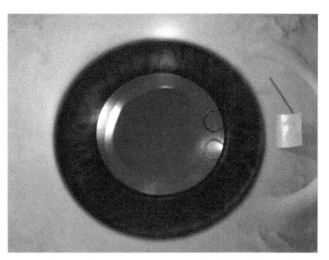

Fig. 18.2 A coat-hanger configured intrascleral Scharioth tunnel and tuck are shown.

18.3 Technique

18.3.1 Surgical Procedure

The degree of subluxation is assessed and if more than one quadrant, a Jacob capsule stabilizer is used. A scleral flap is created, centered on the area of dialysis. Phaco incisions are created. Intravitreal preservative-free triamcinolone acetonide is injected to identify any prolapsed vitreous and if present, a vitrectomy is done to remove it. A rhexis is made in such a way so as to leave an adequate rim of capsule on the side of dialysis. The retroiridal space is expanded by injecting viscoelastic into the eye and a sclerotomy is then made either in an ab interno or an ab externo fashion using a 23-G needle. A gentle hydrodissection is done, and under cover of viscoelastic, the paper clip capsule stabilizer is inserted into the AC by introducing the haptic in first. Alternately, an AC maintainer with balanced salt solution irrigation may also be used to maintain the AC well formed. After again expanding the retroiridal space with viscoelastic, a 23-G microforceps is inserted through the sclerotomy behind the iris and anterior to the anterior capsule and the haptic of the Jacob capsule stabilizer is grasped and externalized through the sclerotomy. Additional translimbal capsular hooks may be placed at this stage to give extra intraoperative support. The paper clip element of the capsule stabilizer

is then grasped and then engaged onto the rhexis rim. Once this is done, pulling the haptic centers the bag into place. The haptic is then trimmed and is tucked into an intrascleral Scharioth tunnel. The tunnel may be made with a gentle slant towards the limbus in a coat-hanger configuration so as to give additional stability. This is easily achieved by initiating the tunnel from the outer corner of the scleral bed (▶ Fig. 18.2). The degree of centration of the tuck determines the degree of centration of the capsular bag. A greater pull is obtained by increasing the degree of tuck. The Jacob capsule stabilizer as well as conventional translimbal capsular hooks, if applied, provide the intraoperative support required for various steps of the cataract surgery. A capsular tension ring may be inserted at any stage that is comfortable to the surgeon either before nucleus removal or before cortex aspiration. This provides additional forniceal expansion during all steps of cataract surgery. Phacoemulsification of the nucleus and cortex aspiration are then performed as conventionally described for subluxated cataracts. The IOL is then implanted into the bag, all additional translimbal capsular hooks that were placed are removed, and final tuck of the haptic of the capsule stabilizer is once again adjusted if required. The scleral flap and the conjunctiva are closed with fibrin glue at the end of surgery (▶ Fig. 18.3, ▶ Fig. 18.4, ▶ Fig. 18.5, and ▶ Fig. 18.6).

The Jacob capsule stabilizer may also be used very effectively to fixate the capsular bag in case of intraoperative zonular dialysis.

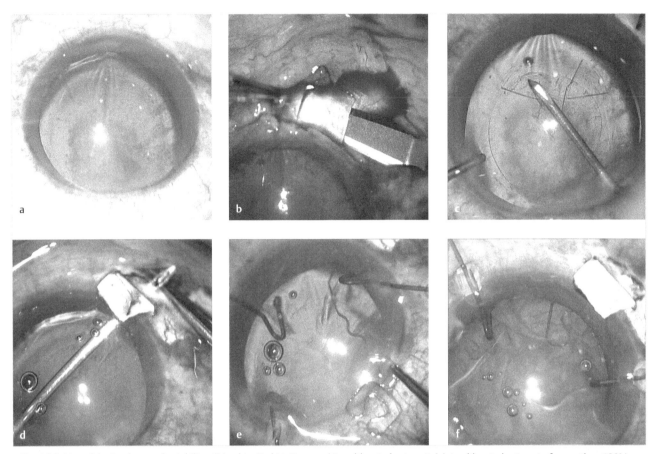

Fig. 18.3 Use of the Jacob capsule stabilizer (Morcher GmbH, Germany) in subluxated cataract. **(a)** A subluxated cataract of more than 180° is seen. **(b)** A partial-thickness scleral flap is created, centered on the area of dialysis. **(c)** A rhexis is created, leaving an adequate rim on the side of dialysis. **(d)** An ab interno sclerotomy is made using a 23-G needle. An ab externo sclerotomy may also be made. **(e)** The Jacob capsule stabilizer is introduced into the AC and the tip of the haptic is grasped by an end-gripping forceps. **(f)** The fixation element of the capsule stabilizer is grasped and engaged onto the rhexis rim. AC, anterior chamber.

18.4 Advantages of the Jacob Capsule Stabilizer

This device allows easier and faster surgery and also makes surgery safer. The surgeon requires less maneuvering than sutured segments to be able to anchor the capsular bag to the scleral wall. The lack of sutures also removes all postoperative suture-related complications that may happen. Intraoperative centration and adjustment of the position of the IOL may be done easily by simply adjusting the degree of tuck of the haptic. For larger degrees of subluxation, two capsule stabilizers may be used.

18.5 Use in Subluxated Intraocular Lenses

Subluxated in-the-bag IOLs[15,16,17] may also be refixated easily and simply using the Jacob capsule stabilizer. This is done in a similar manner as subluxated cataract by making a scleral flap centered on the zone of dialysis followed by a sclerotomy through which the haptic of the Jacob capsule stabilizer is externalized. The fixation element is then used to engage the rhexis rim and the IOL is pulled into position. In larger subluxations, more than one capsule stabilizer may be used. The degree of tuck of the haptic will determine the centration of the IOL.

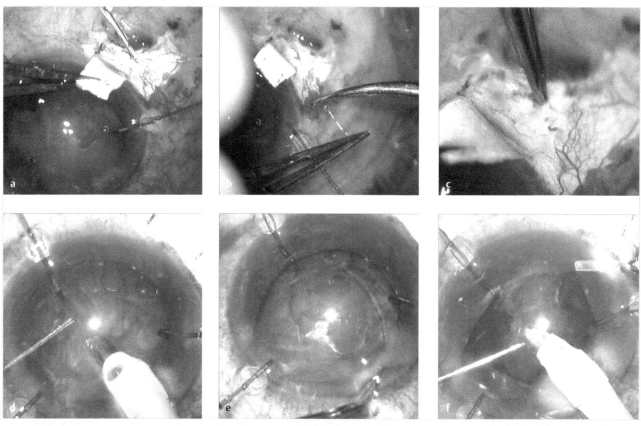

Fig. 18.4 Use of the Jacob capsule stabilizer (Morcher GmbH, Germany) in subluxated cataract. **(a)** A 26-G needle is used to create an intrascleral Scharioth tunnel. **(b)** The haptic of the Jacob capsule stabilizer is trimmed to the desired size. **(c)** The haptic is then tucked into the intrascleral Scharioth tunnel. **(d)** Phacoemulsification of the nucleus is then performed with additional translimbal capsular hooks inserted, if needed for added intraoperative support. **(e)** A capsular tension ring is inserted into the capsular bag for forniceal expansion. **(f)** Cortex aspiration performed.

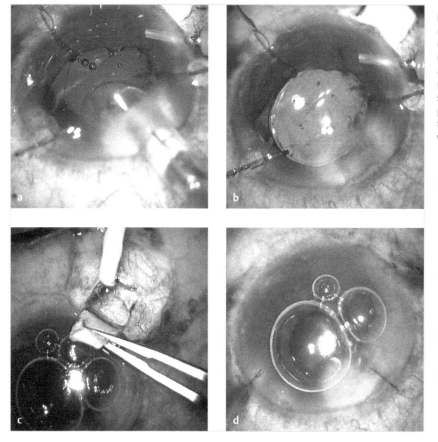

Fig. 18.5 Use of the Jacob capsule stabilizer (Morcher GmbH, Germany) in subluxated cataract. **(a)** The IOL is inserted into the bag. **(b)** The position of IOL is checked and additional translimbal capsular hooks are removed. **(c)** The haptic of the Jacob capsule stabilizer is adjusted to the final desired position and the scleral flap is closed with fibrin glue. **(d)** Conjunctiva is also closed with fibrin glue. IOL, intraocular lens.

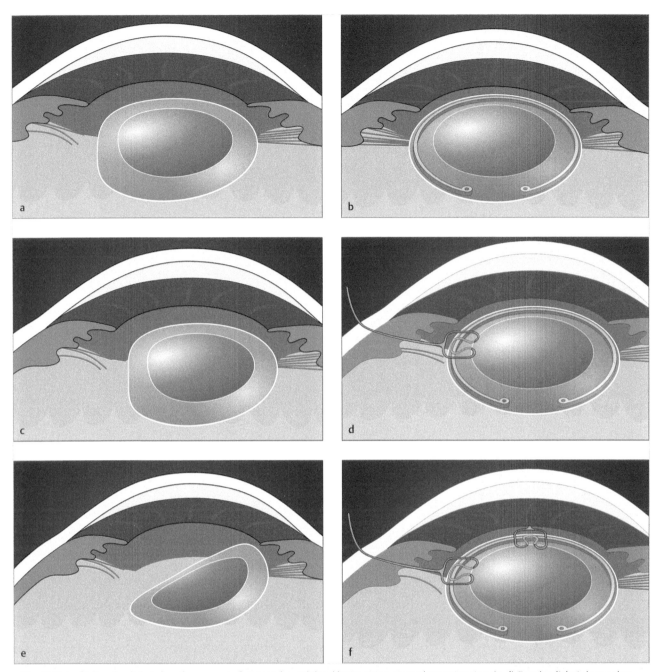

Fig. 18.6 (a, b) Zonular dialysis less than one quadrant can be stabilized by inserting a capsular tension ring. **(c, d)** Zonular dialysis larger than one quadrant needs scleral fixation of the capsular bag. This is achieved in a sutureless manner using the Jacob capsule clip stabilizer (Morcher GmbH). A capsular tension ring is inserted for forniceal expansion. **(e, f)** Very large subluxations may also be managed by inserting two capsule stabilizers together with a capsular tension ring.

References

[1] Davis D, Brubaker J, Espandar L, et al. Late in-the-bag spontaneous intraocular lens dislocation: evaluation of 86 consecutive cases. Ophthalmology 2009;116(4):664–670

[2] Fernández-Buenaga R, Alio JL, Pérez-Ardoy AL, et al. Late in-the-bag intraocular lens dislocation requiring explantation: risk factors and outcomes. Eye (Lond) 2013;27(7):795–801, quiz 802

[3] Jacob S, Agarwal A, Agarwal A, Agarwal S, Patel N, Lal V. Efficacy of a capsular tension ring for phacoemulsification in eyes with zonular dialysis. J Cataract Refract Surg 2003;29(2):315–321

[4] Hara T, Hara T, Yamada Y. "Equator ring" for maintenance of the completely circular contour of the capsular bag equator after cataract removal. Ophthalmic Surg 1991;22(6):358–359

[5] Cionni RJ, Osher RH. Management of profound zonular dialysis or weakness with a new endocapsular ring designed for scleral fixation. J Cataract Refract Surg 1998;24(10):1299–1306

[6] Hasanee K, Ahmed IIK. Capsular tension rings: update on endocapsular support devices. Ophthalmol Clin North Am 2006;19(4):507–519

[7] Assia El, Ton Y, Michaeli A. Capsule anchor to manage subluxated lenses: initial clinical experience. J Cataract Refract Surg 2009;35(8):1372–1379

[8] Jacob S, Agarwal A, Agarwal A, Sathish K, Prakash G, Kumar DA. Glued endocapsular hemi-ring segment for fibrin glue-assisted sutureless transscleral

fixation of the capsular bag in subluxated cataracts and intraocular lenses. J Cataract Refract Surg 2012;38(2):193–201

[9] Jacob S, Agarwal A. Fibrin glue assisted trans-scleral fixation of an endocapsular device for sutureless trans-scleral capsular bag fixation in traumatic subluxations: the glued endocapsular ring/segment. Med Hypothesis Discov Innov Ophthalmol 2013;2(1):3–7

[10] Jacob S, Agarwal A, Agarwal A, Agarwal A, Narasimhan S, Ashok Kumar D. Glued capsular hook: technique for fibrin glue-assisted sutureless transscleral fixation of the capsular bag in subluxated cataracts and intraocular lenses. J Cataract Refract Surg 2014;40(12):1958–1965

[11] Glued Capsular Hook Soosan Jacob. https://www.youtube.com/watch?v=M8A-HOMVCz4k. Accessed January 8, 2018

[12] Glued Capsular Hook for subluxated cataract Soosan Jacob [with audio 5 min]. https://www.youtube.com/watch?v=sz4DiMnHDCk. Accessed January 8, 2018

[13] New Glued Capsular Hook Soosan Jacob [with audio 54 min final]. https://www.youtube.com/watch?v=O3KLj5I2ijY. Accessed January 8, 2018

[14] Glued capsular hook in subluxated IOL Soosan Jacob [32 min with audio]. https://www.youtube.com/watch?v=DOu45glwHOE. Accessed January 8, 2018

[15] Hayashi K, Hirata A, Hayashi H. Possible predisposing factors for in-the-bag and out-of-the-bag intraocular lens dislocation and outcomes of intraocular lens exchange surgery. Ophthalmology 2007;114(5):969–975

[16] Jehan FS, Mamalis N, Crandall AS. Spontaneous late dislocation of intraocular lens within the capsular bag in pseudoexfoliation patients. Ophthalmology 2001;108(10):1727–1731

[17] Jakobsson G, Zetterberg M, Lundström M, Stenevi U, Grenmark R, Sundelin K. Late dislocation of in-the-bag and out-of-the-bag intraocular lenses: ocular and surgical characteristics and time to lens repositioning. J Cataract Refract Surg 2010;36(10):1637–1644

19 Double-Needle Iris/Intraocular Lens Fixation

John C. Hart Jr

Summary

Previously described techniques for fixating an intraocular lens (IOL) to the iris commonly result in distortion of the pupil and iris. Double needle iris/IOL fixation is a technique that addresses the surgical issues which contribute to iris and pupil irregularity. The first needle lifts the iris near the cornea, stretches it away from the iris root, and fixates it to the cornea. This maneuver improves visualization by overcoming total internal reflection from the cornea and improves sectility of the peripheral iris by placing it under tension. Smaller, more peripheral bites of iris can be achieved when suturing the IOL to the iris with the second needle. Optic capture within the pupil distorts the iris and masks distortion caused by fixating sutures. Therefore, suture knots are not locked until after the optic is positioned in the posterior chamber and any pupil distortion caused by the sutures is addressed. The result is iris/IOL fixation without distortion of the iris or pupil.

Keywords: Iris, IOL fixation, sutured IOL, secondary IOL

19.1 Introduction

In the setting of absent capsular or zonular support, IOL fixation to the iris can be an attractive alternative for the anterior segment surgeon. This technique can be used for aphakia or to repair a dislocated IOL. McCannel was the first to describe suture fixation of an IOL to the iris in 1976.[1] The McCannel suture technique requires corneal paracenteses overlying the knots to externalize the sutures. Stark and coauthors described iris fixation of posteriorly dislocated IOLs using the McCannel suture technique in 1980.[2] Siepser published his innovative slip knot technique in 1994.[3] This suture technique allowed knot tying within a closed anterior chamber and did not require additional paracenteses. Condon[4] and later Chang[5] employed the Siepser technique when fixating IOLs to the iris. These techniques all use a single suture needle pass to fixate the haptics of an IOL to the iris. Although these techniques are extremely useful for IOL fixation, often the iris and pupil are left distorted (▶ Fig. 19.1).

In contrast, double-needle iris/IOL fixation uses a suture needle, like a third hand within the anterior chamber, to lift and stretch the peripheral iris prior to suture fixation. This technique allows the surgeon to support the IOL with suture bites, which are smaller and more peripherally positioned in the iris, thereby minimizing iris and pupillary distortion. Suture fixation of a dislocated IOL is primarily reserved for IOLs, which are not within the capsular bag and are of a three-piece design. Iris fixation of single-piece polymethyl methacrylate IOLs is possible but technically more difficult, especially if the IOL is planar in design.

19.2 Description of the Technique

Prior to fixation of a dislocated IOL to the iris, the surgeon must assess the status of the vitreous in relation to the IOL. Appropriate limbal or pars plana vitrectomy should be performed if there is vitreous in the anterior segment or adherent to a dislocated IOL to avoid creating vitreous traction on the retina.

Assessment of the IOL position within the eye is a critical first step in managing IOL dislocation. If the IOL is in the anterior vitreous, a pars plana posterior-assisted levitation[6] may be necessary to bring the IOL into the anterior chamber. It is also critical to determine whether the IOL is right side up (▶ Fig. 19.2). If the IOL is inverted, it should be flipped so that it is right side up prior to fixation. This maneuver should be performed after appropriate vitrectomy.

For dislocated IOLs located in the capsular bag or ciliary sulcus, an anterior approach through two paracenteses is sufficient to deliver the optic anterior to the pupil. The 1-mm paracenteses are created at the superior temporal and inferior temporal limbus. A miotic agent (Miochol) is injected into the anterior chamber. After miosis of the pupil, a dispersive ophthalmic viscosurgical device (OVD) is instilled into the anterior chamber. The optic of the IOL is visualized by retracting the iris with a Kuglen hook. A 27-G OVD cannula is passed through the pupil and then beneath the optic of the IOL. The optic is elevated through the pupil with the 27-G cannula. The

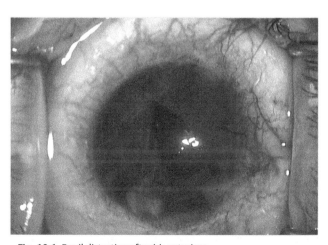

Fig. 19.1 Pupil distortion after iris suturing.

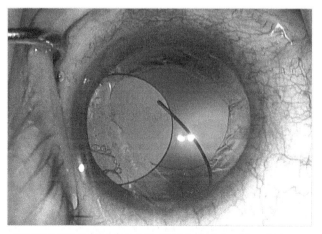

Fig. 19.2 Luxated and decentered intraocular lens with posterior capsular rupture. Orientation of the intraocular has to be determined before suturing to iris.

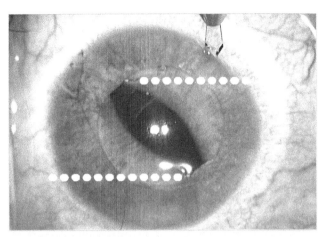

Fig. 19.3 Illustrated picture showing the proper placement of paracentesis by drawing an imaginary line (*yellow, dotted*) parallel to the haptic.

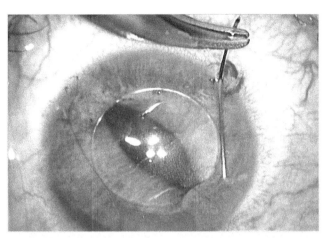

Fig. 19.4 Intraoperative image showing the free needle passed through the oblique paracentesis then through and through the iris capturing the underlying haptic.

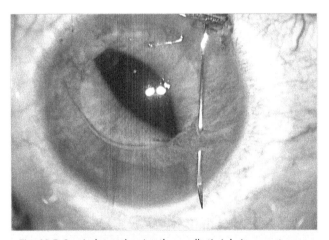

Fig. 19.5 Surgical step showing the needle tip is being swept away from the iris root and then driven into the peripheral cornea.

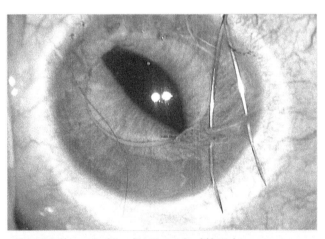

Fig. 19.6 The suture bite of iris tissue should be taken perpendicular to the underlying haptic of the intraocular lens.

iris is pushed off the opposite side of the optic with a Kuglen hook. This maneuver captures the optic anterior to the iris while the haptics remain posterior. Equal amounts of iris should be distributed between the two haptics. An oblique paracentesis is created approximately 90° away from where the haptic is located beneath the iris. The proper placement of this paracentesis is best visualized by drawing an imaginary line parallel to the haptic (▶Fig. 19.3). The internal opening of the paracentesis should touch this line. A 10–0 Prolene suture double armed with CTC-6L needles (Ethicon) is used for this technique. One needle is cut free. This free needle is passed through the oblique paracentesis then through and through the iris capturing the underlying haptic (▶Fig. 19.4). The needle tip is swept away from the iris root and then driven into the peripheral cornea (▶Fig. 19.5). This maneuver achieves four important objectives: it decreases the angle between the iris and the cornea, stretches the iris away from the iris root, fixates the stretched iris to the cornea, and drapes the iris over the haptic highlighting the area for suture fixation. The CTC-6L needle with attached 10–0 Prolene suture (Ethicon) is then passed through the oblique paracentesis,

posterior to the first needle. As the iris has been placed on stretch by the first needle, and more of the peripheral iris is visible, the second needle can be passed more peripherally into the iris for haptic fixation. Keeping the peripheral iris under tension allows the second needle to take a smaller, more controlled bite of iris tissue. The bite of iris tissue should be taken perpendicular to the underlying haptic (▶Fig. 19.6). Both needles are then removed from the eye. The same suturing technique is performed on the second haptic. Both sutures are tied with a double overhand knot using the Siepser sliding knot technique.[3] It is important to not finish or lock the knots at this point. The optic of the IOL is then prolapsed through the pupil. Once the optic is posterior to the pupil, the distorting effects of the sutures on the iris and pupil can be evaluated. As the sutures are not locked, iris tissue can be mobilized through the knots by pulling on the pupil margin with micrograspers if iris or pupillary distortion is present. If this maneuver does not relieve iris distortion, the suture should be removed and double-needle iris/IOL fixation may be repeated for that haptic. The knots are then locked with two single overhand knots utilizing the Siepser sliding knot technique.

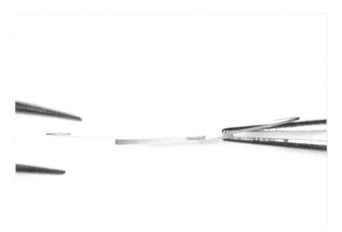

Fig. 19.7 The intraocular lens showing the optic and the haptics. Note that the most anterior portion is where the straight portion of the haptic transitions into the distal curved portion.

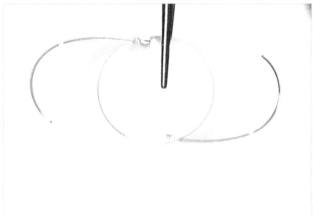

Fig. 19.8 The fixating suture should be placed near the end of the straight portion of the haptic as shown as *yellow vertical line*.

19.3 Discussion

Why does distortion of the iris and pupil occur with previously described iris/IOL fixation techniques? The iris is a diaphanous tissue that is normally planar between the iris root and the pupil margin. Not all parts of the iris move equally. The peripheral iris moves less than the more central collarette. When fixating an IOL to the iris, fixation sutures should be placed as far as possible in the peripheral iris to minimize IOL movement as well as distortion of the iris and pupil. Ultimately, the sutures, which fixate the IOL to the iris, will also limit mydriasis; therefore, the more peripheral the sutures, the greater the pupil can dilate for future retinal examination.

In contrast, the haptic is rigid and angulated anteriorly with respect to the optic. The most posterior portion of the haptic is at the haptic–optic junction. The most anterior portion is where the straight portion of the haptic transitions into the distal curved portion (▶Fig. 19.7). If the fixating suture is placed too close to the haptic–optic junction, iris distortion will occur because the iris will be drawn downward out of the normal plane of the iris. The closer the suture is placed to the haptic–optic junction, the greater the distortion of the iris. Optimal suture placement is dictated by the anatomy of the IOL haptic. The fixating suture should be placed near the end of the straight portion of the haptic (▶Fig. 19.8). This position is approximately 3 mm distal to the point of insertion of the haptic into the optic. Suture fixation beyond this point risks that the haptic can slip out of the suture, resulting in IOL dislocation.

Incarceration of too much iris within the fixating suture also contributes to iris and pupil distortion when fixating an IOL to the iris. This occurs if the bite of iris tissue is too large or the bite of iris is larger on one haptic than the other. Alternatively, iris tissue can become bunched within the knots as the fixating suture is tied. When suturing an IOL to the iris, bunching excess iris tissue within the sutures should be avoided.

The direction of the iris suture can also have an influence on iris distortion. Iris sutures placed perpendicular to the haptic cause less distortion than bites that are parallel to the haptic. Iris sutures placed more parallel to the haptic tend to foreshorten the iris, drawing the pupil margin towards the limbus.

Failure to properly center the IOL on the iris prior to IOL fixation can also contribute to iris and pupil distortion when fixating an IOL to the iris. Care must be taken to ensure that the iris is equally distributed between the haptics before suture fixation. Most often, this occurs due to iris abnormalities such as partial traumatic mydriasis, large iridotomy, iris atrophy, or membrane formation on the pupil margin. If these conditions are present in the iris preoperatively, fixation of an IOL to the iris without causing iris distortion can be extremely challenging.

The first needle improves visualization and sectility of the peripheral iris. A significant amount of the peripheral iris is not visualized through the operating microscope due to total internal reflection from the cornea. Gonioscopy allows visualization of the angle and peripheral iris by optically eliminating total internal reflection from the cornea. Likewise, the first needle in this technique eliminates total internal reflection from the cornea by mechanically reducing the angle between the iris and the cornea below the critical angle for total internal reflection. Overcoming total internal reflection from the cornea allows visualization of the more peripheral iris.

Moreover, visualization of the peripheral iris is frequently obscured due to opacification of the peripheral cornea. Arcus senilis, peripheral corneal ulcers, and penetrating keratoplasty are common corneal conditions, which impair visualization of the underlying iris. However, visualization of iris detail through these lesions is improved when the iris is brought closer to the cornea by the first needle.

The flaccid and loosely folded nature of the iris makes taking small controlled bites with a single needle technically challenging. Tissue sectility describes how easily an instrument can pass through a given tissue. Tissue sectility for the iris can be improved by using a sharp cutting needle and by placing the iris under tension. CTC-6L needles (Ethicon) are utilized for this technique because the spatula design of the tip is significantly sharper than the CIF-4 (Ethicon) needle with its "taper point" design that is commonly used in other techniques.[4,5] The first needle in the double-needle iris/IOL fixation technique not only stretches the iris but also keeps the peripheral iris under tension. Tension removes folds in the peripheral iris

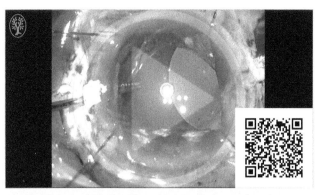

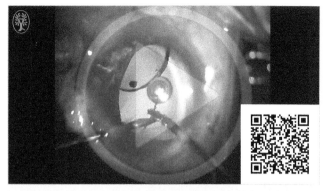

Video 20.2 Sutured scleral fixated intraocular lens with eyelet. https://www.thieme.de/de/q.htm?p=opn/tp/311890101/9781684200979_video_20_02&t=video

Video 20.3 Sutured subluxated posterior chamber intraocular lens to glued intraocular lens. . https://www.thieme.de/de/q. htm?p=opn/tp/311890101/9781684200979_video_20_03&t=video

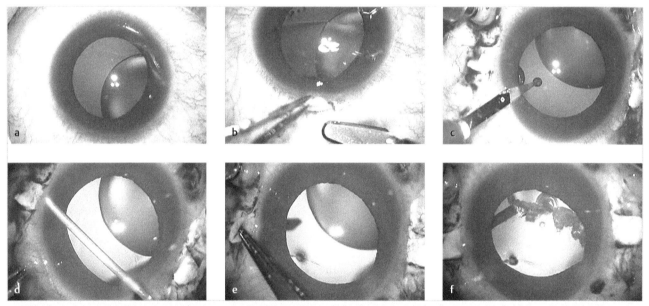

Fig. 20.1 Glued intraocular lens technique. **(a)** Massive subluxation of the crystalline lens is seen. **(b)** Two partial-thickness scleral flaps are made 180° opposite to each other. The flaps here are made at 6 and 12 o'clock positions. **(c)** The surgeon sits temporally so that the flaps are aligned horizontally for easy maneuverability. Fluid infusion is introduced inside the eye. **(d)** Vitrector-assisted peripheral iridectomy is performed at the proposed site of sclerotomy to avert iris complications. **(e)** Anterior sclerotomy is performed with 22-G needle that smoothly passes through the iris base without causing any traction on the iris tissue. **(f)** Lensectomy is performed.

- Sclerotomy: Sclerotomy is made beneath the scleral flaps with a 22-G needle at a distance of 0.5 to 1 mm from limbus and the needle is directed obliquely into the midvitreous cavity (▶Fig. 20.1e).
- Vitrectomy: A 23-G vitrectomy cutter is introduced from the sclerotomy site (▶Fig. 20.1f) and thorough vitrectomy is performed into the retropupillary zone and AC to cut down all the vitreous strands. A high cutter rate with moderate vacuum suffices the need well. Triamcinolone staining can be done to enhance the visualization of the vitreous.
- Haptic externalization: A corneal tunnel incision is made and a three-piece foldable IOL is loaded. The tip of the leading haptic is made to slightly protrude from the cartridge by rotating the injector. This facilitates grasping the tip of the haptic while the IOL is being injected. The end-opening glued IOL forceps is introduced from the left sclerotomy site and the tip of the leading haptic is grasped (▶Fig. 20.2a). The IOL is slowly unfolded

inside the AC and the cartridge is withdrawn a bit so that the trailing haptic lies at the corneal incision. The tip of the leading haptic is then pulled and externalized (▶Fig. 20.2b). The trailing haptic is then held with end-opening glued IOL forceps and is flexed inside the AC (▶Fig. 20.2c); meanwhile, the assistant holds the leading haptic and prevents it from slipping inside the AC. A glued IOL forceps is introduced from the side port incision and the surgeon then transfers the trailing haptic from right hand to left hand (▶Fig. 20.2d). The right-hand glued IOL forceps is withdrawn from the eye and it re-enters the eye from the right sclerotomy incision. The surgeon again transfers the trailing haptic from left hand to right hand (▶Fig. 20.2e). This transfer of haptics from one hand to another is known as *handshake technique*.[8] The tip of the trailing haptic is then grasped and it is pulled and externalized (▶Fig. 20.2f).
- Intrascleral tuck: Scleral pockets are created with a 26-G needle along the edge of the base of flaps parallel to

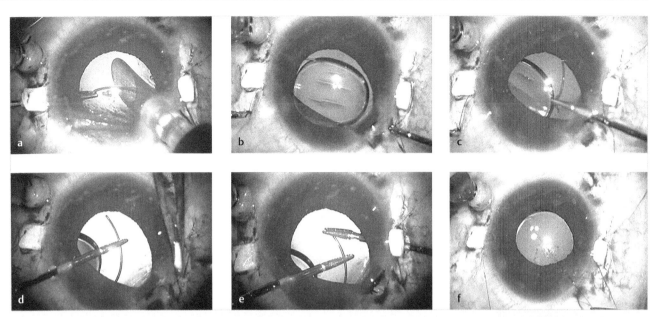

Fig. 20.2 Glued IOL technique. **(a)** A three-piece foldable IOL is loaded onto the cartridge and the tip of the leading haptic is held with an end-opening forceps introduced from the left sclerotomy site. **(b)** The tip of the leading haptic is pulled and externalized while the trailing haptic is held. **(c)** The trailing haptic is flexed inside the eye towards 6 o'clock position, thereby crossing the mid-pupillary plane. **(d)** An end-opening forceps is introduced from the left side port incision and the trailing haptic is transferred to the left hand. Note that the leading haptic does not slip inside the eye and it is known as no-assistant technique. **(e)** Handshake technique being performed. **(f)** Both haptics externalized. IOL, intraocular lens.

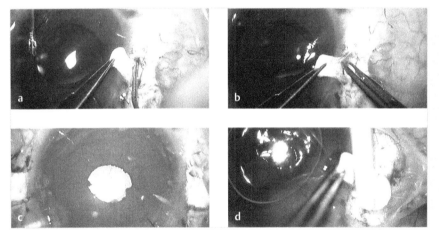

Fig. 20.3 Glued IOL technique. **(a)** Scleral pocket created with 26-G needle. **(b)** Haptic being tucked into the scleral pockets. **(c)** Haptic tucked on both the sides. **(d)** Fluid infusion is removed and fibrin glue is applied to seal the flaps.

the sclerotomy site (▶Fig. 20.3a). The haptics are tucked into these scleral pockets with around 2 to 3 mm of haptic length being entrapped into the length of the pockets (▶Fig. 20.3b, c). Vitrectomy is again performed at the sclerotomy site to prevent any vitreous being incarcerated into the wound.

• Fibrin glue-assisted flap sealing: The fluid infusion is stopped; fibrin glue is applied beneath the flaps and along the conjunctival peritomy site to seal it (▶Fig. 20.3d).

20.3.1 No-Assistant Technique (NAT)

NAT is a modified method of haptic externalization where the surgeon does not need an assistant to hold the leading haptic.[3] The technique works on the principle of direction of vector forces. Once the leading haptic is eternalized, the surgeon grasps the trailing haptic and flexes it more towards 6 o'clock position. At this juncture, the vector forces act in a way that the leading haptic is extruded more from the sclerotomy site and it does not need an assistant to hold the haptic as there is no tendency for the haptic to slip back inside the eye (▶Fig. 20.2). Meanwhile, the surgeon performs handshake technique for externalization of the trailing haptic (▶Video 20.4).

20.4 Other Modifications in Glued Intraocular Lens Surgery

Beiko and Steinert suggested a technique where they used the tire of iris hooks to club onto the IOL haptic to prevent it from slippage inside the eye.[5] Ohta et al suggested making Y- and T-shaped flaps for performing the glued IOL procedure.[6]

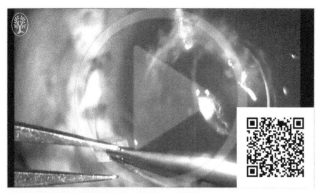

Video 20.4 No-assistant technique in glued intraocular lens. https://www.thieme.de/de/q.htm?p=opn/tp/311890101/9781684200979_video_20_04&t=video

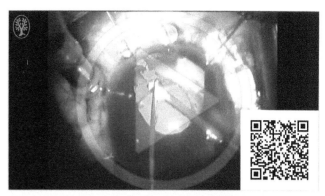

Video 20.5 Soemmering ring. https://www.thieme.de/de/q.htm?p=opn/tp/311890101/9781684200979_video_20_05&t=video

20.5 Combination Procedures

20.5.1 Glued Intraocular Lens Scaffold

This technique combines the glued IOL procedure (▶ Video 20.5) that is performed initially followed by an IOL scaffold procedure as a single-stage procedure.[9,10,11] This technique is done in cases with no capsular support wherein performing a glued IOL initially helps to form the IOL optic as an artificial posterior capsule. IOL scaffold can then be performed on this barrier that helps to emulsify the residual nuclear fragments. This technique has been found helpful in cases with Soemmering ring associated with aphakia and in cases with massive subluxated lens.[11]

20.5.2 Pre-Descemet's Endothelial Keratoplasty (PDEK) with Glued Intraocular Lens

Aphakic and pseudophakic bullous keratopathy is a known entity and often the clinical scenario requires an EK procedure to be performed to enhance the visual potential of the patient. PDEK is our treatment of choice for an EK procedure.[12] In addition to this, single-pass four-throw pupilloplasty is also performed with the combined procedure as it prevents the escape of air into the posterior chamber (PC) and also helps to maintain the effective air tamponade.

20.5.3 Triumvirate Technique

This technique is applicable in cases with sinking nucleus associated with deficient capsular support.[13] The technique comprises performing modified posterior-assisted levitation (PAL), IOL scaffold, and glued IOL procedure. When a sinking nucleus is encountered, a spatula or a rod is passed through the sclerotomy site and the nuclear fragments are levitated into the AC. The advantage of performing modified PAL is that

two sclerotomy sites are available for nucleus levitation that get finally covered by the scleral flaps at the end of the procedure. It also obviates the need to create an extra sclerotomy at pars plana, thereby negating any chances of damaging the peripheral retina.

Once the fragments are in AC, a three-piece foldable IOL is injected inside the AC and the haptics are made to lie on the anterior surface of the iris tissue. The nuclear fragments are emulsified with the phacoemulsification probe following which the haptics are transferred behind the iris plane and with the help of handshake technique, the haptics are externalized through the respective sclerotomy sites. Tucking the haptics and sealing the flaps with fibrin glue then conclude the glued IOL procedure.

20.6 Variations Adopted in Glued Intraocular Lens Surgery

20.6.1 Vertical Glued Intraocular Lens

The vertical corneal diameter is always less than the horizontal diameter. Hence, in cases with larger WTW diameter, scleral flaps are made at 6 and 12 o'clock positions in an attempt to externalize greater haptic length.[14]

20.6.2 Peripheral Iridectomy (PI) for Glued Intraocular Lens

A vitrector-assisted PI is performed beneath the scleral flaps at the prospective site of sclerotomy.[15] It is performed in association with anterior sclerotomy in cases with large eyes undergoing glued IOL fixation.[16] This technique facilitates haptic externalization by ensuring smooth passage of the 22-G needle and the glued IOL end-opening forceps through the sclerotomy site, thereby minimizing the chances of iris damage.

20.6.3 Quintet in Glued Intraocular Lens

This procedure combines five different techniques, namely, vertical glued IOL, trocar ACM, PI, anterior sclerotomy, and pupilloplasty.[17] Quintet in glued IOL comprises assimilation of all surgical procedures that would be valuable in eyes with greater WTW diameter.

20.7 Discussion

Peer review studies demonstrate the postoperative outcomes and the surgical results of glued IOL procedure for short, interim, and long term as satisfactory.[18,19,20] However, for results to be optimal, there are various nuances of the surgery that needs to be understood and executed properly (▶ Video 20.6). The correct positioning of the surgeon with respect to the scleral flaps is extremely important due to the fact that the movement of the surgical hands for handshake technique for effective haptic externalization should be assigned correctly.[21] The surgeon should always be positioned perpendicular to the plane of scleral flaps and to the plane of haptic maneuver.[6] The surgery should be performed under fluid infusion and the use of viscoelastic should be minimized. Gentle handling of the haptics along with proper tucking is essential to prevent any postoperative issue of decentration or subluxation of the IOL. The surgery has varied applications in cases of decentered IOLs (▶ Fig. 20.4 and ▶ Fig. 20.5) and subluxated bag–IOL complex (▶ Fig. 20.6) where the IOL can be either repositioned or explanted and a glued IOL can be fixed inside the eye.

The additional benefit of performing glued IOL surgery is that pseudophacodonesis is not observed in intrascleral haptic fixation that indirectly translates to the lesser vitreous disturbance in the postoperative period.[22] Thus, glued IOL surgery when performed in accordance with the protocol helps to enhance the visual potential of the patient (▶ Fig. 20.7) and curtail all the possible eventualities and complications.

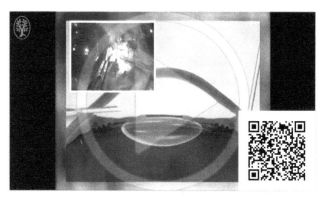

Video 20.6 Lessons learned: complications of glued introcular lens. https://www.thieme.de/de/q.htm?p=opn/tp/311890101/9781684200979_video_20_06&t=video

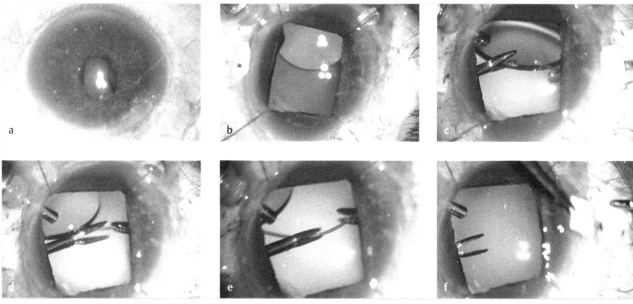

Fig. 20.4 Refixation of a decentered multifocal IOL. **(a)** Decentered multifocal IOL. **(b)** Scleral flaps made for glued IOL surgery and iris hooks are employed for better visualization. **(c)** The IOL is held and limited vitrectomy is performed beneath and around the IOL. **(d)** The trailing haptic is held. **(e)** Handshake technique is performed and the tip of the haptic is grasped. **(f)** The tip of haptic is pulled and externalized. IOL, intraocular lens.

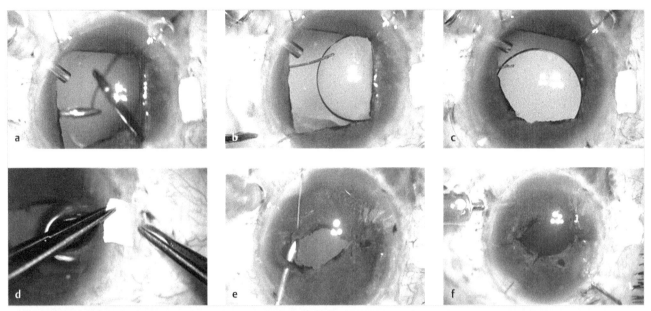

Fig. 20.5 Refixation of a decentered multifocal IOL. **(a)** The other haptic is localized and the tip of the haptic is held. **(b)** The tip is pulled and externalized. **(c)** Both haptics are externalized. **(d)** The haptics are tucked into the scleral pockets. **(e)** Single-pass four-throw pupilloplasty is performed to prevent optic capture. **(f)** Suture is taken and the corneal incision is closed. IOL, intraocular lens.

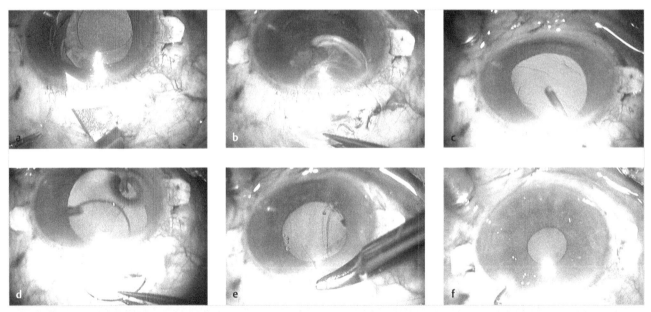

Fig. 20.6 Subluxated bag–IOL complex. **(a)** Two scleral flaps are made for glued IOL in subluxated bag–IOL complex. A scleral tunnel incision is made for explantation of the complex. **(b)** The bag–IOL complex is explanted. **(c)** Vitrectomy is performed in the anterior chamber and in pupillary zone. **(d)** A three-piece IOL is introduced and the tip of the haptic is held. **(e)** Both haptics externalized. **(f)** Both haptics tucked into the scleral pockets followed by sealing of the flaps with fibrin glue. IOL, intraocular lens.

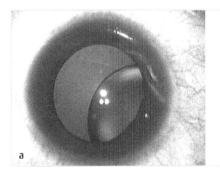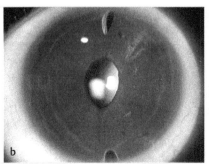

Fig. 20.7 Pre- and postoperative image. **(a)** Preoperative image with decentered crystalline lens. **(b)** Postoperative image after glued IOL surgery. IOL, intraocular lens.

References

[1] Gabor SG, Pavlidis MM. Sutureless intrascleral posterior chamber intraocular lens fixation. J Cataract Refract Surg 2007;33(11):1851–1854

[2] Agarwal A, Kumar DA, Jacob S, Baid C, Agarwal A, Srinivasan S. Fibrin glue-assisted sutureless posterior chamber intraocular lens implantation in eyes with deficient posterior capsules. J Cataract Refract Surg 2008;34(9): 1433–1438

[3] Narang P. Modified method of haptic externalization of posterior chamber intraocular lens in fibrin glue-assisted intrascleral fixation: no-assistant technique. J Cataract Refract Surg 2013;39(1):4–7

[4] Narang P. Postoperative analysis of glued intrascleral fixation of intraocular lens and comparison of intraoperative parameters and visual outcome with 2 methods of haptic externalization. J Cataract Refract Surg 2013;39(7):1118–1119

[5] Beiko G, Steinert R. Modification of externalized haptic support of glued intraocular lens technique. J Cataract Refract Surg 2013;39(3):323–325

[6] Ohta T, Toshida H, Murakami A. Simplified and safe method of sutureless intrascleral posterior chamber intraocular lens fixation: Y-fixation technique. J Cataract Refract Surg 2014;40(1):2–7

[7] Agarwal A, Narang P, Kumar DA, Agarwal A. Trocar anterior chamber maintainer: Improvised infusion technique. J Cataract Refract Surg 2016; 42(2):185–189

[8] Agarwal A, Jacob S, Kumar DA, Agarwal A, Narasimhan S, Agarwal A. Handshake technique for glued intrascleral haptic fixation of a posterior chamber intraocular lens. J Cataract Refract Surg 2013;39(3):317–322

[9] Agarwal A, Jacob S, Agarwal A, Narasimhan S, Kumar DA, Agarwal A. Glued intraocular lens scaffolding to create an artificial posterior capsule for nucleus removal in eyes with posterior capsule tear and insufficient iris and sulcus support. J Cataract Refract Surg 2013;39(3):326–333

[10] Narang P, Agarwal A, Kumar DA, Agarwal A. Clinical outcomes of the glued intraocular lens scaffold. J Cataract Refract Surg 2015;41(9):1867–1874

[11] Narang P, Agarwal A, Kumar DA. Glued intraocular lens scaffolding for Soemmerring ring removal in aphakia with posterior capsule defect. J Cataract Refract Surg 2015;41(4):708–713

[12] Narang P, Agarwal A, Dua HS, Kumar DA, Jacob S, Agarwal A. Glued Intrascleral Fixation of Intraocular Lens With Pupilloplasty and Pre-Descemet Endothelial Keratoplasty: A Triple Procedure. Cornea 2015;34(12): 1627–1631

[13] Narang P, Agarwal A. Modified posterior-assisted levitation with intraocular lens scaffold and glued IOL for sinking nucleus in eyes with inadequate sulcus support. J Cataract Refract Surg 2017;43(7):872–876

[14] Ladi JS, Shah NA. Vertical fixation with fibrin glue-assisted secondary posterior chamber intraocular lens implantation in a case of surgical aphakia. Indian J Ophthalmol 2013;61(3):126–129

[15] Narang P, Agarwal A. Peripheral iridectomy for atraumatic haptic externalization in large eyes having anterior sclerotomy for glued intraocular lens. J Cataract Refract Surg 2016;42(1):3–6

[16] Jacob S, Agarwal A, Agarwal A, Narasimhan S. Closed-chamber haptic reexternalization for posteriorly displaced sclerotomy and inadequate haptic tuck in glued posterior chamber intraocular lenses. J Cataract Refract Surg 2015;41(2):268–271

[17] Narang P, Agarwal A. Pupilloplasty for pupil size attenuation to prevent pupillary capture: Theory of quintet in glued IOL. J Cataract Refract Surg 2017;43(1):3–7

[18] Kumar DA, Agarwal A, Packiyalakshmi S, Jacob S, Agarwal A. Complications and visual outcomes after glued foldable intraocular lens implantation in eyes with inadequate capsules. J Cataract Refract Surg 2013;39(8): 1211–1218

[19] Kumar DA, Agarwal A. Glued intraocular lens: a major review on surgical technique and results. Curr Opin Ophthalmol 2013;24(1):21–29

[20] Kumar DA, Agarwal A, Agarwal A, Chandrasekar R, Priyanka V. Long-term assessment of tilt of glued intraocular lenses: an optical coherence tomography analysis 5 years after surgery. Ophthalmology 2015;122(1):48–55

[21] Narang P, Agarwal A. The "correct shake" for "handshake" in glued intrascleral fixation of intraocular lens. Indian J Ophthalmol 2016;64(11):854–856

[22] Narang P, Agarwal A, Sanu AS. Detecting subtle intraocular movements: Enhanced frames per second recording (slow motion) using smartphones. J Cataract Refract Surg 2015;41(6):1321–1323

21 Flanged Intrascleral Intraocular Lens Fixation with Double-Needle Technique

Shin Yamane

Summary

Flanged intraocular lens (IOL) technique is a simple method for achieving firm haptic fixation. Haptics of the IOL are fixed into the scleral tunnel made by 30-gauge needle. The tip of the haptics are cauterized to make flange for firm fixation.

Keywords: Flange, double-needle technique, sutureless, 30-gauge laceration repair

21.1 Introduction

Scharioth and Agarwal reported the intrascleral IOL fixation technique as a sutureless technique for IOL fixation.[1,2] This technique has become a popular procedure because it has some advantages over conventional trans-scleral suturing of the IOL.[3,4,5,6,7] Flanged IOL fixation is a new surgical procedure that can be carried out via the conjunctiva in which the haptics of the IOL are strongly fixed to the sclera without using suture or glue.[8] This technique is simple but not easy. The surgeon needs to understand some key points of the technique (▶ Video 21.1).

21.2 Surgical Technique

- Pars plana vitrectomy or anterior vitrectomy.
- Subluxated crystalline lens or dislocated IOL removal.
- A three-piece IOL insertion into the anterior chamber. The trailing haptic must be kept outside to prevent the IOL from falling into the vitreous cavity.
- Angled sclerotomies made with a 30-G thin-wall needle through the conjunctiva at 2 mm from the limbs (▶ Fig. 21.1 and ▶ Fig. 21.2).
- Insertion of the leading haptic into the lumen of the needle using a forceps (▶ Fig. 21.3).
- A second sclerotomy made with a 30-G thin-wall needle at 180° from the first sclerotomy.
- Insertion of the trailing haptic into the lumen of the second needle while the first needle was put on the conjunctiva (double-needle technique; ▶ Fig. 21.4).
- Externalization of the haptics onto the conjunctiva with the needles (▶ Fig. 21.5).

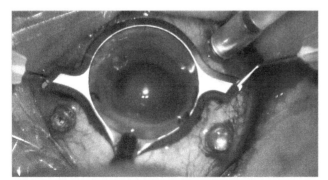

Video 21.1 Yamane technique. https://www.thieme.de/de/q.htm?p=opn/tp/311890101/9781684200979_video_21_01&t=video

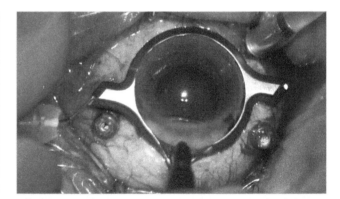

Fig. 21.1 A 30-G thin-wall needle is inserted 2.0 mm from the limbus using the needle stabilizer.

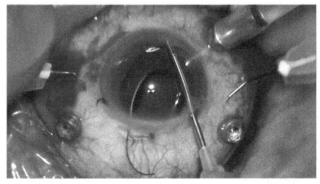

Fig. 21.2 The second needle is inserted on the opposite site of the first needle.

Fig. 21.3 Introduction of the leading haptic into the lumen of the 30-G needle.

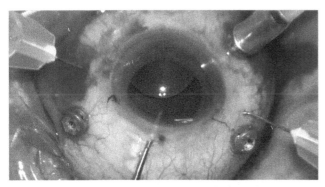

Fig. 21.4 Introduction of the trailing haptic into the lumen of the 30-G needle using the double-needle technique.

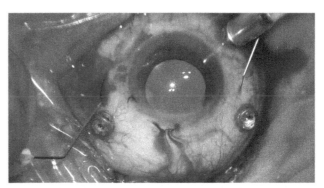

Fig. 21.5 Externalization of the haptics with two needles.

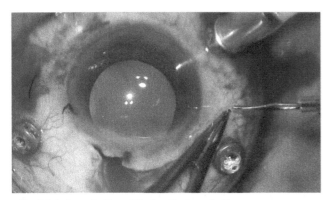

Fig. 21.6 Cauterization of the haptics to make flanges.

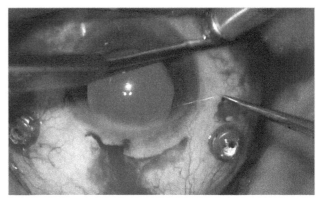

Fig. 21.7 Pushing back of the haptics to fix the flanges in the scleral tunnel.

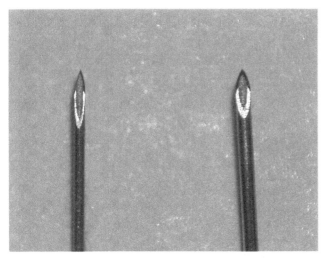

Fig. 21.8 Thin-wall needle. A 30-G thin-wall needle **(left)** has larger lumen than normal 30-G needle **(right)**.

- Cauterization of the ends of the haptics using an ophthalmic cautery device (Accu-Temp Cautery, Beaver Visitec) to make a flange with a diameter of 0.3 mm (▶ Fig. 21.6).
- Fixation of the flange of the haptics into the scleral tunnels (▶ Fig. 21.7).
- Peripheral iridotomy using the vitrectomy cutter after miosis.

21.3 Key Points

- A 30-G thin-wall needle (▶ Fig. 21.8): This needle (TSK ultrathin-wall needle) is available in Japan (Tochigi Seiko), the United States (Delasco Dermatologic Lab and Supply, Inc.), and Netherlands (TSK Laboratory Europe). The inner diameter of the needle must be 0.18 mm or more. The outer diameter of the needle should not be larger than flange of the IOL haptics. A 27-G needle is available if the diameter of the flange is over 0.4 mm.
- The positional relationship of the wounds: It is appropriate for the wound where the IOL is inserted and the site where the 30-G needle is inserted to be in positions that are separated by approximately 90° (▶ Fig. 21.9).
- Double-needle technique: Placing the leading haptic in the inner cavity of the 30-G needle makes the positional relationship of the trailing haptic and the second 30-G needle appropriate and facilitates easy insertion. If the leading haptic is pulled out together with the 30-G needle, the IOL will rotate in the anticlockwise direction. It is difficult to insert the tip of the trailing haptic into a 30-G needle in this situation (▶ Fig. 21.10).
- The insertion angle of the 30-G needle: To avoid IOL tilt and dislocation, the haptics must be fixed symmetrically. We have developed a device to stabilize the direction of the needles that will help us to fix the IOL with perfect positioning (not commercially available yet).

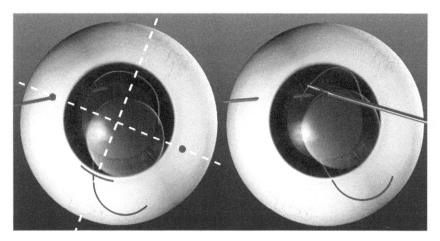

Fig. 21.9 The positional relationship of the wounds. It is easy to insert the leading haptic into the needle if the positional relationship of the wounds is appropriate **(left)**. If the wounds are too distant, the haptic hits the cornea **(right)**.

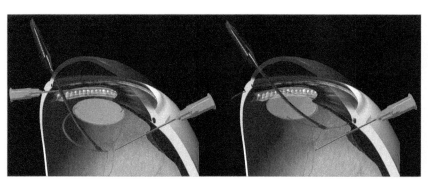

Fig. 21.10 Double-needle technique. The correct position **(left)**. The leading haptic is in the needle. It is difficult to insert the tip of the trailing haptic into a 30-G needle after pulling out of the leading haptic from the needle **(right)**.

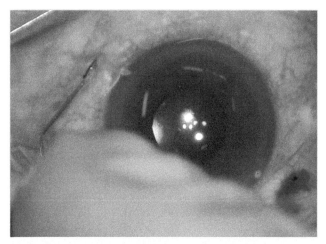

Fig. 21.11 Enlargement of the entry site of the scleral tunnel. It makes easy to insert the flange into the scleral tunnel by enlarging the entry site of the scleral tunnel with a 30-G needle.

• Making and fixation of flange: The cautery should not touch the haptic while cauterization to avoid adhesion. The haptic should be dry to avoid twisted flange. The appropriate length of the haptic to cauterize is 0.5 to 1.0 mm. If the size of the flange was too large to insert into the scleral tunnel, the entry site of the scleral tunnel should be enlarged using 30-G needle (▶ Fig. 21.11).

21.4 Conclusion

The flanged IOL fixation technique is simple and minimally invasive and provides firm haptic fixation. Although it is a simple procedure, there are some key points for making this surgery a success.

References

[1] Gabor SG, Pavlidis MM. Sutureless intrascleral posterior chamber intraocular lens fixation. J Cataract Refract Surg 2007;33(11):1851–1854

[2] Agarwal A, Kumar DA, Jacob S, Baid C, Agarwal A, Srinivasan S. Fibrin glue-assisted sutureless posterior chamber intraocular lens implantation in eyes with deficient posterior capsules. J Cataract Refract Surg 2008;34(9): 1433–1438

[3] Yamane S, Inoue M, Arakawa A, Kadonosono K. Sutureless 27-gauge needle-guided intrascleral intraocular lens implantation with lamellar scleral dissection. Ophthalmology 2014;121(1):61–66

[4] Kumar DA, Agarwal A, Prakash G, Jacob S, Saravanan Y, Agarwal A. Evaluation of intraocular lens tilt with anterior segment optical coherence tomography. Am J Ophthalmol 2011;151(3):406–412.e2

[5] Hayashi K, Hayashi H, Nakao F, Hayashi F. Intraocular lens tilt and decentration, anterior chamber depth, and refractive error after trans-scleral suture fixation surgery. Ophthalmology 1999;106(5):878–882

[6] Durak A, Oner HF, Koçak N, Kaynak S. Tilt and decentration after primary and secondary transsclerally sutured posterior chamber intraocular lens implantation. J Cataract Refract Surg 2001;27(2):227–232

[7] Sinha R, Bansal M, Sharma N, Dada T, Tandon R, Titiyal JS. Transscleral suture-fixated versus intrascleral haptic-fixated intraocular lens: a comparative study. Eye Contact Lens 2017;43(6):389–393

[8] Yamane S, Sato S, Maruyama-Inoue M, Kadonosono K. Flanged intrascleral intraocular lens fixation with double-needle technique. Ophthalmology 2017;124(8):1136–1142

22 Iris Claw Lens

Ravijit Singh, Kiranjit Singh, Indu Singh, Harmit Kaur

Summary

Implantation of intraocular lens (IOL) inside the capsular bag is the "standard of care" to correct aphakia. However, when we are dealing with complex situations involving anterior segment reconstruction and lens implantation, the capsular bag may either be not available at all or be inadequate or some other clinical situation makes it difficult, precarious, or impossible for posterior chamber lens implantation. It could be a case of inadvertent posterior capsule rupture during phacoemulsification, grossly subluxated capsular bag due to trauma, congenital, aphakia, traumatized iris, or any other condition with absent or deficient capsular support. Angle-supported IOLs have historically been known to cause a lot of problems in the long term but end up getting implanted for lack of a popular alternative.[1,2] Scleral-fixated lens implantation techniques are generally time-consuming and require a lot of instrumentation and manipulation.[2,3]

In such conditions, the Artisan lens, also known as the iris claw lens, may come to the rescue of the surgeon. All that the iris claw lens requires is available iris tissue that may provide for two points where the claws of the lens may be anchored. Implantation of the iris claw lens may be done on the anterior surface of the iris (classical way of fixation) or the posterior surface of the iris, also known as the retropupillary implantation.[4,5] Long-term results with iris claw lens implantation are very encouraging. Every anterior segment surgeon needs to have a backup system in case a posterior chamber lens implantation is not possible. The iris claw lens is the best design for this purpose. In this chapter, we shall learn about the iris claw lens design, instrumentation, and technique of implantation of this unique lens in a variety of clinical situations.

Keywords: Iris claw lens, retropupillary, absent posterior capsule, aphakia, trauma

22.1 Introduction

Iris claw lens or the Artisan lens is an entirely unique genre of IOLs, which does not need the angle of the anterior chamber, the ciliary sulcus, the sclera, or the capsular bag for support. Instead, it is fixated to the iris muscle either to the front surface or to its back surface. Fixation to the back surface of the iris is referred to as retropupillary fixation. Classically, this lens had been designed to be fixated to the anterior surface of the iris. In this chapter, we shall be discussing the versatility of implantation of the iris claw in a variety of situations, both on anterior as well as on the posterior surface of the iris according to the situation at hand.

22.2 History and Design of the Iris Claw Lens

Before we say anything else, it is important that we briefly delve into the history of the lens. Designed by legendary Dutch ophthalmologist Dr. J. G. F. Worst in the early 1970s, the basic design of the iris claw lens has remained unchanged for nearly four and a half decades. This lens has weathered the eventful years of revolution in cataract surgery technology from the era of primitive lens designs to the present day. The iris claw lens is a single-piece all-polymethyl methacrylate design (▶ Fig. 22.1 and ▶ Fig. 22.2). It is a planoconvex lens with an optic in the center and two oval openings in the haptic on either side of the optic, which are split in the middle to form a pincer-/claw-like mechanism, which the surgeon uses to fixate the lens to the iris tissue. Dr. Daljit Singh of India modified this design, which was known as the Singh–Worst design, in which the claws instead of being at 180° were positioned at 45 and 135°. We shall be discussing primarily about the original design of the iris claw lens with claws at 180° in this chapter.

22.3 Size of the Iris Claw Lens

The design of iris claw lens is primarily of the same as the original Artisan lens that Prof. Dr. J. G. F. Worst designed. However, the comparison ends here. The overall dimensions of the original lens manufactured by Ophtec, Netherlands (8.5-mm overall length and 5-mm optic diameter) are much bigger than

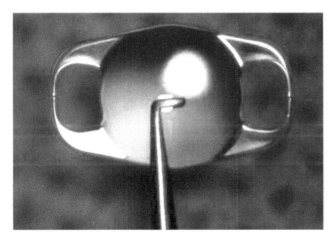

Fig. 22.1 The iris claw lens.

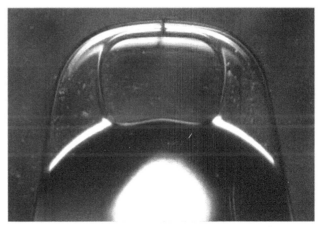

Fig. 22.2 The claw of the lens in magnification.

the lenses currently being used. The larger size of the lens was meant to achieve peripheral iris fixation and to avoid distorting the pupil. However, this brought the haptic of the lens perilously close to the endothelium. Perpetual iridodonesis and pseudophacodonesis led to intermittent endothelial touch and persistent cell loss.

However, if the lens is fixated to the iris tissue just outside the collarette (both anterior and posterior), pupillary distortion does not occur and this also does not impede the dilatation of the pupil; hence, smaller sized lenses were chosen over the original sized lenses.

The sizes of iris claw lenses (▶ Fig. 22.3) used are manufactured in India and are available in the following dimensions:
• Size 1: Overall length 7.25 mm × 4.20-mm optic diameter.
• Size 2: Overall length 6.4 mm × 4.00-mm optic diameter.
• Size 3: Overall length 5.5 mm × 3.50-mm optic diameter.
• Size 4: Overall length 4.0 mm × 2.00-mm optic diameter (special order).

The only reason why these lenses can be implanted in small sizes is because this lens does not require the support of the external shell of the eyeball for its fixation. This is also precisely the reason that implantation can be carried out in eyes of all diameters ranging from microcornea to megalocornea.

22.4 Implantation of the Iris Claw Lens

All lens designs in principle derive their fixation support by way of their springy haptics, which lean against the angle of the anterior chamber, the ciliary sulcus, the capsular bag, or the sclera. The iris claw lens is the only design that uses the iris tissue for its fixation. As the name implies, the lens is fixed to the iris. The lens can be implanted horizontally, vertically, or obliquely to suit any clinical situation according to the availability of the iris tissue, the accessibility of the surgeon, or the availability of an optical window. The lens can be implanted centrally over the pupil or eccentrically, something which is unique to this lens design. The iris claw lens can be fixated to the anterior surface as well as to the posterior surface of the iris.

22.4.1 Biometry

IOL power calculation is done using the standard calculation formulae. For implantation of the iris claw lens to the anterior surface of the iris, a constant of 115.5 is used and for posterior fixation, a constant of 116.5 is used with the SRK/T formula.

22.4.2 Instrumentation for Implantation of the Iris Claw Lens

• A set of two Clayman forceps (right- and left-sided).
• A bent 27-G, 0.5-in steel cannula mounted on a 1-mL syringe.
• The 0.6-mm trifacet diamond keratome.

The 0.6-mm diamond keratome is used to make paracentesis openings. The Clayman forceps (▶ Fig. 22.4) steadies the iris claw lens inside the eye, while the 27-G, 0.5-in cannula is used to enclave/push the iris tissue through the claw of the iris claw lens. A bent 26- or 27-G needle can also be used to enclave the iris for anterior fixation of the IOL.

22.4.3 Endothelial Cell count

It must be made sure that endothelial cell count is adequate before embarking upon iris claw lens implantation in complicated and often compromised cases so that you know how much surgical trauma the eye can tolerate. The patient has to be counseled about the possibility of corneal decompensation in borderline cases and the need for penetrating keratoplasty or Descemet's stripping endothelial keratoplasty (DSEK) just in case corneal decompensation takes place.

22.4.4 Training for Iris Claw Lens Implantation

Iris claw lens implantation is not difficult but just different. This is a skill that needs to be acquired and learnt properly in the wet lab from someone who has good experience in its use. Moreover, the use of correct instruments helps in mastering the technique correctly and quickly.

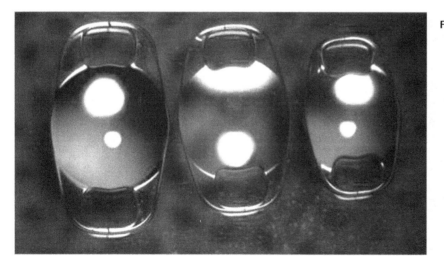

Fig. 22.3 Iris claw lens sizes available.

22.4.5 Anesthesia

Iris claw lens implantation is easily performed under perilimbal subconjunctival injection of lignocaine 2%; however, beginner surgeons may consider using a peribulbar or retrobulbar block. Akinesia is a must in eyes with nystagmus.

22.5 Unique Indications for the Use of Iris Claw Lens

22.5.1 Posterior Capsule Tear during Cataract Surgery

Inadvertent posterior capsule tear during cataract surgery is one of the most unnerving moments for a cataract surgeon. Provided there is no lens material lost into the vitreous, vitreous has been managed properly and an intact anterior capsular rim is available; a three-piece IOL may be implanted into the ciliary sulcus. However, if capsular support is not available or

not reliable, traditionally available options are very few. The choice is between leaving the patient aphakic and then planning a secondary IOL later, implanting an angle-supported lens or a scleral-fixated IOL in the same sitting. An iris claw lens is a lifesaver in such a situation. Its implantation procedure is definite, clean, quick, and hassle-free. A retropupillary-fixated iris claw lens is an extremely safe solution for the long term.

22.5.2 Secondary Lens Implantation in the Absence of Capsular Support

Perhaps the only lens design that is best suited for rehabilitation of an aphakic patient as a secondary lens implant is the iris claw lens. This lens can be implanted both in the anterior (▶Fig. 22.5) as well as in the posterior surfaces of the iris (▶Fig. 22.6), though our preferred recommendation is a retropupillary fixation (▶Fig. 22.7). For anterior fixation, a smaller sized IOL is preferred. Moreover, the enclavation with a good amount of iris tissue keeps the lens firmly in place.

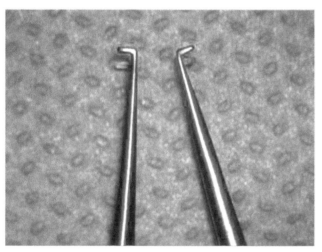

Fig. 22.4 A set of two Clayman forceps for fixing right and left claws.

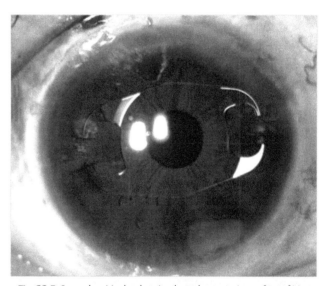

Fig. 22.5 Secondary iris claw lens implanted on anterior surface of iris.

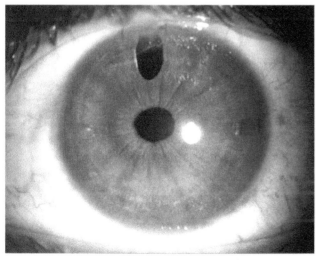

Fig. 22.6 Retropupillary implanted secondary iris claw lens.

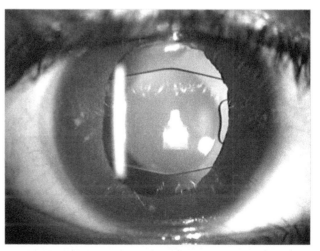

Fig. 22.7 Pupil dilated after retropupillary iris claw lens implantation.

22.5.3 Iris Claw Lens Implantation in Megalocornea

All available lens designs would be unsuitable in patients with extreme megalocornea because of sizing issues. As iris claw is fixed to the iris, this is the only design (▶ Fig. 22.8) that can be safely implanted in such cases.

22.5.4 Iris Claw Lens Implantation in Microcornea

This is another clinical situation where an iris claw lens finds indication for implantation because this lens is available in smaller sizes. A lens with an overall length 5.5 mm and optic diameter 3.5 mm would be suitable for most cases of microcornea (▶ Fig. 22.9 and ▶ Fig. 22.10). For extreme cases of microcornea, a lens with dimension of 4-mm overall length and optic diameter 2 mm can be implanted. Implantation may be done on either surface of the iris as the situation allows.

22.5.5 Iris Claw Lens in Cases of Trauma

Cases of blunt and penetrating trauma may present in a variety of ways such as corneal scars, iris tissue tear or loss, irregular pupil, traumatic cataract, traumatic mydriasis, iridodialysis, subluxated lens, dislocated lens in the vitreous, and so forth. Every case is challenging in its own way for visual rehabilitation with lens implantation. Iris claw lens allows the surgeon to be imaginative in the use of this lens in varied situations like secondary anterior-fixated iris claw lens post trauma (▶ Fig. 22.11); secondary retropupillary-fixated iris claw lens post trauma (▶ Fig. 22.12), with pupilloplasty for traumatic mydriasis (▶ Fig. 22.13), and with subluxated cataract extraction and anterior vitrectomy (▶ Fig. 22.14); and iridodialysis repair.

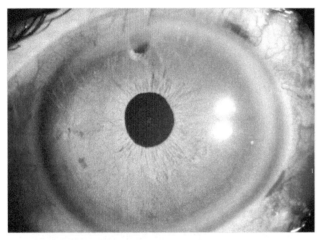

Fig. 22.8 Secondary retropupillary iris claw lens implantation in megalocornea.

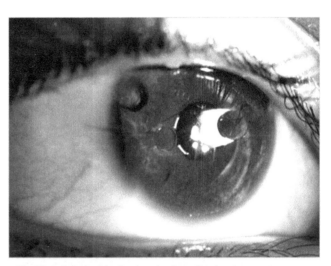

Fig. 22.9 Anterior iris claw lens implantation in microcornea (4.0 mm × 2.0 mm).

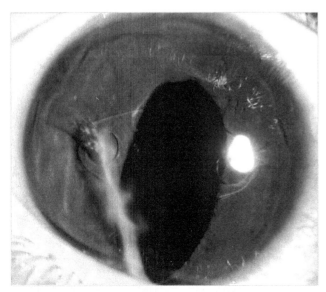

Fig. 22.10 Iris claw lens implantation in microcornea with coloboma.

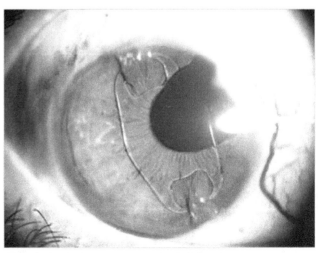

Fig. 22.11 Secondary anterior-fixated iris claw lens post trauma.

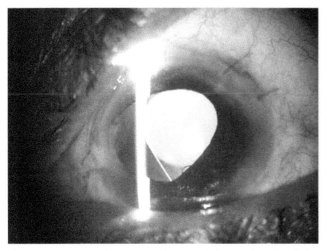

Fig. 22.12 Secondary retropupillary-fixated iris claw lens post trauma.

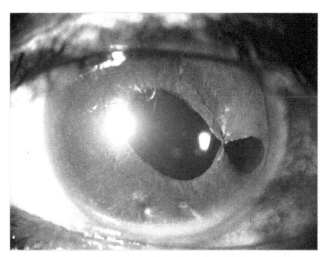

Fig. 22.13 Secondary retropupillary-fixated iris claw lens with pupilloplasty for traumatic mydriasis.

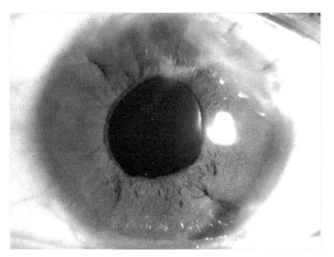

Fig. 22.14 Subluxated cataract extraction, anterior vitrectomy, and retropupillary-fixated iris claw lens.

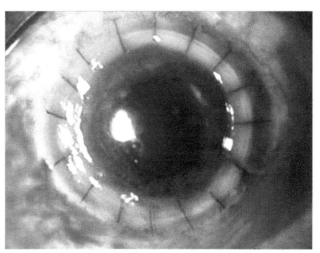

Fig. 22.15 Retropupillary-fixated iris claw lens in penetrating keratoplasty.

22.5.6 Iris Claw Lens Implantation in Conjunction with Penetrating Keratoplasty or Descemet's Stripping Endothelial Keratoplasty

A retropupillary-fixated iris claw lens is the most elegant technique to address aphakia while performing a penetrating keratoplasty (▶ Fig. 22.15) or a DSEK procedure. A medium-sized lens may be implanted on the anterior surface of the iris or may perform retropupillary fixation. A properly performed fixation does not hamper with the steps of DSEK involving graft positioning with air bubble. The iris claw lens is very easy to implant and is a safe alternative to an angle-supported lens or a scleral-fixated IOL.

22.5.7 Iris Claw Concept for Treatment of Unrelenting Angle Closure

There are times when either due to trauma or inflammation or after VR surgery, the peripheral iris gets plastered into the angle of the anterior chamber leading to glaucoma, which refuses to get controlled with antiglaucoma medicines or traditional glaucoma filtration procedures. Surgical separation of the extensive peripheral anterior synechiae gives temporary relief in intraocular pressure reduction but these synechiae tend to form again after a few days, leading to glaucoma once again. Is there a way to prevent these peripheral anterior synechiae from forming? With this question in mind, a device was developed with five to six claws, to be implanted into the anterior chamber. This device has no optic and has primarily been designed to take

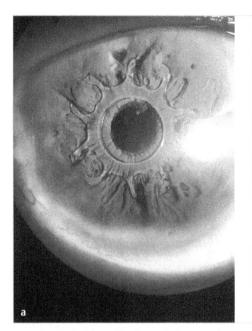
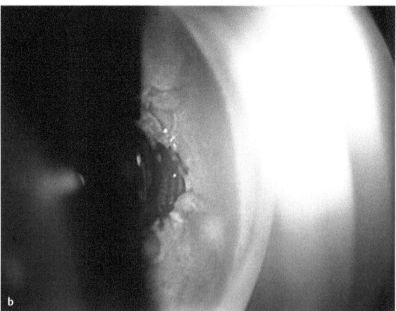

Fig. 22.16 (a, b) Iris claw device for keeping the iris root from closing the angle.

care of glaucoma in the aforementioned conditions. Pilot study is being done in painful blind eyes in an effort to control glaucoma. At first, synechiae are released from all around the angle and then the iris tissue is pulled and enclaved into the claws to prevent it from crowding up the angle again (▶ Fig. 22.16 a, b). Initial results have been very encouraging with this procedure. Initial response seems encouraging.

22.5.8 Iris Claw Lens Implantation in Corneal Opacity

This is the only IOL design that can be intentionally implanted eccentrically to avoid a corneal opacity and to allow some vision to the patient through the clear part of the cornea.

22.6 Complications with Iris Claw Lens

The lens is well tolerated over a long period of time. Patients operated more than three decades ago continue to enjoy good vision till now. However, there have been problems with this lens, the most significant of which is pseudophakic bullous keratopathy. This complication is attributed to the size mismatch of the anterior chamber and overall length of the lens and this complication has been fixed with smaller size lenses. Earlier lenses were approximately 8.5 mm in overall length in trying to achieve peripheral iris fixation and allow the pupil freedom of movement. This size brought the lens precariously close to the endothelial surface where it would rub intermittently over many decades causing slow but persistent cell loss, which would ultimately end up with pseudophakic bullous keratopathy. The present approach is to use smaller sized lenses according to the size of the anterior chamber diameter and try to err on the smaller size. Iris enclavation into the claw done just outside the collarette does not impede the normal functioning of the pupil

and fairly good pharmacological dilatation is also possible to achieve. Smaller sized lenses and retropupillary-fixated lenses have ensured endothelial cell health. Rarely, one claw of the lens may subluxate if the initial fixation was not so good or after trauma. Such a lens can be refixed or explanted and exchanged if need be. While considering all that has been mentioned above, one cannot discount the fact that iris claw lenses are being used in extraordinary circumstances, often in previously compromised eyes, which also contributes to the overall results.

22.7 Conclusion

The iris claw lens is a wonderful device that has stood the test of time. The reduced size of the iris claw lens has made this lens design very safe for both anterior and retropupillary implantation. Implantation of this lens anteriorly or posteriorly is a matter of personal choice or as per the circumstances at hand. The versatility of this lens design makes it absolutely necessary to be in every ophthalmic operation theater. This lens helps the surgeon in managing a variety of circumstances, which are out of the ordinary.

References

[1] Dadeya S, Kamlesh, Kumari Sodhi P. Secondary intraocular lens (IOL) implantation: anterior chamber versus scleral fixation long-term comparative evaluation. Eur J Ophthalmol 2003;13(7):627–633

[2] Wagoner MD, Cox TA, Ariyasu RG, Jacobs DS, Karp CL; American Academy of Ophthalmology. Intraocular lens implantation in the absence of capsular support: a report by the American Academy of Ophthalmology. Ophthalmology 2003;110(4):840–859

[3] Sindal MD, Nakhwa CP, Sengupta S. Comparison of sutured versus sutureless scleral-fixated intraocular lenses. J Cataract Refract Surg 2016;42(1):27–34

[4] De Silva SR, Arun K, Anandan M, Glover N, Patel CK, Rosen P. Iris-claw intraocular lenses to correct aphakia in the absence of capsule support. J Cataract Refract Surg 2011;37(9):1667–1672

[5] Gonnermann J, Klamann MK, Maier AK, et al. Visual outcome and complications after posterior iris-claw aphakic intraocular lens implantation. J Cataract Refract Surg 2012;38(12):2139–2143

23 Purkinje Images for Tracking Pseudophacodonesis

Dhivya Ashok Kumar, Athiya Agarwal, Ashvin Agarwal, Ashar Agarwal, Amar Agarwal

Summary

Pseudophacodonesis can be clinically seen by observing the motion of Purkinje images on the intraocular lens (IOL). Comparison of pseudophacodonesis of capsular IOLs and non-capsular secondary fixated IOLs has been reported in this chapter. The different types of IOL including the anterior chamber IOL, the iris claw lenses, the scleral fixated IOL, the posterior chamber IOL, and the glued IOL were compared. Iris claw IOLs had the highest incidence of pseudophacodonesis among the non-capsule fixated IOLs. We have shown that the pseudophacodonesis can be quantified and documented for all IOLs by using the simple image analysis software without sophisticated instrumentation.

Keywords: Pseudophacodonesis , purkinje images, capsular IOLs, non-capsular secondary fixated IOLs, image analysis software

23.1 Introduction

Purkinje images are reflections from light source formed on the surfaces of the ocular structures. In total there are four, named as Purkinje 1 to 4. P1 is the first corneal reflection and it reflects from the outer surface of the cornea. P2 reflects off the inner surface of the cornea, and P3 reflects off the outer surface of the lens. P4 reflects off the inner surface of the lens. Of the four images, P4 is the only inverted image, while the others are erect images due to how it reflects from the inner surface of the lens. Purkinje Sanson images have distinctive clinical applications like the clinical Hirschberg test, the keratometer, the videokeratography, the dual Purkinje tracker, and the biometric analysis.[1,2,3,4,5,6,7,8,9,10,11] Purkinje images have been utilized in IOL position and tilt determination as well. The technological advancements in managing the complicated ocular conditions with newer IOL designs have demanded the understanding of the possible effects of IOL oscillations in relation to their position in vivo and their effect on optical performance. The oscillations of the IOL implant after saccadic eye movements have been rarely quantified by Purkinje images in the literature.[12,13,14]

23.2 Detection of Pseudophacodonesis Using Purkinje Images

Purkinje images were observed through the digital slit lamp photography and video recorder (Topcon, DC-3, Tokyo, Japan) by a single examiner (DAK). Purkinje image 1 (PI) and image 2 (PII) were seen overlapped, defined, and bright. Purkinje image 4 (PIV) from the IOL was less intense, inverted, and diffuse. The motion of Purkinje image was recorded continuously at fixed frames per second while focusing on the target illumination for about 30 seconds on fixing at a fixed target and also following a horizontal saccade (▶ Video 23.1).

The video was then streamed in the video editor software (Pinnacle, Studio 15, Corel Corporation) in Windows XP and the image frames showing PIV and PI were grabbed (▶ Fig. 23.1). The JPEG file format was followed and evaluated by ImageJ analysis (http://rsb.info.nih.gov/ij/) software for the difference in the position of PIV in relation to PI. After correction of geometric distortion and the preliminary edge detection, the grabbed three randomized image frames of the overall 30 seconds were included (▶ Fig. 23.2). Scaling has been performed as 1 mm to be equivalent to 200 pixels using the set scale option (▶ Fig. 23.3). Following this, the files for the patient were selected and the difference in positions of PIV in relation to P1 was calculated using the line tool. Measurement of the distance between PI and PIV was determined for each eye at all the three time frames (TF). The time taken for the dampening of the oscillations after the abduction saccade in seconds were also determined.

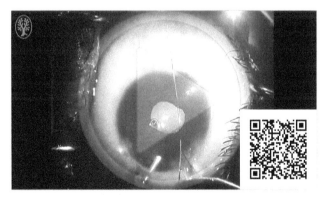

Video 23.1 Purkinje images. https://www.thieme.de/de/q.htm?p=opn/tp/311890101/9781684200979_video_23_01&t=video

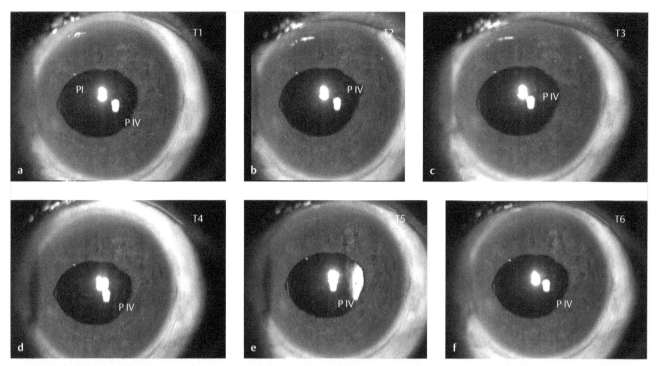

Fig. 23.1 (a–f) Purkinje image 4 (PIV) position in relation to Purkinje image 1 (PI) was determined at various time frames for 30 seconds.

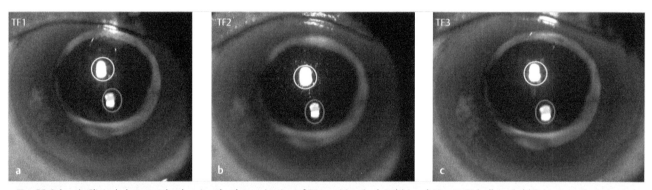

Fig. 23.2 (a–c) Clinical photographs showing the determination of PIV position (*red circle*) in relation to PI (*yellow circle*) in systematic randomized time frames (TF1, TF2, and TF3). PIV, Purkinje image 4; TF, time frame.

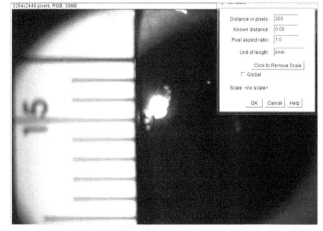

Fig. 23.3 Scaling has been performed as 1 mm to be equivalent to 200 pixels using the set scale option.

23.3 Pseudophacodonesis among Various Intraocular Lens

Out of 127 eyes included in the trial, there were capsule-fixed posterior chamber (PC) IOL, anterior chamber (AC) IOL, retropupillary iris-fixated IOL, glued trans-scleral-fixated IOL, and sutured scleral-fixated (SF) IOL. There was no statistically significant difference in PIV positions at various time points in PC IOL, AC IOL, SF IOL, and glued IOL. Iris claw lens showed a statistically significant difference in the position of Purkinje PIV at various time frames, F(2,38) = 3.80 and *p* = 0.0418 (▶Fig. 23.4).

The median difference in the range of movements of PIV was noted to be higher for the iris claw IOL and least for the PC IOL (▶Fig. 23.5). In comparison, of the range of difference in the PIV movements between the five groups, there was

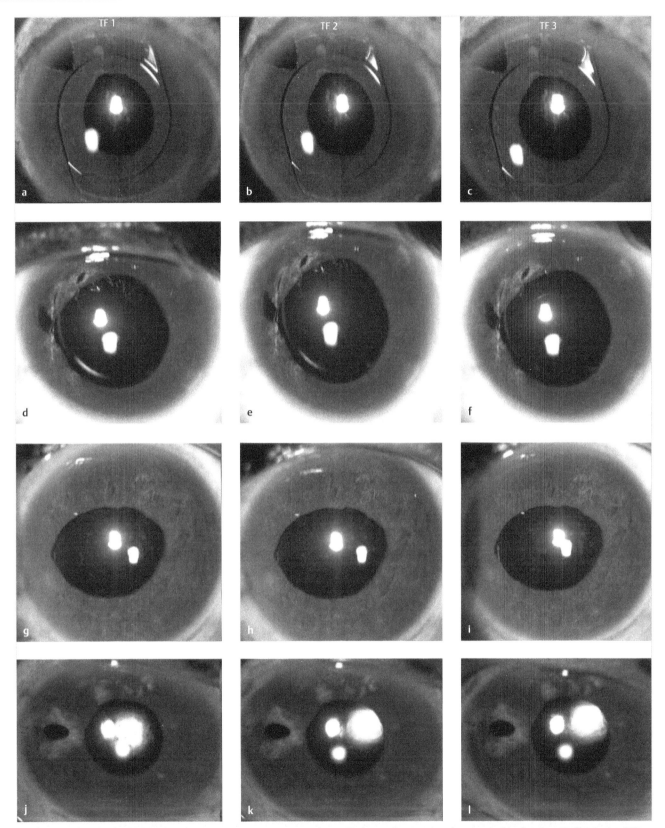

Fig. 23.4 Image comparing the PIV position in different IOLs at random time frames (TF1, TF2, and TF3). Anterior chamber IOL **(a–c)**, glued IOL **(d–f)**, iris claw IOL **(g–i)**, and sutured scleral-fixated IOL **(j–l)**. IOL, intraocular lens.

a statistically significant difference in median PIV position between the five groups, chi-square = 25.863, p = 0.0001. In subsequent comparison of post hoc analysis (Dunne test with Bonferroni correction) between the individual groups, there was a significant difference between the PC IOL and the iris claw IOL (p = 0.0001), the glued IOL and the iris claw IOL (p = 0.0020), and the AC IOL and the iris claw IOL (p = 0.0302) (▶ Fig. 23.6). On comparison of the difference in the movement of PIV at rest and motion, there was a significant exaggeration of the position of PIV noted in iris claw IOL (p = 0.0395). However, there were no differences noted among PC IOL, glued IOL, AC IOL, or SF IOL. There was spontaneous suppression of oscillations noted in PC IOL, glued IOL, and AC IOL; iris claw and SF IOL showed mild delay in (1–2 seconds) after motion saccade. On dividing the IOL oscillations in relation to the movement of PIV difference as < 0.5 mm (low frequency), 0.5 to 1 mm (moderate), and ≥1 mm (severe), PC IOL about 68% (n = 34) had movement < 0.5 mm and only 2% (n = 1) had ≥1 mm. Iris claw IOL recorded the difference ≥1 mm in 55% (n = 11) and 0.5 to 1 mm in 30% (n = 6) eyes.

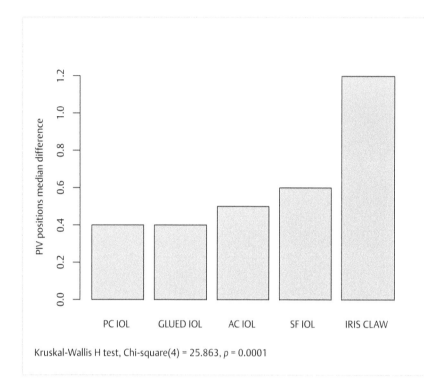

Kruskal-Wallis H test, Chi-square(4) = 25.863, p = 0.0001

Fig. 23.5 Bar diagragm showing the difference in the range of movement of PIV image in various IOLs. AC IOL, anterior chamber intraocular lens; IOL, intraocular lens; PIV, Purkinje image 4; PC IOL, posterior chamber intraocular lens; SF IOL, sutured scleral-fixated intraocular lens.

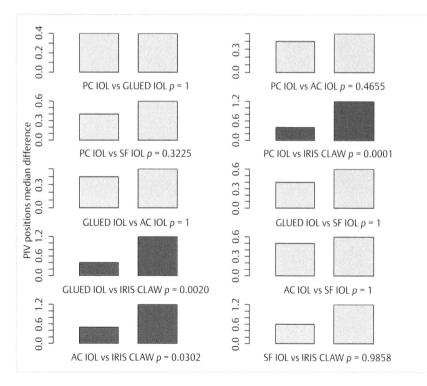

Fig. 23.6 Post hoc analysis between the five groups comparing the change in the position of PIV. AC IOL, anterior chamber intraocular lens; PIV, Purkinje image 4; PC IOL, posterior chamber intraocular lens; SF IOL, sutured scleral-fixated intraocular lens.

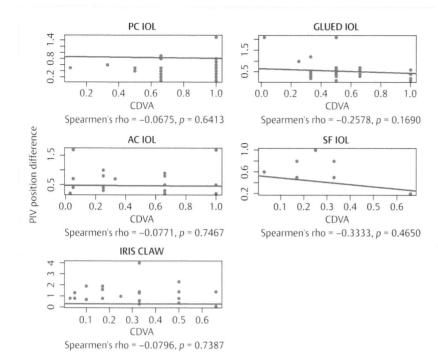

Fig. 23.7 The correlation of CDVA with a PIV mean position difference. AC IOL, anterior chamber intraocular lens; CDVA, corrected distance visual acuity; PIV, Purkinje image 4; PC IOL, posterior chamber intraocular lens; SF IOL, sutured scleral-fixated intraocular lens.

23.4 Pseudophacodonesis and Ocular Clinical Changes

On comparison of corrected distance visual acuity (CDVA) among the different IOLs, there was significant difference noted (Kruskal–Wallis H-test, $p = 0.0001$) between the IOL groups. There was no statistically significant correlation with CDVA and Purkinje PIV movements among the IOLs (►Fig. 23.7). The normal PC IOL showed higher CDVA as compared to other IOLs. The mean specular count was highest in PC IOL (2090.7 ± 398.6 cells/mm²) followed by SF IOL (1847.6 ± 490.5 cells/mm²) and glued IOL (1716.4 ± 459.7 cells/mm²). Clinically, the central corneal thickness was highest in the AC IOL with a mean of 566.8 ± 53.1 μm and the central foveal thickness was highest in SF IOL 325.3 ± 61.7 μm. There was no significant statistical difference in IOP among the IOLs ($p = 0.0801$).

23.5 Clinical Implications

Monestam et al have shown 0.7 and 1.4% risk of severe and moderate pseudophacodonesis after uneventful phacoemulsification with IOL in the capsular bag.[15] IOL types that are placed in the abnormal position apart from the capsular bag always have the propensity to produce abnormal oscillations as there is pre-existing disruption of capsule and anterior hyaloid face. Aqueous oscillates back and forth about its normal position until the energy of the system has dissipated.[16,17] Therefore, the implant directly in relation to the internal ocular fluids has higher risk of oscillations as compared to the one that is protected by the underlying capsule. Similarly, we noted that the retropupillary iris claw has shown a high incidence of pseudophacodonesis among all the IOLs. Moreover, as it is attached to the overlying iris, there is frequent risk of pigment chaffing and rarely IOL drop due to loss of grip because of loss of iris stroma on long term.[18,19,20]

The early clinical predicting sign of future IOL subluxation is the severity of pseudophacodonesis.[15,18,19] Various methods have been used to document the IOL oscillations.[4,5,6,7,8,9,10,20,21,22] Optical quality degradation can occur in gross oscillations of the IOL as it can induce transient microtilt and may induce momentary aberrations. Microtilts usually adjust as the IOL comes back to its original position, as this can be compared to a damped harmonic oscillation. The eyes with <0.5 mm of PIV differences have been classified as mild or low frequency and the same has been noted to be high in PC IOL. This showed that the low frequency of the oscillations is not affecting the visual performance and may not cause structural abnormality. However, in iris claw, high frequency oscillations (≥1 mm) were higher (55%), indicating greater pseudophacodonesis, which correlated with CDVA.

Glued IOL has shown pseudophacodonesis similar to the AC and the PC IOL and no significant difference in the CDVA as compared to other IOLs. Iris claw IOLs have been in use for more than two decades either as anterior enclavation or as retropupillary. The known complications of iris claw are the iris chaffing, late dislocation, and inflammation. Pseudophacodonesis in iris claw is the risk factor for chronic iris stromal loss and inflammation and vice versa.

23.6 Conclusion

Clinically, pseudophacodonesis is often observed as a quick oscillation of the PIV reflection with respect to the already stationary PI. Obtaining commercial trackers for pseudophacodonesis is unlikely for all surgeons; however, utilizing the image tracking method to calculate the incidence of phacodonesis in their patients for follow-up analysis is possible. Further analysis of the effect of the retinal image movement due to the IOL oscillations in the secondary fixated IOL has to be studied in the future.

References

[1] Tabernero J, Benito A, Nourrit V, Artal P. Instrument for measuring the misalignments of ocular surfaces. Opt Express 2006;14(22):10945–10956

[2] Guyton DL, Uozato H, Wisnicki HJ. Rapid determination of intraocular lens tilt and decentration through the undilated pupil. Ophthalmology 1990;97(10):1259–1264

[3] Korynta J, Cendelín J, Bok J. [Relation between postoperative refraction errors and decentration of the intraocular lens] Cesk Oftalmol 1994;50(4):219–225

[4] Mester U, Sauer T, Kaymak H. Decentration and tilt of a single-piece aspheric intraocular lens compared with the lens position in young phakic eyes. J CataractRefract Surg 2009;35(3):485–490

[5] Mutlu FM, Erdurman C, Sobaci G, Bayraktar MZ. Comparison of tilt and decentration of 1-piece and 3-piece hydrophobic acrylic intraocular lenses. J Cataract Refract Surg 2005;31(2):343–347

[6] Nishi Y, Hirnschall N, Crnej A, et al. Reproducibility of intraocular lens decentration and tilt measurement using a clinical Purkinje meter. J Cataract Refract Surg 2010;36(9):1529–1535

[7] Phillips P, Pérez-Emmanuelli J, Rosskothen HD, Koester CJ. Measurement of intraocular lens decentration and tilt in vivo. J Cataract Refract Surg 1988;14(2):129–135

[8] Auran JD, Koester CJ, Donn A. In vivo measurement of posterior chamber intraocular lens decentration and tilt. Arch Ophthalmol 1990;108(1):75–79

[9] Kirschkamp T, Dunne M, Barry J-C. Phakometric measurement of ocular surface radii of curvature, axial separations and alignment in relaxed and accommodated human eyes. Ophthalmic Physiol Opt 2004;24(2):65–73

[10] Dunne MCM, Davies LN, Mallen EAH, Kirschkamp T, Barry JC. Non-invasive phakometric measurement of corneal and crystalline lens alignment in human eyes. Ophthalmic Physiol Opt 2005;25(2):143–152

[11] Belin MW, Khachikian SS. An introduction to understanding elevation-based topography: how elevation data are displayed - a review. Clin Exp Ophthalmol 2009;37(1):14–29

[12] de Castro A, Rosales P, Marcos S. Tilt and decentration of intraocular lenses in vivo from Purkinje and Scheimpflug imaging. Validation study. J Cataract Refract Surg 2007;33(3):418–429

[13] Tabernero J, Artal P. Lens oscillations in the human eye. Implications for post-saccadic suppression of vision. PLoS One 2014;9(4):e95764

[14] Rosales P, De Castro A, Jiménez-Alfaro I, Marcos S. Intraocular lens alignment from Purkinje and Scheimpflug imaging. Clin Exp Optom 2010;93(6):400–408

[15] Mönestam EI. Incidence of dislocation of intraocular lenses and pseudophakodonesis 10 years after cataract surgery. Ophthalmology 2009;116(12):2315–2320

[16] Jagger WS, Jacobi KW. An analysis of pseudophakodonesis and iridodonesis. J Am Intraocul Implant Soc 1979;5(3):203–206

[17] Jacobs PM, Cheng H, Price NC. Pseudophakodonesis and corneal endothelial contact: direct observations by high-speed cinematography. Br J Ophthalmol 1983;67(10):650–654

[18] Jing W, Guanlu L, Qianyin Z, et al. Iris-claw intraocular lens and scleral-fixated posterior chamber intraocular lens implantations in correcting aphakia: a meta-analysis. Invest Ophthalmol Vis Sci 2017;58(9):3530–3536

[19] Moran S, Kirwan C, O'Keefe M, Leccisotti A, Moore T. Incidence of dislocated and subluxed iris-fixated phakic intraocular lens and outcomes following re-enclavation. Clin Exp Ophthalmol 2014;42(7):623–628

[20] Shen C, Elbaz U, Chan CC. Late spontaneous dislocation of a silicone iris-claw phakic intraocular lens. Can J Ophthalmol 2014;49(4):e92–e94

[21] Narang P, Agarwal A, Sanu AS. Detecting subtle intraocular movements: enhanced frames per second recording (slow motion) using smartphones. J Cataract Refract Surg 2015;41(6):1321–1323

[22] Kumar DA, Agarwal A, Packialakshmi S, Agarwal A. In vivo analysis of glued intraocular lens position with ultrasound biomicroscopy. J Cataract Refract Surg 2013;39(7):1017–1022

24 Reconstructing the Posterior Capsular Barrier

Priya Narang, Amar Agarwal

Summary

Posterior capsule forms a protective barrier to segregate the anterior and posterior segment structures. Posterior capsular rupture (PCR) is a dreaded complication of cataract surgery that is often associated with nonemulsified nuclear fragments and often with sinking nucleus that may advance into a dropped nucleus if not managed properly. The chapter highlights the procedure and techniques that can be adopted to restrain the extension of PCR and the effective placement of an intraocular lens.

Keywords: Decentration, glued IOL, IOL exchange, subluxation, repositioning, capsular bag–IOL complex, IOL explant, posterior capsule rupture, vitrectomy, three-piece IOL, triumvirate technique, IOL scaffold, posterior-assisted levitation, modified PAL, trocar AC maintainer

24.1 Introduction

Posterior capsule rupture (PCR) is an infrequent but a known complication of cataract surgery and it can also be iatrogenically induced during a vitreoretinal surgery.[1,2,3] PCR can lead to significant ocular morbidity and suboptimal outcomes with permanent vision loss if not handled judiciously. Recognition of an intraoperative PCR in early stages is extremely important to limit the extent of complication and prevent it from being detrimental to a greater extent.

Loss of followability of the nuclear fragments, sudden deepening of the anterior chamber (AC) with pupil dilation, or sudden appearance of red glow is one of the early sign of a PCR. At this stage, the surgeon should lower down the machine parameters and try to assess the clinical scenario. Before the phacoemulsification probe is withdrawn from the eye, an ophthalmic viscosurgical device (OVD) is injected onto the AC from the side port incision. This helps to prevent sudden shallowing of the AC and further extension of the PCR. Subsequent to PCR, the initial objective is the safe and thorough removal of vitreous and lens fragments from the AC followed by the next prime objective of the stable placement of an intraocular lens (IOL) selected for best refractive outcomes.

Newer techniques available to anterior and posterior segment surgeons in the setting of PCR allow the surgeons to manage the nuclear fragments with the simultaneous placement of an IOL that acts as scaffold and can be used as a pupillary barrier that blocks the subsequent drop of nuclear fragment into the vitreous cavity during its removal through phacoemulsification (▶Video 24.1, ▶Video 24.2, ▶Video 24.3, ▶Video 24.4, ▶Video 24.5, ▶Video 24.6, ▶Video 24.7, ▶Video 24.8, and ▶Video 24.9).

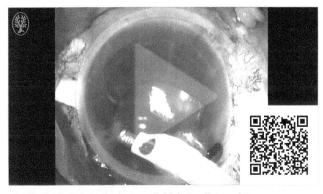

Video 24.1 Intraocular lens scaffold. https://www.thieme.de/de/q.htm?p=opn/tp/311890101/9781684200979_video_24_01&t=video

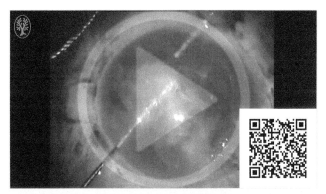

Video 24.2 Intraocular lens scaffold: iridodialysis and dislocations. https://www.thieme.de/de/q.htm?p=opn/tp/311890101/9781684200979_video_24_02&t=video

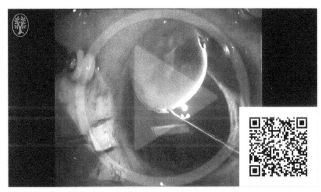

Video 24.3 Glued Intraocular lens scaffold. https://www.thieme.de/de/q.htm?p=opn/tp/311890101/9781684200979_video_24_03&t=video

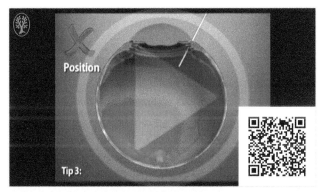

Video 24.4 Extrusion cannula assisted levitation of an intraocular lens. https://www.thieme.de/de/q.htm?p=opn/tp/311890101/9781684200979_video_24_04&t=video

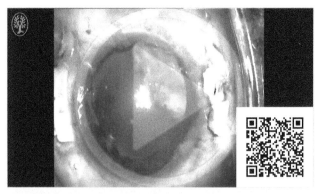

Video 24.5 Traumatic subluxated cataract. https://www.thieme. de/de/q.htm?p=opn/tp/311890101/9781684200979_video_ 24_05&t=video

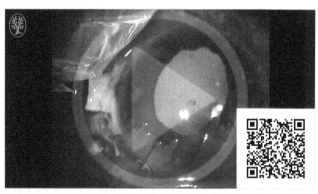

Video 24.6 The longest day. https://www.thieme.de/de/q. htm?p=opn/tp/311890101/9781684200979_video_24_06&t=video

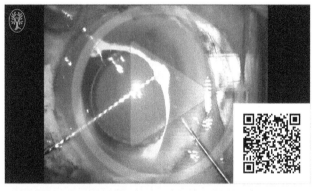

Video 24.7 The longest day part 10. https://www.thieme. de/de/q.htm?p=opn/tp/311890101/9781684200979_ video_24_07&t=video

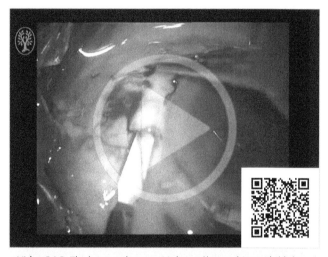

Video 24.8 The longest day part 11. https://www.thieme.de/de/q. htm?p=opn/tp/311890101/9781684200979_video_24_08&t=video

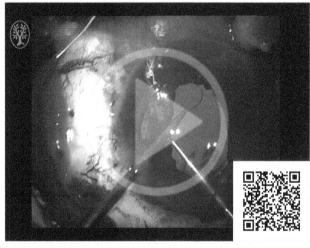

Video 24.9 The longest day part 12. https://www.thieme.de/de/q. htm?p=opn/tp/311890101/9781684200979_video_24_09&t=video

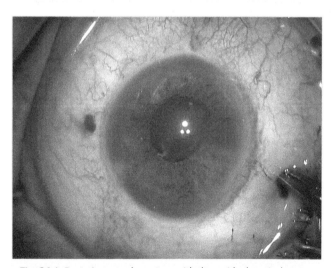

Fig. 24.1 Posterior capsule rupture with the residual cortical matter.

24.2 Management

The management of PCR depends upon the stage at which the PCR occurred and also upon the extent of posterior capsule (PC) opening. PCR in the initial stages of surgery entails the management of entire nucleus/nuclear fragments along with the vitreous and PC opening management, whereas in the later stages, it involves managing the cortical matter and the vitreous prolapse (▶ Fig. 24.1). Often with big PC opening, nucleus drop also may occur that involves the management from a vitreoretinal surgeon.

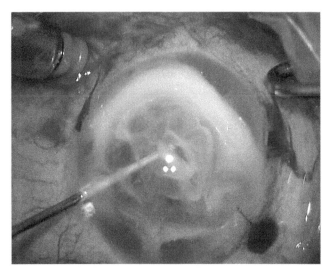

Fig. 24.2 Triamcinolone staining for detection of the vitreous strands in the anterior chamber.

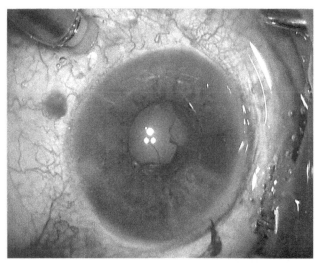

Fig. 24.3 Fluid infusion is introduced into the eye to perform vitrectomy.

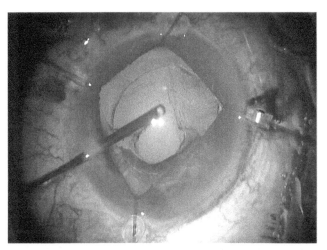

Fig. 24.4 Vitrectomy being performed after pupil dilation with iris hooks.

24.3 Vitrectomy and Its Importance

Disruption of the anterior vitreoretinal barrier can enhance the rate of postoperative complications like endophthalmitis, retinal detachment, and cystoid macular edema (CME).[4,5] Along with this, complete removal of the vitreous from the AC is equally essential as it can lead to traction and also it can be detrimental to the corneal endothelium along with the rise of IOP. Staining of the transparent vitreous can help a lot in optimizing the visual outcomes as the stained vitreous strands can be easily visualized and managed by the surgeon.[6,7,8]

Triamcinolone staining (▶ Fig. 24.2) is the most common method employed for enhancing the visualization of the prolapsed vitreous.[9,10] Triamcinolone acetonide aids in the visualization of transparent ocular structures by attachment to the collagen matrix of vitreous.[11,12] Before starting anterior vitrectomy, triamcinolone acetonide can be instilled into the AC. This enhances the visibility of vitreous and ensures adequate vitreous cutting with the vitrector along with appropriate judgment of the endpoint of vitrectomy.

Introduction of infusion into the eye is essential (▶ Fig. 24.3 and ▶ Fig. 24.4) before performing vitrectomy. The basic principle of vitreous cutting should be adopted: "Cutting should be more than suction." In other words, the vitrectomy cutter rate should be set higher, whereas the suction should be at moderate levels as if we do not follow this rule and have a suction rate more than the cutting rate, a lot of vitreous gets aspirated even before the vitreous strands have been completely cut. This can lead to vitreous traction and all its sequential complications.

24.4 Posterior Assisted Levitation

Packard and Kinnear described the technique of levitating the sinking nucleus with a spatula[13] that was later named as posterior assisted levitation (PAL) by Kelman.[14,15] Chang et al[16] described Viscoat-assisted PAL where a Viscoat-filled cannula is introduced through the pars plana site and the Viscoat is injected beneath the nucleus so that it helps to cushion the nuclear fragments that are then lifted with the cannula of the Viscoat-filled syringe into the AC.

Following a PCR, the corneal tunnel incision is sutured, as it is essential to secure the wound. The sclerotomy incision for PAL can be made with a microvitreoretinal (MVR) blade or with a trocar at a distance of 3 to 3.5 mm away from the limbus in the region of pars plana. Trocars have an advantage of creating a self-sealing incision without the need of conjunctival peritomy.

A rod is passed through the trocar and the nuclear fragments are manipulated and are lifted with the rod into the AC (▶ Fig. 24.5a, b). While doing PAL, another rod can also be passed from the side port incision so as to support the fragments when they are present in the AC and prevent them from falling back into the vitreous cavity (▶ Fig. 24.5c, d). Once the fragments are in the AC, they are made to rest on the anterior surface of the iris tissue.

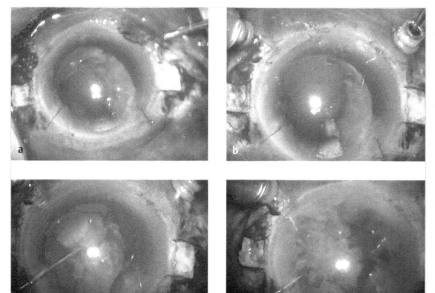

Fig. 24.5 Posterior-assisted levitation. (a) Nuclear fragment seen lying in the pupillary zone. (b) Standard pars plana incision made with trocar. A rod is inserted through the trocar to lift the nucleus. (c) The rod is placed beneath the nuclear fragment and the nuclear pieces are pushed forward and placed into the AC. Another rod inserted from the side port incision can be used to support the nuclear pieces that are being levitated into the AC. (d) All the nuclear pieces are resting into the AC. AC, anterior chamber.

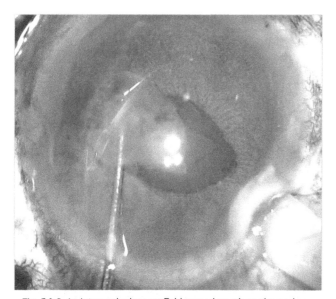

Fig. 24.6 An intraocular lens scaffold procedure where the nucleus is levitated into anterior chamber.

Fig. 24.7 A three-piece foldable IOL is injected beneath the nuclear fragments and is placed above the iris tissue. The nucleus is emulsified with a phaco probe. IOL, intraocular lens.

24.5 Intraocular Lens Scaffold

The word scaffold is derived from the Medieval Latin word "scaffuldus" of Old French origin that means "a temporary platform." As the name suggests, an IOL is used as a scaffold to compartmentalize the eye into anterior and posterior segment with the placement of an IOL that seals the posterior capsular opening.[17,18]

As soon as the PCR is recognized, the surgery is halted and OVD is injected from the side port incision to stabilize the AC. The phaco probe is then withdrawn and all the nuclear fragments are levitated into the AC (▶ Fig. 24.6). A trocar or an AC maintainer is introduced into the eye and fluid is switched ON with care being taken that the flow of fluid does not push the nuclear pieces into the vitreous cavity. A limited vitrectomy is done at moderate settings and a three-piece foldable IOL is injected beneath the nuclear fragments. The haptics are made to rest either on the anterior surface of the iris tissue or in the sulcus above the margin of capsulorhexis. Phacoemulsification probe is then introduced and the remaining nuclear fragments are emulsified with phaco machine set at low parameters (▶ Fig. 24.7).

Once the nuclear fragments are emulsified (▶ Fig. 24.8), the IOL is dialed into the sulcus if placed previously on the iris tissue. With the preplacement of an IOL, a barrier is created between the AC and the posterior chamber. The IOL also prevents the nucleus drop and also facilitates emulsification procedure by acting as a scaffold. IOL scaffold allows the management of PCR without enlargement of the corneal incision, thereby passing all the advantages of a closed chamber incision surgery.

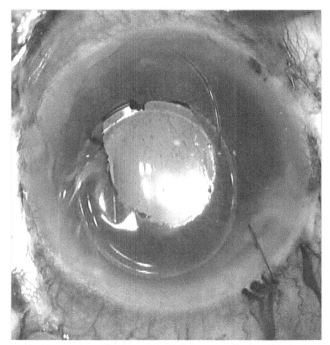

Fig. 24.8 All the nuclear fragments are emulsified and the IOL is seen resting on the anterior surface of the iris tissue. This IOL is then dialed into the sulcus. IOL, intraocular lens.

The limitation with this technique is that it cannot be adopted for very hard cataract as the nucleus is emulsified in AC close to the corneal endothelium and doing so can lead to damage to the corneal endothelial cell count. Due precaution should be taken while performing IOL scaffold and it is recommended to coat the endothelium with an adequate amount of OVD. In cases with dilated pupil, the optic–haptic junction can be manipulated with the dialer so as to block the pupillary aperture with the IOL optic during nuclear emulsification to prevent any nuclear fragment from slipping into the vitreous cavity.

24.6 Triumvirate Technique

This technique is a combination of modified PAL with IOL scaffold and glued IOL (▶ Fig. 24.9, ▶ Fig. 24.10, and ▶ Fig. 24.11) in cases with PCR that have inadequate capsular support and sinking nucleus with residual nuclear remnants to be emulsified.[19]

Following a PCR, two partial-thickness scleral flaps are made as in a glued IOL surgery followed by sclerotomy. A rod is inserted from the sclerotomy and placing the rod posterior to the nuclear fragment retrieves the sinking nucleus. A second rod can also be passed from the opposite sclerotomy site that is created for the glued IOL procedure. Passage of two rods from the opposite direction enables and facilitates the nucleus retrieval into the AC. Once the nucleus is brought into AC, a three-piece foldable IOL is inserted beneath the nuclear fragments and the haptics of the IOL are made to rest on the anterior surface of the iris tissue (▶ Fig. 24.9). Phacoemulsification probe is introduced

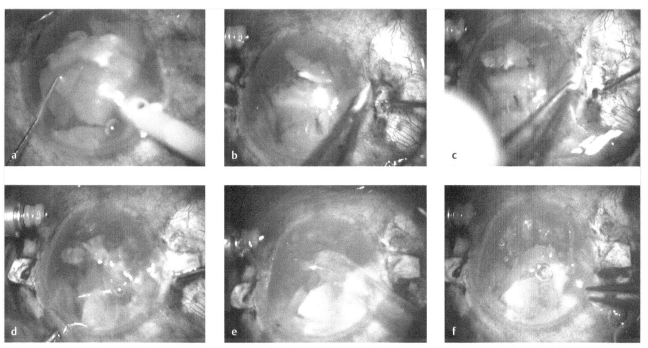

Fig. 24.9 Triumvirate technique: modified PAL with IOL scaffold with glued IOL. **(a)** A PCR is noted during a phacoemulsification procedure. **(b)** Two partial-thickness scleral flaps are made 180° opposite to each other as in glued IOL surgery. Sclerotomy is done with a 22-G needle 1 mm away from the limbus beneath the scleral flaps. **(c)** A rod is being inserted through the sclerotomy site. **(d)** The nuclear fragments are levitated into the AC with modified PAL technique. **(e)** A three-piece foldable IOL is injected beneath the nuclear fragments. **(f)** The IOL rests on the anterior surface of the iris tissue with nuclear pieces in the AC. AC, anterior chamber; IOL, intraocular lens; PAL, posterior assisted levitation; PCR, posterior capsule rupture.

into the AC and the nucleus is emulsified. Phacoemulsification is done at low to moderate settings and the fragments are fed into the port of phaco probe to prevent any slippage of the fragments into the vitreous cavity from around the edges of the IOL (▶ Fig. 24.10).

The haptic of the IOL is then grasped with an end-opening glued IOL forceps and handshake technique is done till the tip of the haptic is grasped. The haptics are then pulled from the tip and are externalized (▶ Fig. 24.11). The haptics are tucked into the scleral pockets created with 26-G needle and vitrectomy is

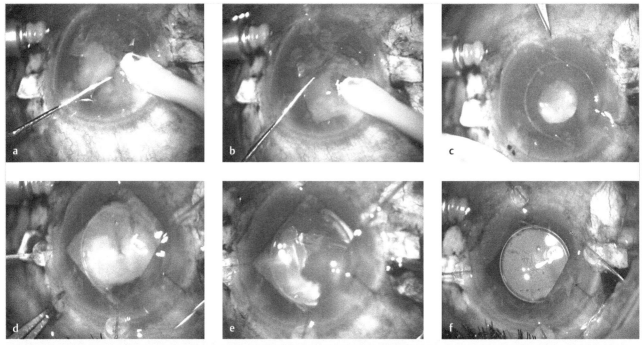

Fig. 24.10 Triumvirate technique: modified PAL with IOL scaffold with glued IOL. **(a)** Emulsification of the nuclear pieces being performed. **(b)** All the nuclear pieces are emulsified. **(c)** Corneal suture taken; IOL in AC with cortical matter seen lying in the pupillary area. **(d)** Iris hooks are applied to enhance visualization. **(e)** Vitrectomy probe passed through the sclerotomy site and the cortical matter is cleaned up. **(f)** Entire cortical matter is cleaned. AC, anterior chamber; IOL, intraocular lens; PAL, posterior assisted levitation.

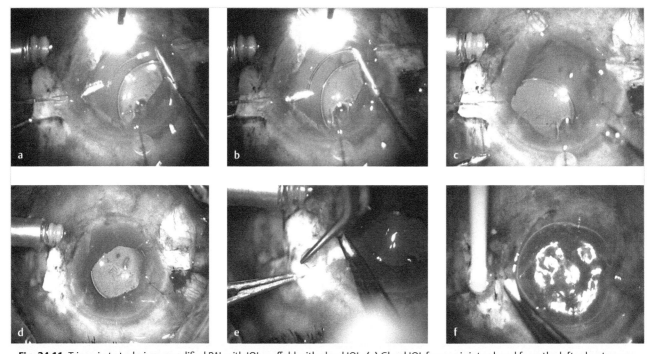

Fig. 24.11 Triumvirate technique: modified PAL with IOL scaffold with glued IOL. **(a)** Glued IOL forceps is introduced from the left sclerotomy site and the leading haptic is held with another glued IOL end-opening forceps. **(b)** The tip of the haptic is grasped to facilitate externalization. **(c)** The leading haptic is pulled and externalized. **(d)** Both haptics externalized. **(e)** The haptics are tucked into the scleral pockets. **(f)** Fibrin glue is applied beneath the scleral flaps. IOL, intraocular lens; PAL, posterior assisted levitation.

performed at the sclerotomy site. Fibrin glue is applied beneath the scleral flaps and the conjunctival incisions are sealed.

In cases with dropped nucleus, triumvirate comprises sleeveless phaco tip-assisted levitation (SPAL)[20] with IOL scaffold and glued IOL. In SPAL, the sleeveless phaco tip is passed from pars plana sclerotomy and the nucleus is lifted from the surface of the retina by vacuum from the tip of the phaco probe. Once the nucleus is levitated and is in the midvitreous cavity, a short burst of phacoemulsification is applied, leading to embedment of phaco probe into the nucleus. The nucleus is then brought into the pupillary area and is lifted and placed onto the surface of iris. A three-piece foldable IOL is then injected beneath it as in an IOL scaffold procedure followed by glued fixation of the IOL.

24.7 Sleeveless Extrusion Cannula-Assisted Levitation for Dropped Intraocular Lens

Agarwal et al started this technique wherein the sleeve of the extrusion cannula is removed before managing the dropped IOL (▶ Fig. 24.12). Removal of the silicone sleeve exposes wider access of the bore of the cannula, which helps to create an effective suction around the IOL.[21]

In this technique, after adequate vitrectomy, the sleeveless extrusion cannula is connected to the vitreotome and the vacuum is set to 300 mm Hg with the cutting function turned off. As the IOL rests flat on the retina, the sleeveless extrusion cannula is made to face the center of the optic and suction is initiated that can be dynamically controlled with the foot pedal. The linear control of the foot pedal helps to increase the vacuum as and when needed during the levitation of IOL. Ineffective apposition of the lumen of the cannula to the surface of the IOL optic can lead to loss of vacuum. The IOL is lifted from the surface of the retina and is brought into the anterior vitreous in the mid-pupillary area. The end-opening forceps introduced from the corneal incision under direct visualization through the microscope grasps the IOL; the extrusion cannula is then removed as the forceps grasps the IOL. The IOL can then be subsequently managed depending on the surgical scenario. It can be either replaced or repositioned in the sulcus or it can be explanted.

The advantage of this technique is that it is safe, reliable, and reproducible. Moreover, it is effective for dislocation of any type of IOL, including the plate haptic IOLs, which are often difficult to grasp with a retinal forceps.

24.8 Sleeveless Phaco Tip-Assisted Levitation of Dropped Nucleus

Dislocation of crystalline lens fragments into the vitreous cavity is a potentially serious complication of cataract surgery and can lead to marked intraocular inflammation resulting in CME, glaucoma, and retinal detachment. Various techniques have provided new ways of managing a dropped nucleus with improved visual outcomes and fewer complications. After successful management of the dropped nucleus, IOL implantation is needed to achieve good visual rehabilitation. As far as visual output is concerned, the surgeon faces a dual challenge of managing a complication like dropped nucleus and simultaneously striving to achieve the expectations of a routine postcataract surgery patient.

In 1999, we described a technique called *FAVIT*, meaning "fallen in vitreous" for levitating dropped nucleus. This technique has undergone several modifications by us and is currently named as SPAL of dropped nucleus (▶ Fig. 24.13, ▶ Fig. 24.14, and ▶ Fig. 24.15). SPAL along with the application of IOL scaffold and glued IOL technique allows a complete closed chamber intraocular manipulation of dropped nucleus and an IOL implantation, thereby providing all the benefits of a small incision cataract surgery without the use of any special surgical adjuncts.

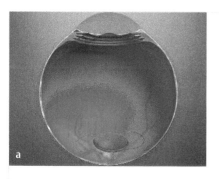
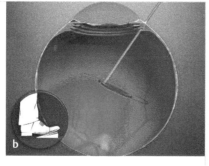
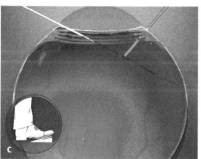
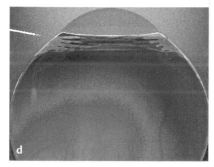
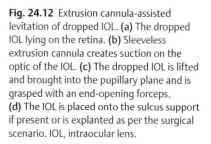

Fig. 24.12 Extrusion cannula-assisted levitation of dropped IOL. **(a)** The dropped IOL lying on the retina. **(b)** Sleeveless extrusion cannula creates suction on the optic of the IOL. **(c)** The dropped IOL is lifted and brought into the pupillary plane and is grasped with an end-opening forceps. **(d)** The IOL is placed onto the sulcus support if present or is explanted as per the surgical scenario. IOL, intraocular lens.

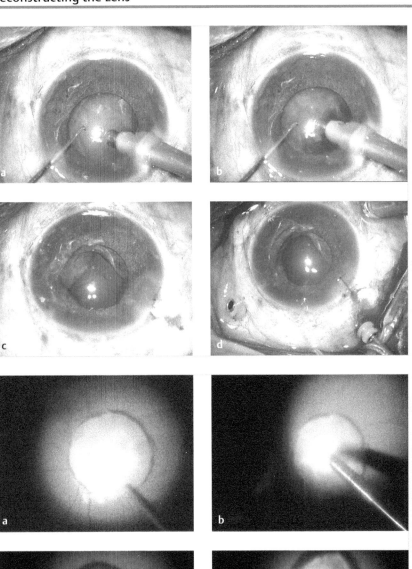

Fig. 24.13 Surgical steps of sleeveless phaco tip-assisted levitation. **(a)** Phacoemulsification being performed. **(b)** Posterior capsule rupture. **(c)** Dropped nucleus. **(d)** Standard three-port pars plana vitrectomy incisions framed.

Fig. 24.14 Surgical steps of SPAL for dropped nucleus. **(a)** Vitrectomy being performed and all adhesions surrounding the dropped nucleus are removed. **(b)** Sleeveless phaco tip is introduced and is brought near the dropped fragment. **(c)** The dropped nucleus is lifted from the surface of the retina into the vitreous cavity. **(d)** The nucleus is embedded with a short burst of phaco power. This prevents the nucleus from falling down back onto the surface of retina. SPAL, sleeveless phaco tip-assisted levitation.

The technique comprises framing a standard three-port pars plana vitrectomy incisions and performing a thorough vitrectomy to remove all the cortical matter in the pupillary plane to enhance visualization, followed by a complete posterior chamber vitrectomy and removal of all vitreolenticular adhesions. An endoilluminator or a chandelier system can be used to improve visualization in the posterior chamber (▶ Video 24.10). The trocar cannula on the dominant hand side is removed and the incision is enlarged with the passage of an MVR blade to facilitate the entry of a 20-G sleeveless phaco tip.

When the phaco tip lies close to the dropped nucleus, a suction mode is initiated and the dropped nucleus is lifted from the surface of retina with the help of phaco tip. As the nucleus is elevated and is brought into the midvitreous cavity, phaco energy mode is initiated to embed the nucleus, which is then effectively levitated and brought into the AC and is placed above the surface of iris. A three-piece foldable IOL is injected beneath the nuclear fragments and an IOL scaffold procedure is performed. In cases of adequate sulcus support, the same IOL can then be placed above the support of anterior capsulorhexis, whereas in cases of inadequate sulcus support, glued IOL procedure can be performed to facilitate IOL fixation. At the end of the case, the periphery of retina is meticulously inspected for breaks and if any cortical matter is present, it is removed with the vitrectomy probe. Stromal hydration is done and all the corneal wounds are secured. A

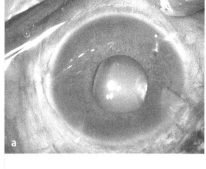
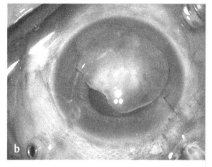

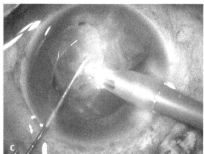
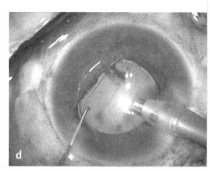

Fig. 24.15 Surgical steps of scaffold for dropped nucleus with SPAL. **(a)** The nucleus is levitated and brought into the pupillary plane. **(b)** The nucleus is manipulated into the AC. **(c)** A three-piece foldable IOL is injected beneath the nucleus and is placed into the sulcus. The nuclear fragment is being emulsified. **(d)** Nucleus emulsification complete. AC, anterior chamber; IOL, intraocular lens; SPAL, sleeveless phaco tip-assisted levitation.

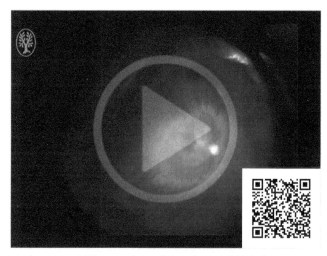

Video 24.10 Cliff Hanger. https://www.thieme.de/de/q.htm?p=opn/tp/311890101/9781684200979_video_24_10&t=video

4–0 Vicryl suture is used to close the sclerotomy site enlarged for the introduction of phaco needle.

SPAL technique offers various advantages such as to minimize the amount of phaco energy delivered in the vitreous cavity. Levitating the dropped nucleus followed by its emulsification in the AC encompasses an ideal surgical scenario. This technique does not necessitate the use of any special surgical instrument like phacofragmatome or surgical adjuvant like perfluorocarbon liquid, without compromising on the patients' safety concern.

Moreover, there is no strong intravitreal fluid current or inadvertent suction of residual vitreous gel resulting from the larger port of the phaco needle as vacuum is initiated when the phaco tip is very close to the dropped nucleus. In addition to this, prior adequate vitrectomy ensures that the vitreous cavity is filled with fluid. SPAL, when coupled with IOL scaffold, offers a very good alternative towards proper emulsification of nucleus and when coupled with glued IOL technique, it offers

an ideal scenario for IOL fixation in cases of inadequate sulcus support. Apart from all this, it simultaneously maintains all the advantages of a small incision, closed chamber intraocular surgery even in a complicated surgical scenario.

References

[1] Asaria RHY, Wong SC, Sullivan PM. Risk for posterior capsule rupture after vitreoretinal surgery. J Cataract Refract Surg 2006;32(6):1068–1069

[2] Novak MA, Rice TA, Michels RG, Auer C. The crystalline lens after vitrectomy for diabetic retinopathy. Ophthalmology 1984;91(12):1480–1484

[3] Faulborn J, Conway BP, Machemer R. Surgical complications of pars plana vitreous surgery. Ophthalmology 1978;85(2):116–125

[4] Gimbel HV. Posterior capsule tears using phacoemulsification causes, prevention and management. Eur J Implant Refract Surg 1990;2:63–69

[5] Arbisser LB, Charles S, Howcroft M, Werner L. Management of vitreous loss and dropped nucleus during cataract surgery. Ophthalmol Clin North Am 2006;19(4):495–506

[6] Angunawela RI, Liyanage SE, Wong SC, Little BC. Intraocular pressure and visual outcomes following intracameral triamcinolone assisted anterior vitrectomy in complicated cataract surgery. Br J Ophthalmol 2009;93(12):1691–1692

[7] Fine HF, Spaide RF. Visualization of the posterior precortical vitreous pocket in vivo with triamcinolone. Arch Ophthalmol 2006;124(11):1663

[8] Gillies MC, Simpson JM, Billson FA, et al. Safety of an intravitreal injection of triamcinolone: results from a randomized clinical trial. Arch Ophthalmol 2004;122(3):336–340

[9] Burk SE, Da Mata AP, Snyder ME, Schneider S, Osher RH, Cionni RJ. Visualizing vitreous using Kenalog suspension. J Cataract Refract Surg 2003;29(4):645–651

[10] Kasbekar S, Prasad S, Kumar BV. Clinical outcomes of triamcinolone-assisted anterior vitrectomy after phacoemulsification complicated by posterior capsule rupture. J Cataract Refract Surg 2013;39(3):414–418

[11] Peyman GA, Cheema R, Conway MD, Fang T. Triamcinolone acetonide as an aid to visualization of the vitreous and the posterior hyaloid during pars plana vitrectomy. Retina 2000;20(5):554–555

[12] Enaida H, Hata Y, Ueno A, et al. Possible benefits of triamcinolone-assisted pars plana vitrectomy for retinal diseases. Retina 2003;23(6):764–770

[13] Packard RBS, Kinnear FC. Manual of Cataract and Intraocular Lens Surgery. Edinburgh: Churchill Livingstone; 1991:47

[14] Kelman C. Posterior capsular rupture: PAL technique. J Cataract Refract Surg 1996 ;12:30

[15] Kelman CD. Posterior assisted levitation. In: Burrato L, ed. Phacoemulsification: principles and techniques. Thorofare: Slack Incorporated; 1998:511–512

[16] Chang DF, Packard RB. Posterior assisted levitation for nucleus retrieval using Viscoat after posterior capsule rupture. J Cataract Refract Surg 2003;29(10):1860–1865

[17] Kumar DA, Agarwal A, Prakash G, Jacob S, Sivagnanam S. IOL scaffold technique for posterior capsule rupture. J Refract Surg 2012;28(5): 314–315

[18] Narang P, Agarwal A, Kumar DA, Jacob S, Agarwal A, Agarwal A. Clinical outcomes of intraocular lens scaffold surgery: a one-year study. Ophthalmology 2013;120(12):2442–2448

[19] Narang P, Agarwal A. Modified posterior-assisted levitation with intraocular lens scaffold and glued IOL for sinking nucleus in eyes with inadequate sulcus support. J Cataract Refract Surg 2017;43(7):872–876

[20] Agarwal A, Narang P, Kumar DA, Agarwal A. Clinical outcomes of sleeveless phaco tip-assisted levitation of dropped nucleus. Br J Ophthalmol 2014;98(10):1429–1434

[21] Agarwal A, Narang P, Agarwal A, Kumar DA. Sleeveless-extrusion cannula for levitation of dislocated intraocular lens. Br J Ophthalmol 2014;98(7):910–914

Section V

Miscellaneous

V

25 Anterior Segment Repair and Reconstruction in Traumatic Cases

Fasika A. Woreta, James T. Banta, Ferenc Kuhn, J. Fernando Arevalo

Summary

Ocular trauma is a leading cause of monocular blindness worldwide. Injuries isolated to the anterior segment have a better prognosis than injuries with posterior segment involvement. Meticulous primary repair of open-globe injuries is essential to restore globe integrity and minimize long-term sequelae such as corneal scarring and irregular astigmatism. Careful preoperative planning and adherence to key principles of corneal suturing as outlined in this chapter can help achieve successful outcomes. After primary repair, secondary surgeries to reconstruct the anterior segment may be necessary depending on the nature and severity of the initial injury. Trauma to the iris, angle, or lens can result in sequelae such as traumatic mydriasis, iridodialysis, a cyclodialysis cleft, cataract, or lens subluxation or dislocation. This chapter reviews key procedures in anterior segment reconstruction such as corneal transplantation, traumatic cataract removal, iris reconstruction, goniosynechialysis, cyclodialysis repair, and the management of vitreous from an anterior approach. Ocular surface reconstruction after severe chemical injuries, including the use of amniotic membrane early on and limbal stem cell transplants, are reviewed. Finally, special considerations in pediatric eye injuries such as the healing response, pearls in traumatic cataract removal, and amblyopia, are discussed.

Keywords: Anterior segment trauma, anterior segment reconstruction, ocular trauma, corneal laceration repair

25.1 Introduction

Ocular trauma is an important cause of vision loss worldwide, with an estimated 19 million people unilaterally blind and 1.6 million bilaterally blind from eye injuries.[1] Moreover, eye injuries disproportionately affect young people, with the peak incidence occurring in young adult and adolescent males.[2] While the prevention of ocular trauma should be the primary goal, optimizing post-traumatic surgical repair and reconstruction is of utmost importance. Injuries limited to the cornea and anterior segment generally have a better prognosis than those with posterior segment involvement.[3]

The management of anterior segment trauma can be classified into three stages: the initial management of acute trauma, the intermediate care, and the definitive anterior segment reconstruction.[4] In cases of open-globe injuries, careful preoperative planning and attention to microsurgical suturing techniques during the primary repair may minimize the need for secondary surgeries. The primary goal of the initial repair is to restore globe integrity and achieve a watertight closure. Intermediate care should focus on the prevention of infection, control of inflammation, and stabilization of the ocular surface with medical therapy. Although certain situations may require early urgent surgical intervention, elective cases of anterior segment reconstruction are typically delayed to allow adequate time for inflammation control, wound healing, and assessment of the patient's visual potential. In some cases, one or more reconstructive surgeries may be necessary to improve visual outcomes and prevent secondary complications. Just as with the primary repair, secondary reconstruction requires careful planning and meticulous anatomic restoration to achieve excellent outcomes.

This chapter will focus on the principles of primary repair and secondary reconstruction of corneal and anterior segment injuries.

25.2 Primary Repair

Ocular injuries are classified as either an *open-* or *closed*-globe injury.

The term open globe denotes a full-thickness wound of the eyewall due to either a laceration by a sharp object or a rupture due to a blunt object. The initial surgical repair of open-globe injuries is performed promptly after the initial injury, as delays may be associated with a worse visual prognosis. The primary surgical goal is to restore globe integrity with watertight wound closure. Secondary goals are to restore normal anatomical relationships, conserve viable tissue, minimize cornea scarring and astigmatism, and prevent future complications.

The sutures necessary for anterior segment repair and reconstruction are summarized in ▶ Table 25.1. Spatulated microsurgical needles are ideal for corneal closure as they allow for passage of the suture with minimal tissue damage.

When suturing a laceration, the first step is to identify the edges of the wound. Tissue loss is rare, and it is imperative to avoid removal of any viable cornea or sclera, which can complicate wound closure. A paracentesis opposite the wound is used to inject the minimum amount of viscoelastic necessary and reposition any incarcerated iris. Iris tissue should be carefully preserved for future reconstruction and resected only if necrotic, infected, or epithelialized. Anatomic landmarks such as the limbus or an angle in the wound should be reapproximated first.

The following principles should be followed for corneal suturing:[5]
- Entry and exit with the needle should be perpendicular to the corneal surface.
- Suture depth should be 90% deep in the stroma; full thickness also acceptable.

Table 25.1 Sutures required for various anterior segment surgeries

Tissue	Suture type
Conjunctiva	7–0 or 8–0 Vicryl
Cornea	10–0 nylon
Limbus	9–0 nylon
Sclera	8–0 or 9–0 nylon
Iris repair and iris-sutured IOL	9–0 or 10–0 polypropylene
Scleral-sutured IOL	9–0 or 10–0 polypropylene 7–0 polytetrafluoroethylene
Amniotic membrane	10–0 Vicryl or 10–0 nylon

Abbreviation: IOL, intraocular lens.

- Suture length should be equal length and depth on both sides of the wound.
- Sutures should be placed radial to the axis of the wound.

If the wound transects the entire cornea, it should be closed from the periphery to the center. Placing long, tighter sutures near the limbus and shorter bites near the central cornea will help maintain the natural prolate shape of the cornea. Suture placement in the center of the visual axis should be avoided. All suture knots should be buried into the cornea, away from the visual axis. Proper suturing is essential to minimize corneal astigmatism and achieve good closure (▶Fig. 25.1). Stepwise removal of sutures following the injury may help reduce astigmatism.

In a wound with multiple angles, each linear aspect is individually closed. Stellate lacerations can be difficult to repair and may require a combination of suture, tissue adhesive, and a bandage contact lens. A star-shaped technique described by Akkin can also be considered.[6]

If an avulsed piece of viable corneal tissue is still present, it should be sutured back into place. Areas of large tissue loss are repaired with a full-thickness patch graft using donor tissue or a lamellar graft using gamma-irradiated corneas.[7] A full-thickness penetrating keratoplasty (PK) is rarely necessary for the primary repair of ocular trauma but may be necessary for secondary anterior segment reconstruction.

Corneal lacerations are frequently accompanied by trauma to the iris and lens. Iris incarcerated in the wound should be freed and repositioned in the eye. Excess iris manipulation during primary repair is avoided until the eye is less inflamed. If there is no anterior or posterior capsular violation, cataract surgery can be delayed until the cornea has healed and the initial trauma-related inflammation has subsided. Removal of the lens is indicated at the time of initial repair if there is violation of the anterior capsule with lens material in the anterior chamber. If the corneal laceration is large, it may be difficult to maintain a stable anterior chamber during removal of the lens. In these cases, the free lens material should be removed from the anterior chamber at the time of initial repair with plans for cataract removal when the corneal laceration is adequately stable, typically 5 or more days later. If there is a posterior capsular violation, an anterior or posterior approach can be used to the remove the cataract. The advantage of the posterior approach is that anterior chamber stability is improved. When possible, the sulcus should be salvaged for future intraocular lens (IOL) placement.

25.3 Anterior Segment Reconstruction

Definitive anterior segment reconstruction following ocular trauma is delayed until adequate healing from the initial trauma has occurred, the ocular inflammation has subsided, and treatment of the ocular surface is maximized. The patient's visual potential is assessed to determine if the patient is a candidate for further surgery. If there is damage to the optic nerve or retina with limited vision potential, the decision to defer any further surgery may be appropriate.

The secondary complications of severe ocular trauma can be as devastating as the initial injury and include:[8]

- Disruption of eyelid anatomy.
- Conjunctival scarring with ocular surface damage and symblepharon.
- Corneal scarring and neovascularization.
- Intraocular fibrosis.
- Epithelial downgrowth.
- Pupillary or cyclitic membranes.
- Lens-related injuries such as traumatic cataract, lens particle glaucoma, or lens subluxation.
- Glaucoma secondary to peripheral anterior synechiae (PAS) or angle recession.

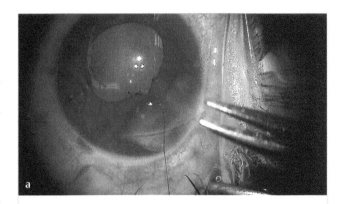

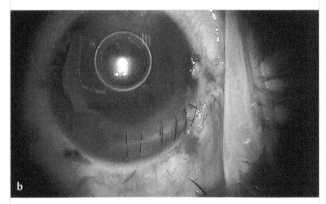

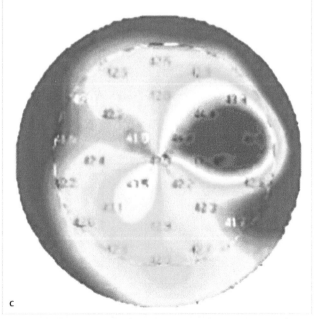

Fig. 25.1 (a) Full-thickness corneal laceration following tree branch trauma. (b) One month after surgical repair, visual acuity without correction is 20/30. (c) Axial/sagittal map on Pentacam demonstrates steepening in the area of injury.

- Vitreous incarceration within ocular wounds leading to chronic inflammation, cystoid macular edema, or retinal detachment.
- Infections such as corneal ulceration or endophthalmitis.

The sequelae of ocular trauma that may be amenable to reconstruction are summarized in ▸ Table 25.2. A rigid gas permeable (RGP) contact lens may be useful in the management of decreased vision from irregular corneal astigmatism or aphakia, which can coexist in a patient following anterior segment trauma. If medical management alone is not able to restore vision, additional anterior segment reconstruction may be warranted and include any combination of the following procedures:

- PK.
- Removal of anterior segment membranes.
- Cataract extraction.
- IOL implantation.
- Goniosynechialysis.
- Iris reconstruction.
- Cyclodialysis cleft repair.
- Anterior vitrectomy.

25.3.1 Penetrating Keratoplasty

Although lamellar techniques are being performed more frequently, full-thickness PK remains integral in the management of anterior segment trauma. Irregular astigmatism can generally be managed with an RGP. If an RPG fails to improve vision because of significant corneal scarring or persistent corneal edema, corneal transplantation is considered. If the injury was full thickness and the scarring involves the central visual axis, PK will be necessary. Partial-thickness injuries may be amenable to deep anterior lamellar keratoplasty. To optimize graft survival, corneal transplantation should be delayed until there is no intraocular or extraocular inflammation and the IOP is well controlled.

The size of the corneal button should be large enough to remove any central corneal scarring, and a size of about 7.5 mm is often sufficient.[8] The donor corneal button should be oversized 0.5 mm more than the host bed to help preserve anterior chamber depth and prevent the development of PAS and glaucoma postoperatively.[9,10] In eyes with shallow anterior chambers or broad PAS, trephination should be performed with great care. Dry cellulose sponges and smooth forceps should be used to gently separate the cornea from posterior adhesions. Vannas scissors

should be used sparingly, taking great care not to excise or damage tissue that may be utilized for subsequent iris reconstruction.[4]

It is often necessary to perform other anterior segment reconstructive techniques in conjunction with PK. ▸ Fig. 25.2

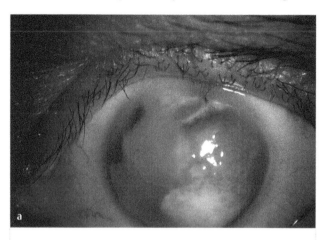

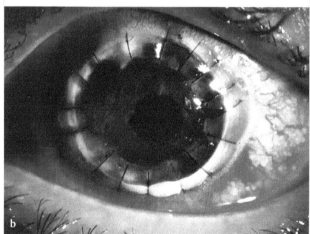

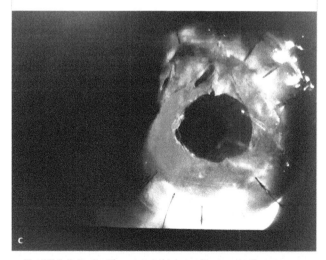

Fig. 25.2 Patient with a remote history of trauma to the eye presents for consideration of reconstructive surgery. **(a)** At baseline, his vision was hand motions with corneal opacification and a severely damaged anterior chamber. **(b, c)** Postoperative day 1 following an open sky PK, cataract removal, sulcus intraocular lens implantation, and iris reconstruction, his VA is 20/70. PK, penetrating keratoplasty; VA, visual acuity. (These images are provided courtesy of Yassine Daoud, Wilmer Eye Institute.)

Table 25.2 Sequelae of ocular trauma requiring anterior segment reconstruction

Cornea	Irregular astigmatism Scar Persistent edema Retrocorneal membrane
Iris	Pupillary membrane Iris sphincter tears Traumatic mydriasis Iridodialysis
Angle	Cyclodialysis cleft Cyclitic membrane
Lens	Traumatic cataract Aphakia Subluxation or dislocation

illustrates a case of iris and anterior chamber reconstruction in conjunction with a PK in a patient with a remote history of trauma. The health of the ocular surface should be maximized prior to PK. In cases where there is still neovascularization in the host, cautery is sometimes used to ablate vessels in hopes of decreasing the risk of rejection. If the host cornea is vascularized, 16 or more interrupted sutures should be used to suture the graft instead of running sutures.

Open sky goniosynechialysis can be performed if significant PAS is present. Organized fibrovascular or cellophane-like hyaline membranes can form over the anterior surface of the iris, angle, and posterior cornea.[4] Dry cellulose sponges or 0.12 forceps can be used to identify the edge and peel the membranes away from the iris and angle to avoid synechiae and compromise of the angle. Any vitreous should be removed manually with Westcott scissors and a dry cellulose sponge or with automated vitrectomy.

If cataract extraction with posterior chamber IOL (PCIOL) implantation is planned in combination with PK, intravenous mannitol and a Honan balloon may be used to decrease posterior pressure. A Flieringa ring can also be used to maintain scleral rigidity and prevent an expulsive hemorrhage. If there is a view through the cornea at the beginning of the case, the capsulorhexis can be created under a closed system to minimize the chance of radialization and the cataract removed with an open sky technique. For IOL calculations, an average keratometry of 45 can be used to estimate the post-PK corneal curvature.

In aphakic patients without capsular support in whom PK is planned, suturing of a PCIOL to the iris or sclera at the time of transplantation can be considered, when appropriate.

In cases with severe anterior and posterior segment trauma, vitreoretinal surgery can be performed with the use of a temporary keratoprosthesis.[11] The decision to suture a donor cornea versus the patient's trephined corneal button after the vitrectomy should be based on the expected prognosis given the posterior segment findings.[12]

In a review of 39 patients who underwent PK and anterior segment reconstruction after severe ocular trauma, 49% achieved a visual acuity of 20/100 or better compared with 10% preoperatively and 80% of grafts remained clear at a mean follow-up of 23 months.[8] It is important to note that chronically elevated IOP occurred in 46% patients postoperatively and was more common in eyes with preoperative glaucoma and persistent PAS. Thus, glaucoma management before and after reconstructive surgery is imperative.

25.3.2 Traumatic Cataract Removal and Intraocular Lens Placement

Trauma to the lens may occur after contusive or penetrating ocular trauma. Following contusive injury, a subcapsular, stellate-shaped lens opacity is most commonly seen. The cataract may remain small and focal, but in some cases may rapidly progress and become intumescent, as shown in ▶ Fig. 25.3. Lens subluxation or dislocation can also occur following trauma, and one should always carefully examine the patient for evidence of phacodonesis or zonular weakness.

Preoperative assessment includes careful examination for anterior or posterior capsular violation, zonular injury, or vitreous in the anterior chamber. If there is no anterior capsule violation, cataract surgery is delayed until the cornea has stabilized and there is no evidence of any anterior chamber inflammation. If violation of the anterior capsule is present, lens material will often escape into the anterior chamber, necessitating lens removal during primary repair of the open globe to avoid IOP elevation and inflammation. IOL placement can be deferred until there is improved visualization through the cornea, the anterior chamber is more stable, and there is no evidence of infection. IOL placement in an inflamed eye may lead to worsening uveitis, pupillary membranes, or posterior synechiae. In addition, corneal trauma will limit the ability to obtain accurate keratometry measurements for IOL calculations.[13] Waiting until the cornea has healed and removing the sutures before obtaining corneal topography will enable more accurate measurements. In the presence of significant irregular corneal astigmatism, an RGP is a good option to correct both the aphakia and irregular astigmatism.

When there is no capsular injury, a continuous curvilinear capsulorhexis (CCC) is performed, noting any signs of zonular weakness during completion, such as capsular folds or lens movement. In purely traumatic cataracts in young patients, the cataract can often be removed with aspiration only. If no zonular weakness is noted, an IOL can be inserted into the bag.

If there is an anterior capsular violation but the posterior capsule is intact, trypan blue can be used to visualize the injury to the anterior capsule intraoperatively. If the violation is small, it can sometimes be incorporated into a routine CCC. However, capsular fibrosis often makes a CCC challenging. Curved microscissors are an excellent tool to create or continue a capsular opening in the region of injury and fibrosis (▶ Fig. 25.4). Viscodissection can facilitate the prolapse of the lens material into

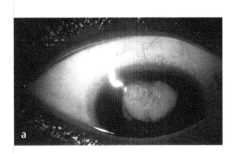
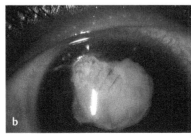

Fig. 25.3 (a, b) A 10-year-old hit with a dart in the right eye. The corneal laceration was repaired with 10–0 nylon sutures and cyanoacrylate glue. One week after closure, an intumescent cataract with lens material in the anterior chamber was noted. A capsulorhexis was created, incorporating the anterior capsule defect. The soft lens material was removed with bimanual irrigation and aspiration and the IOL was placed in the sulcus. At 1-month follow-up, best corrected VA is 20/20. IOL, intraocular lens; VA, visual acquity.

the anterior chamber. Capsular or sulcus IOL placement is then performed, depending on the stability of the capsular bag.

If there is a posterior capsular violation with limited vitreous in the anterior chamber, bimanual automated vitrectomy can be used to trim back prolapsed vitreous and sometimes remove the cataract if the lens is soft. Viscoelastic is used to tamponade and compartmentalize prolapsed vitreous and viscodissect the lens material from the capsule. If the cataract is too dense for removal with the vitreous cutter, phacoemulsification with slow-motion settings (low infusion pressure, low vacuum, and low aspiration) is utilized. If the posterior capsular defect is large with significant vitreous prolapse, a pars plana lensectomy and vitrectomy by a vitreoretinal specialist may be necessary.

Damage to the zonules is common, following contusive trauma to the eye. A capsular tension ring (CTR) can be used to stabilize the bag in cases of limited zonular dehiscence (less than 3–4 clock hours) and works by redistributing the forces on the intact zonules to support the area of zonular loss (▶ Fig. 25.5). Of note, a CTR should not be used if the capsulorhexis is not continuous or there is a defect in posterior capsule.

In the absence of sufficient capsular support, the options for secondary placement include an anterior chamber IOL (ACIOL) or fixation of a PCIOL to the iris or sclera.

ACIOL placement is often not ideal after trauma due to the presence of a PAS or pupillary irregularities. ACIOL should also be avoided if there is any potential for corneal transplantation in the future. Iris fixation can be achieved by using an iris claw IOL or suture fixation of a three-piece foldable IOL but should be avoided if there is severe iris atrophy or extensive transillumination defects. For suture fixation, 9–0 or 10–0 polypropylene

sutures are used with a McCannel technique or Siepser sliding knots to secure the haptics to the iris.

Scleral fixation can be performed when there is insufficient iris tissue but should be avoided in patients with significant injuries to the sclera. There are numerous techniques that be used for scleral fixation and this procedure is often combined with a pars plana vitrectomy.

The CZ70BD (Alcon Laboratories, Fort Worth, TX, USA), a one-piece polymethyl methacrylate IOL with islets in the haptics, was a popular choice for scleral fixation in the past. In this technique, a double-armed 9–0 or 10–0 polypropylene suture on a long, straight needle is tied around the islets and the needles are passed through the ciliary sulcus and exit beneath a scleral flap or scleral groove. The main disadvantages of this technique are the large 7-mm incision, an IOL that is neither foldable or cuttable, and postoperative IOL tilt or torque that is sometimes encountered with a 2-point fixation.

Newer surgical techniques that allow for a smaller incision with a foldable IOL have gained popularity. Sutureless techniques rely on the creation of intrascleral tunnels to fixate the haptics of a three-piece IOL such as the CT Lucia 602 (Carl Zeiss Meditec AG, Jena, Germany).[14]

The Akreos AO60 (Bausch & Lomb, Rochester, NY) is a foldable single-piece IOL with four eyelets in the haptic feet. Passing 7–0 polytetrafluoroethylene (Gore-Tex, W. L. Gore & Associates, Newark, DE) suture through the haptics in a mattress fashion allows 4-point fixation, as shown in ▶ Fig. 25.6, which minimize tilt and allows for a full-thickness scleral bite. Of note, the ophthalmic use of Gore-Tex sutures is "off-label," but it is a resilient suture frequently used in cardiac surgery, and studies

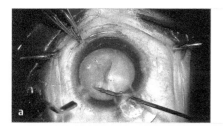
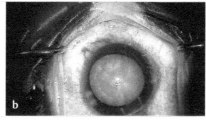
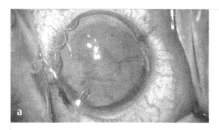
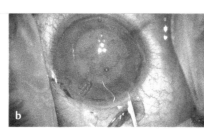
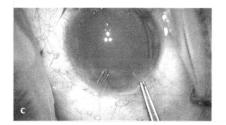
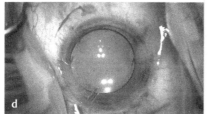

Fig. 25.4 **(a)** Traumatic cataract, 23-G curved microscissors necessary to cut anterior capsular plaque. **(b)** Continuous curvilinear capsulorhexis completed with microscissors.

Fig. 25.5 **(a)** Patient with a distant history of trauma presents with decreased vision secondary to traumatic cataract. He had a history of prior glaucoma tube shunt surgery. Note the traumatic mydriasis and folds in the anterior capsule. Three clock hours of zonular weakness were also noted with the patient lying down. **(b)** A CCC was completed. **(c)** Given 3 clock hours of zonular weakness, a capsular tension ring was placed in the bag, followed by injection of a three-piece IOL into the bag. **(d)** Postoperative day 1, the IOL is well centered and stable, and the VA is 20/30. CCC, continuous curvilinear capsulorhexis; IOL, intraocular lens; VA, visual acquity.

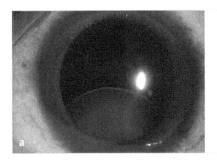
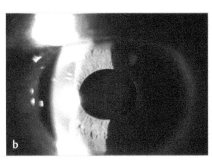

Fig. 25.6 (a) Crystalline lens subluxation following contusive trauma. **(b)** Postoperative month 1 after 4-point scleral fixation with an Akreos IOL. VA is 20/20. IOL, intraocular lens; VA, visual acquity.

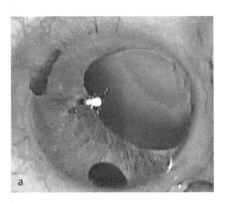
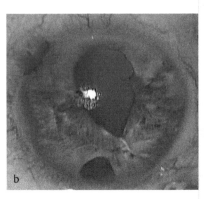

Fig. 25.7 (a) Patient had contusive trauma with a ruptured globe and extrusion of the crystalline lens. The eye underwent vitrectomy with silicone oil implantation, hence the 6 o'clock iridectomy. The iris is drawn towards the scleral wound superotemporally. **(b)** Postoperative image of the same eye. The silicone oil has been removed and during the same surgery, the iris was again gently pulled away from the wound with serrated retinal forceps. A 10–0 Prolene suture was used to perform a pupilloplasty to create a pupil size that is small enough to prevent photophobia but large enough to allow fundus examination in the future.

have shown good short-term safety and efficacy in the eye.[15] The major disadvantage of the Akreos IOL is its hydrophilic composition, and IOL opacification has been reported following gas tamponade.[16]

Other anterior segment reconstruction modalities such as goniosynechialysis, pupilloplasty, or iridodialysis repair may be needed at the time of cataract extraction and will be discussed below.

25.3.3 Goniosynechialysis and Iris Reconstruction

The goal of iris repair is to provide a central, appropriately sized pupil while minimizing glare and monocular diplopia. Opening the anterior chamber angle and providing improved cosmesis are secondary goals.

Lysis of PAS can be performed to improve aqueous outflow, minimize the risk of postoperative glaucoma, and free iris tissue for reconstruction. Viscoelastic allows for gentle blunt dissection, while iris forceps can be used to pull the iris away from the angle. The use of intraocular scissors is typically avoided unless the extent of incarceration does not allow blunt dissection. If bleeding of the iris occurs, the intraocular pressure can be temporarily elevated to staunch the bleeding. If this is unsuccessful, preservative-free intracameral epinephrine diluted 1:10,000 can be injected into the anterior chamber to help achieve hemostasis. If open sky techniques are being used, direct cauterization using a pencil-tip cautery can be considered.

Damage to the iris is common after trauma and can result in traumatic mydriasis, iris sphincter tears, or iridodialysis. Iris trauma can also lead to prolonged inflammation, cystoid macular edema, and synechiae formation. If the patient has glare,

photophobia, or cosmetic disfigurement, surgical intervention may be warranted and can be performed at the time of other reconstructive surgeries (▶Fig. 25.7). Sectoral iris defects can be repaired using 9–0 or 10–0 polypropylene with a McCannel technique or Siepser sliding knots. A diffusely flaccid, atrophic iris is more difficult to fix and may require suture reconstruction or an iris cerclage. In cases of traumatic aniridia, treatment options include a colored contact lens or insertion of an artificial iris device. Currently, the major manufacturers of artificial iris devices available are Morcher (Stuttgart, Germany), Ophtec (Groningen, the Netherlands), and HumanOptics (Erlangen, Germany). The Morcher and Ophtec CTR-based prosthetic iris devices can be implanted within the capsular bag during phacoemulsification surgery. The CustomFlex artificial iris from HumanOptics can be implanted into the bag or suture fixated to the sclera and can be sized and colored for each individual patient.[10] All three devices are available outside of the United States, but the CustomFlex artificial iris is the first and only device that has been approved by the Food and Drug Administration for use in the United States.

Iridodialysis, or disinsertion of the iris from its attachment to the ciliary body at the iris root, often creates glare and monocular diplopia that warrant repair (▶Fig. 25.8). Suturing the iris to the scleral wall can be performed using a double-armed 9–0 or 10–0 polypropylene to create a mattress suture. Techniques vary, but the suture can be secured through full-thickness sclera or under a scleral flap or Hoffman pocket. The sutures should be tied under low tension in a hang-back fashion to prevent distortion of the pupil.

In certain severe cases, fibrosis and scar tissue can cover the visual axis. In these cases, a central pupillary opening can be fashioned with small Vannas scissors.

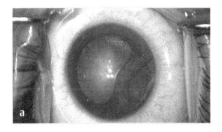
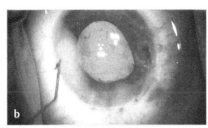

Fig. 25.8 **(a)** Traumatic iridodialysis following a ball bearing (BB) gun injury. **(b)** The iridodialysis was repaired at the time of cataract surgery using a long, straight needle and a Hoffman pocket.

25.3.4 Cyclodialysis Cleft Repair

Traumatic cyclodialysis occurs when the ciliary body is disinserted from the sclera, allowing a direct route of aqueous entry into the suprachoroidal space and subsequent hypotony. On gonioscopy, a visible gap between the sclera and ciliary body is seen. Ultrasound biomicroscopy can be used to confirm and localize the cleft. Initial treatment should include atropine to rotate the ciliary body closer to the scleral spur to promote closure. If medical management fails after 4 to 6 weeks and the IOP is < 4 with hypotony maculopathy and choroidal folds, argon laser can be applied to the ciliary body and scleral sides of the clefts to promote closure. If laser fails, direct cyclopexy, in which the ciliary body is sutured to the cleft under a scleral flap, can be performed.[17] Closure of the cleft typically leads to an acute, transient rise in IOP; therefore, close monitoring is advised.

25.3.5 Anterior Vitrectomy

Vitreous in the anterior chamber can create a multitude of complications. It is imperative to remove any vitreous incarcerated in the wound and relieve anteroposterior vitreous traction, as a vitreous wick or traction may lead to infection, cystoid macular edema, or a retinal detachment. Ideally, automated vitrectomy should be used to remove vitreous to the level of the iris diaphragm. If an automated vitrector is not available, vitreous can be removed manually with Wescott scissors and a dry cellulose sponge, ensuring not to exert traction on the vitreous without cutting. Vitreous can be directly visualized using an intracameral injection of preservative-free triamcinolone acetonide when necessary. At the end of the case, an intracameral miotic can also be administered to shrink the pupil and reveal residual vitreous strands when peaking of the pupil is demonstrated.

25.4 Ocular Surface Reconstruction

Chemical injuries to the eye can lead to extensive damage of the ocular surface with corneal scarring and loss of vision. Alkali burns are most dangerous, as they cause saponification of fatty acids in cell membranes and therefore may penetrate into deeper structures of the eye. The degree of limbal ischemia is directly related to the prognosis. ▶ Fig. 25.9 demonstrates a severe alkali injury secondary to sodium hydroxide, with severe limbal ischemia. The most important step in the initial management of chemical injuries is immediate copious irrigation to remove the offending agent. Initial therapy in the

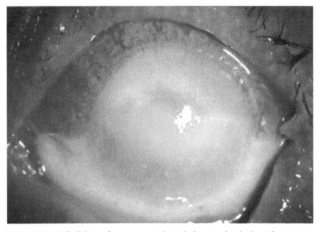

Fig. 25.9 Alkali burn from an accidental chemical splash with sodium hydroxide. Note the limbal ischemia and blanching of vessels from the 3 to 9 o'clock position.

acute stage focuses on reducing inflammation, promoting epithelialization, and preventing cicatricial complications.

In the early stages following the injury, amniotic membrane transplantation (AMT) can be useful in terms of suppressing inflammation, promoting re-epithelialization, and preventing symblepharon formation. The sutureless amniotic membrane with a ring system (ProKera, Bio-Tissue, Miami, FL) is useful in early management but often needs replacement every few days until re-epithelialization occurs.[18] A tarsorrhaphy can frequently accelerate healing. In later stages, conjunctival reconstruction with AMT or a buccal mucosa graft may be needed to reconstruct the fornix.

Limbal stem cell deficiency can occur after severe chemical injuries leading to neovascularization and opacification of the cornea. Ocular surface reconstruction with a limbal stem cell transplant (LSCT) may be necessary. Newer techniques of LSCT such as simple limbal epithelial transplantation have shown promising results.[19] Once the ocular surface has stabilized, PK may be necessary for visual rehabilitation.

25.5 Special Considerations in Pediatric Trauma

Very young patients with severe ocular trauma are at risk for amblyopia and aggressive wound healing which can limit visual outcomes without special attention. Given children have an exaggerated wound healing response, sutures used in the primary repair should be removed as early as possible, typically

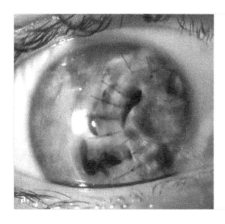 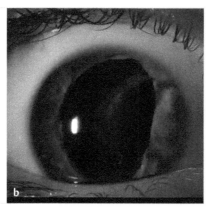

Fig. 25.10 **(a)** A 6-year old with an open-globe injury from a toy arrow. The lens was expulsed at the time of the injury. Primary repair of the corneal laceration was performed. **(b)** One month after the injury, the patient was taken to the operating room for removal of corneal sutures and lysis of iridocorneal adhesions. A postoperative image shows a marked reduction in the corneal scarring.

within 4 to 8 weeks following the initial injury, to avoid vascularization and scarring (▶ Fig. 25.10).

Traumatic cataract surgery in children has unique challenges. The pediatric lens capsule is highly elastic with a greater tendency to radialize. This can be avoided by altering the capsulorhexis technique. A high molecular weight viscoelastic like Healon 5 can help flatten the dome of the anterior lens capsule and trypan blue alters the tearing properties of the anterior capsule, both allowing a modicum of control. Multiple grabs with the capsulorhexis forceps directing the tear centrally on each grab allow slow controlled creation of a round capsulorhexis. Alternately, a vitreous cutter can be used to create a round anterior capsular opening. Some traumatic patients will have a pre-existing anterior capsular violation. Interestingly, anterior capsular violations tend to take on a stable, oval configuration with a circumferential rim of significant fibrosis that often requires sharp instruments to cut. In this scenario, a small defect can be incorporated into the rhexis opening, or if too large or eccentric, scissors can be used to create a flap within the violation that allows creation of a round capsular opening. These violations tend not to radialize. The lens in pediatric patients is uniformly soft and can be removed purely with aspiration. In some cases, it is possible to aspirate the entirety of the lens via a pre-existing traumatic capsular tear, fill the capsule with viscoelastic, and then create the anterior capsular opening as the last step. The absorbable suture should be used to close the clear corneal incisions in children. To aid in visual recovery and potentially prevent amblyopia, primary IOL implantation with a foldable acrylic IOL should be considered. Visually significant posterior capsular opacification is nearly uniform postoperatively in the pediatric population. In patients too young to cooperate with a laser capsulotomy (typically age 7 or younger), a primary posterior capsulorhexis or creation of a posterior capsular opening with a vitreous cutter is vital.[20]

Pediatric corneal transplants are considered high risk and modifications in surgical technique are necessary in the pediatric eye.[21] These include using a Flieringa ring to provide scleral support, providing digital massage or a Honan balloon to decrease posterior pressure, administering intravenous mannitol, and avoiding any open sky time. Corneal suture removal can begin much earlier in children as they heal very quickly and should be complete within 2 months.

Aggressive management of amblyopia with patching in children under the age of 10 is necessary to ensure good outcomes in children, and these patients should be managed in conjunction with a pediatric ophthalmologist.

25.6 Conclusion

Loss of vision is one of the most devastating consequences of trauma. Prevention through safety precautions and consistent use of eye protection should be a worldwide public health effort. Meticulous primary surgical repair to provide definitive closure is imperative as soon as possible after the initial injury. Advances in microsurgical techniques have enhanced the rehabilitation of severely traumatized eyes. Secondary reconstructive surgeries with care across ophthalmic subspecialties can restore vision and prevent late complications of the injured eye.

References

[1] Négrel AD, Thylefors B. The global impact of eye injuries. Ophthalmic Epidemiol 1998;5(3):143–169

[2] Klopfer J, Tielsch JM, Vitale S, See LC, Canner JK. Ocular trauma in the United States. Eye injuries resulting in hospitalization, 1984 through 1987. Arch Ophthalmol 1992;110(6):838–842

[3] Schmidt GW, Broman AT, Hindman HB, Grant MP. Vision survival after open globe injury predicted by classification and regression tree analysis. Ophthalmology 2008;115(1):202–209

[4] Hersh PS, Kenyon KR. Anterior segment reconstruction following ocular trauma. Int Ophthalmol Clin 1988;28(1):57–68

[5] Macsai MS. Ophthalmic microsurgical suturing techniques. Berlin; New York: Springer; 2007

[6] Akkin C, Kayikcioglu O, Erakgun T. A novel suture technique in stellate corneal lacerations. Ophthalmic Surg Lasers 2001;32(5):436–437

[7] Chae JJ, Choi JS, Lee JD, et al. Physical and biological characterization of the gamma-irradiated human cornea. Cornea 2015;34(10):1287–1294

[8] Kenyon KR, Starck T, Hersh PS. Penetrating keratoplasty and anterior segment reconstruction for severe ocular trauma. Ophthalmology 1992;99(3):396–402

[9] Heidemann DG, Sugar A, Meyer RF, Musch DC. Oversized donor grafts in penetrating keratoplasty. A randomized trial. Arch Ophthalmol 1985;103(12):1807–1811

[10] Zimmerman T, Olson R, Waltman S, Kaufman H. Transplant size and elevated intraocular pressure. Postkeratoplasty. Arch Ophthalmol 1978;96(12):2231–2233

[11] Nowomiejska K, Haszcz D, Forlini C, et al. Wide-field landers temporary keratoprosthesis in severe ocular trauma: functional and anatomical results after one year. J Ophthalmol 2015;2015:163675

[12] Chen HJ, Wang CG, Dou HL, et al. Anatomical outcome of vitreoretinal surgery using temporary keratoprosthesis and replacement of the trephined corneal button for severe open globe injuries: one-year result. J Ophthalmol 2014;2014:794039

[13] Chuang LH, Lai CC. Secondary intraocular lens implantation of traumatic cataract in open-globe injury. Can J Ophthalmol 2005;40(4):454–459

[14] Nudleman E, Yonekawa Y, Prenner JL. Sutureless transscleral fixation of secondary intraocular lenses. Curr Opin Ophthalmol 2018;29(3):210–216

[15] Terveen DC, Fram NR, Ayres B, Berdahl JP. Small-incision 4-point scleral suture fixation of a foldable hydrophilic acrylic intraocular lens in the absence of capsule support. J Cataract Refract Surg 2016;42(2):211–216

[16] Kalevar A, Dollin M, Gupta RR. Opacification of Scleral-Sutured Akreos Ao60 intraocular lens after vitrectomy with gas tamponade: case series. Retin Cases Brief Rep 2017

[17] Wang C, Peng XY, You QS, et al. Internal cyclopexy for complicated traumatic cyclodialysis cleft. Acta Ophthalmol 2017;95(6):639–642

[18] Kheirkhah A, Johnson DA, Paranjpe DR, Raju VK, Casas V, Tseng SC. Temporary sutureless amniotic membrane patch for acute alkaline burns. Arch Ophthalmol 2008;126(8):1059–1066

[19] Borroni D, Wowra B, Romano V, et al. Simple limbal epithelial transplantation: a review on current approach and future directions. Surv Ophthalmol 2018;63(6):869–874

[20] Jinagal J, Gupta G, Gupta PC, et al. Visual outcomes of pediatric traumatic cataracts. Eur J Ophthalmol 2019;29(1):23–27

[21] Trief D, Marquezan MC, Rapuano CJ, Prescott CR. Pediatric corneal transplants. Curr Opin Ophthalmol 2017;28(5):477–484

26 Phacocele and Pseudophacocele

Priya Narang, Amar Agarwal

Summary

The terms phacocele and pseudophacocele denote forceful extrusion of the crystalline lens and of the intraocular lens implant respectively into the subconjunctival space. This chapter highlights the investigations and management aspect of this emergency like situation that if left untreated can lead to poor visual prognosis.

Keywords: Phacocele, pseudophacocele, vitrectomy, ocular trauma, scleral tear, uveal prolapse, scleral rupture

26.1 Introduction

Ocular trauma is one of the causes of visual impairment and is commonly encountered in young patients who are associated with sports and recreational activities. Elderly people most commonly report ocular trauma after a fall that can be due to gait disturbances, neurological deficits, or may be accidental. Ocular trauma can be broadly categorized into a blunt or penetrating trauma and it may be a closed or open wound injury. Following blunt ocular trauma, scleral rupture is most commonly observed at superonasal and temporal quadrants. The presence of supraorbital rim and nasal bridge makes the temporal and inferior quadrants more susceptible to trauma.[1,2,3] Hence, post-trauma scleral rupture is commonly observed in the superonasal and temporal quadrants.

As a sequelae to trauma, the *seven rings of ocular tissue* are affected, namely, sphincter pupillae, the iris base, anterior ciliary body, detachment of ciliary body to the spur, trabecular meshwork, zonular detachment, and retinal detachment.[4] Depending upon the type of injury and the impact of trauma, the clinical scenario differs in presentation and prognosis. The terms phacocele and pseudophacocele indicate extrusion of the natural crystalline lens in a phakic eye and of the intraocular lens implant in a pseudophakic eye into the subconjunctival space (▶Video 26.1 and ▶Video 26.2).

26.2 Phacocele

The concussive force due to blunt trauma damages the zonular integrity and pushes the crystalline lens through the ruptured scleral wall[5] into the subconjunctival space (▶Fig. 26.1). Alternatively, the crystalline lens can also be pushed back into the vitreous cavity. The patients typically present with a history of blunt trauma associated with pain and dimness of vision. In patients with phacocele, slit lamp examination (SLE) demonstrates aphakia with subconjunctival or a sub-Tenon's mass, which is probably the extruded crystalline lens. Often the anterior chamber (AC) details are obscured due to hyphema and vitreous hemorrhage.

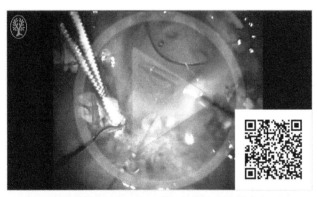

Video 26.1 Bull horn injury. https://www.thieme.de/de/q.htm?p=opn/tp/311890101/9781684200979_video_26_01&t=video

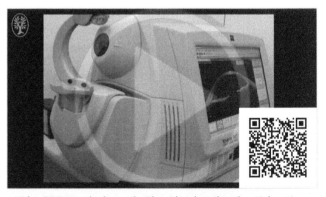

Video 26.2 Pseudophacocele. The video describes the etiology, impact, treatment, and management of cases with pseudophacocele in a concise yet elaborative way. https://www.thieme.de/de/q.htm?p=opn/tp/311890101/9781684200979_video_26_02&t=video

26.3 Pseudophacocele

Biedner et al,[6] who first reported the subconjunctival extrusion of an IOL (▶Fig. 26.2) associated with globe rupture following blunt ocular trauma, formulated the terminology of "pseudophacocele." The traumatic rupture and gaping of the surgical wound have been reported even after 12 years of surgery. The surgical wound healing is a slow process and is often delayed due to associated diseases.[7,8,9,10] Wound healing after cataract extraction is a slow process and traumatic wound rupture is not uncommon.

26.4 Diagnostic Procedures and Examination

26.4.1 Slit Lamp Examination

The SLE broadly helps to assess the anterior segment ocular structures and their relationship to each other. It also gives a brief overview of the further investigations that are essential to rule out the potential visual outcome of a patient.

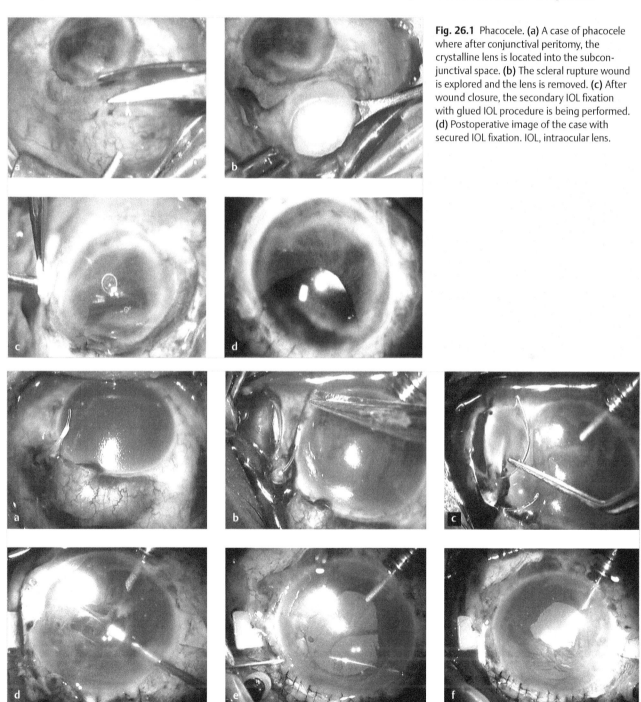

Fig. 26.1 Phacocele. **(a)** A case of phacocele where after conjunctival peritomy, the crystalline lens is located into the subconjunctival space. **(b)** The scleral rupture wound is explored and the lens is removed. **(c)** After wound closure, the secondary IOL fixation with glued IOL procedure is being performed. **(d)** Postoperative image of the case with secured IOL fixation. IOL, intraocular lens.

Fig. 26.2 Pseudophacocele. **(a)** Subconjunctival extrusion of the IOL and uveal tissue with haptic protruding from the conjunctiva. **(b)** Conjunctival peritomy is done and the IOL is detected. **(c)** The IOL is explanted and a broken haptic is detected. **(d)** Two partial-thickness flaps are made at 180° for glued IOL procedure. The scleral wound is sutured and limited anterior vitrectomy is performed to clear the hyphema. **(e)** Glued IOL fixation is done and single-pass four-throw (SFT) pupilloplasty is being performed. **(f)** Intraoperative image of the patient at the end of the procedure. IOL, intraocular lens.

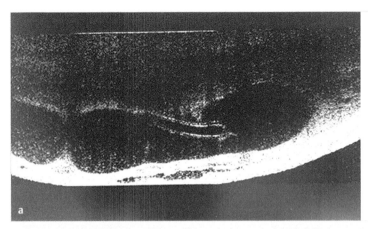
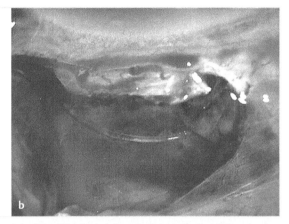

Fig. 26.3 AS-OCT imaging of a case of pseudophacocele. **(a)** AS-OCT shows extrusion of the IOL with breakage in the continuity of the scleral wall. **(b)** IOL optic protruding through the scleral wound. AS-OCT, anterior segment optical coherence tomography; IOL, intraocular lens.

26.4.2 Ultrasound Biomicroscopy

Ultrasound Biomicroscopy (UBM) imaging is the most informative diagnostic tool in cases with massive intraocular damage as it delineates the intraocular structures in hazy media. Care should be taken while performing the examination, as too much pressure on the already compromised globe should be avoided.

26.4.3 Anterior Segment Optical Coherence Tomography

An anterior segment optical coherence tomography (AS-OCT) examination is a noncontact modality and it has been used in the past to delineate the structures in penetrating trauma. It also helps to assess the continuity of sclera and also to assess the relationship between the cornea, angle structures, and the uveal tissue. AS-OCT demonstrates phacocele and pseudophacocele (▶Fig. 26.3) as a heterogeneous reflection in the subconjunctival space.[11]

26.4.4 X-Ray Orbit

The anteroposterior and lateral views of X-ray orbit help to delineate the bony integrity in cases with brutal trauma where orbital roof, floor, or bony structure deformations or fracture is suspected.

26.4.5 Others

Computed tomography scan and magnetic resonance imaging (MRI) can also be employed to delineate the details of ocular trauma, especially in penetrating injuries with foreign bodies. However, MRI should be used cautiously if magnetic foreign bodies are suspected.

26.5 Surgical Technique

The procedure is performed under general anesthesia and exploration of the wound is undertaken. Fluid infusion is first infused inside the eye. A routine anterior chamber maintainer (ACM) or a trocar ACM can be employed for this (▶Fig. 26.4a, b). The conjunctival dissection is done and the wound is explored. The extruded crystalline lens or the IOL is located and is

removed (▶Fig. 26.4c, d). The scleral wound is sutured with 8–0 nylon suture and a closed globe is achieved.

A corneal paracentesis incision is made and limited anterior vitrectomy is performed to clear the vitreous and hyphema in the AC (▶Fig. 26.4e). Two partial-thickness scleral flaps 2 × 2 mm are made 180° apart and sclerotomy is performed beneath the flaps with a 22-G needle. A 23-G vitrectomy probe is again introduced through the sclerotomy and limited vitrectomy is performed in the retropupillary plane. Following this posterior segment, the examination is performed and the clinical entity is dealt with as per the diseased condition of the vitreous and retina (▶Fig. 26.4 f).

A three-piece foldable IOL is introduced inside the AC and the tip of the haptic is grasped with an end-opening forceps introduced from the left sclerotomy site (▶Fig. 26.5a). Once the entire IOL has unfolded, the tip of the leading haptic is pulled and externalized. The tip of the trailing haptic is held and is then flexed inside the AC towards 6 o'clock position. No-assistant technique is performed and this leads to more extrusion of the leading haptic without the tendency to slip back inside the eye. The end-opening forceps is introduced from the stab incision and the tip of trailing haptic is transferred to the left hand. The right-hand forceps is then withdrawn from the eye and is reintroduced from the right sclerotomy incision. This is referred to as the handshake technique following which the tip of trailing haptic is held and externalized (▶Fig. 26.5b).

The haptics are then tucked into the scleral pockets created with 26-G needle and vitrectomy is performed at the sclerotomy site. Pupil shape distortion and iris root damage are often seen as the associated features that need iris repair. Pupilloplasty is performed for pupil shape configuration and our preferred mode of performing pupilloplasty is single-pass four-throw pupilloplasty (▶Fig. 26.5c, d). Once the integrity of intraocular structures is restored, the fluid infusion is stopped and fibrin glue is applied beneath the flaps and they are sealed (▶Fig. 26.5e, f).

The standard postoperative protocol is followed with dosing of topical moxifloxacin four times a day for initial 2 months postoperative period and topical prednisolone acetate 1% every 2 hours for the initial 2 weeks, four times daily for 1 month, twice daily for 2 months, and once daily thereafter for 3 months.

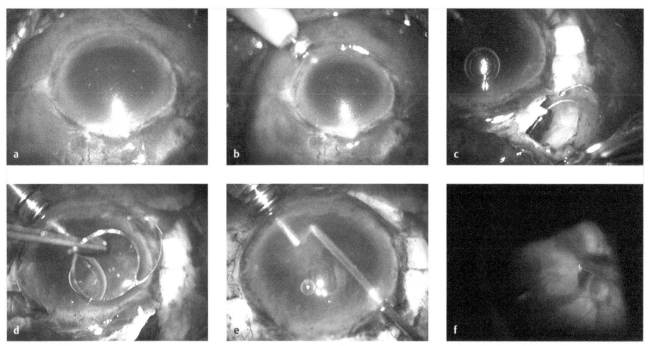

Fig. 26.4 Surgical steps for management of pseudophacocele. **(a)** A case of blunt ocular trauma with hyphema, chemosis, and a possible pseudophacocele. **(b)** A trocar anterior chamber maintainer being introduced for fluid infusion. **(c)** Exploration of the wound following peritomy confirms the possibility of a pseudophacocele. **(d)** The IOL is explanted and a broken haptic is noted. **(e)** The scleral wound is sutured with 8–0 nylon. A corneal paracentesis incision is made and limited anterior vitrectomy is performed to clear hyphema and vitreous in the anterior chamber. **(f)** The posterior segment is examined and core vitrectomy along with the removal of vitreous hemorrhage is done. IOL, intraocular lens.

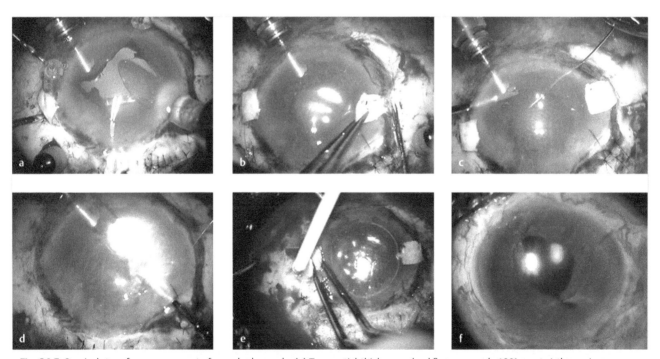

Fig. 26.5 Surgical steps for management of pseudophacocele. **(a)** Two partial-thickness scleral flaps are made 180° apart. A three-piece foldable IOL is loaded and the tip of the leading haptic is held with glued IOL end-opening forceps. **(b)** The leading and trailing haptics are externalized. Scleral pockets are created with a 26-G needle. **(c)** The haptics are tucked into the scleral pockets. A 10–0 suture attached to the long arm of the needle is passed through the proximal iris leaflet. **(d)** The needle is passed through the distal iris leaflet and SFT pupilloplasty is performed. The ends of the knot are then cut with scissors. **(e)** The trocar ACM is removed and fibrin glue is applied beneath the scleral flaps. **(f)** Postoperative image of the patient at 1 week. ACM, anterior chamber maintainer; IOL, intraocular lens; SFT, single-pass four-throw.

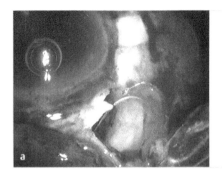 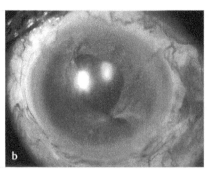

Fig. 26.6 Preoperative and postoperative image of the patient. **(a)** Preoperative image of the case with pseudophacocele. **(b)** Postoperative image of the case managed with glued IOL, SFT pupilloplasty, and vitrectomy. IOL, intraocular lens; SFT, single-pass four-throw.

26.6 Discussion

In phacocele, the scleral rupture is usually seen between the limbus and spiral of Tillaux.[1,2] The inferior-temporal region of the globe is considered to be the most susceptible to trauma as the nasal bridge and supraorbital rim protect the globe in other quadrants. The subconjunctivally extruded lens is reported to get absorbed over a period of few months.[12] Nevertheless, the scleral wound needs to be repaired along with restoring the anatomical configuration of other intraocular structures.

As compared to phacocele, the site of scleral rupture observed in pseudophacocele is usually the postcataract surgical wound. The incidence of pseudophacocele is seen more after extracapsular cataract surgery and manual small incision cataract surgery than phacoemulsification. The probable explanation for this would be that the scleral or limbal wound constructed is of larger dimension and serves as the point of inherent weakness.

The choice of performing the surgical maneuver as a single-stage or a two-stage procedure depends upon the surgeon's preference and also on the associated features and complications. With timely and appropriate surgical intervention,[13] the postoperative outcomes in these devastating injuries of globe rupture are favorable (▶ Fig. 26.6).

References

[1]   Cherry PMH. Rupture of the globe. Arch Ophthalmol 1972;88(5):498–507

[2]   Cherry PM. Indirect traumatic rupture of the globe. Arch Ophthalmol 1978;96(2):252–256

[3]   Fuchs A. Spontaneous internal scleral ruptures and the splitting of the corneasclera. Am J Ophthalmol 1958;46(6):855–864

[4]   Feldman B, Tripathy K. American Academy of Ophthalmology. EyeWiki. http://drkoushik.blogspot.in/2010/11/seven-rings-of-blunt-trauma-to-eye.html

[5]   Duke-Elder A, MacFaul PA. Injuries: mechanical injuries. In: Duke-Elder S, ed. System of Ophthalmology. Vol. 14, Pt. 1. London: Henry Kimpton; 1972:147

[6]   Biedner B, Rothkoff L, Blumenthal M. Subconjunctival dislocation of intraocular lens implant. Am J Ophthalmol 1977;84(2):265–266

[7]   Gliedman ML, Karlson KE. Wound healing and wound strength of sutured limbal wounds. Am J Ophthalmol 1955;39(6):859–866

[8]   Flaxel JT, Swan K. C: Limbal wound healing after cataract extraction. Arch Ophthalmol 1969;81:653

[9]   Flaxel JT. Histology of cataract extractions. Arch Ophthalmol 1970;83(4):436–444

[10] Heller MD, Irvine SR, Straatsma BR, Foos RY. Wound healing after cataract extraction and position of the vitreous in aphakic eyes as studied postmortem. Trans Am Ophthalmol Soc 1971;69:245–262

[11] Prakash G, Ashokumar D, Jacob S, Kumar KS, Agarwal A, Agarwal A. Anterior segment optical coherence tomography-aided diagnosis and primary posterior chamber intraocular lens implantation with fibrin glue in traumatic phacocele with scleral perforation. J Cataract Refract Surg 2009;35(4):782–784

[12] Yurdakul NS, Uğurlu S, Yilmaz A, Maden A. Traumatic subconjunctival crystalline lens dislocation. J Cataract Refract Surg 2003;29(12):2407–2410

[13] Narang P, Agarwal A. Clinical outcomes in traumatic pseudophacocele: a rare clinical entity. Indian J Ophthalmol 2017;65(12):1465–1469

27 Trocar Anterior Chamber Maintainer

Priya Narang, Amar Agarwal

Summary

The trocar anterior chamber maintainer (ACM) helps to maintain fluid infusion. It has an advantage of the ease of insertion as with routine ACM and also of the trocar cannula system as it prevents any incidence of leakage or spontaneous extrusion from the eye.

Keywords: Trocar ACM, anterior chamber maintainer, fluid infusion, trocar, pars plana infusion, limbal infusion

27.1 Introduction

The merits of a closed chamber infusion system that helps to maintain the tonicity of the globe throughout the intraocular surgery cannot be understated. Maintenance of a deep anterior chamber (AC) is a prerequisite for safe, smooth performance of an intraocular surgery as it prevents inadvertent and harmful touch to the corneal endothelium and also to various other structures. For the same reason, sodium hyaluronate was introduced and it served as a major breakthrough for all anterior segment intraocular surgeries.[1,2,3] Although the use of viscoelastic cannot be understated, its role in the maintenance of an AC in corneal surgeries is not a prudent idea, more so with endothelial keratoplasty procedures.

Blumenthal devised a simple and practical method for maintaining the AC with a device that he called as the anterior chamber maintainer (ACM) that was made from a 21-G scalp vein ("butterfly") set. Since the introduction of an ACM, there have been various modifications to the ACM so as to suit the surgical condition of the eye (▶ Video 27.1, ▶ Video 27.2, and ▶ Video 27.3).

27.2 Concept

Fluid is the natural milieu of the eye and constant fluid infusion inside the eye helps to maintain the globe and prevent it from collapsing. Anterior segment surgeons most commonly employ ACM. The advantage with the use of ACM is that it is simple to use, as it needs only a paracentesis incision to set the ACM in place. However, the disadvantage is that the paracentesis incision has to be of an exact size or else forceful introduction can lead to Descemet's membrane detachment, whereas with a slightly larger width of paracentesis incision, the ACM can get extruded from the eye leading to sudden globe collapse.

Posterior segment surgeons primarily employ trocar infusion at pars plana site and it has an inherent advantage of being self-retaining. Initially, the authors published the technique of using routine trocars employed as ACM for fluid infusion wherein the trocars were inserted at a distance of 0.5 mm from the limbus (▶ Fig. 27.1, ▶ Fig. 27.2, and ▶ Fig. 27.3).[4] The disadvantage in using the routine trocars was that the surgeon had to be very careful while introducing it or else there was a

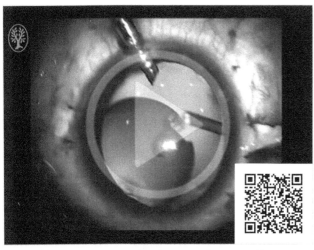

Video 27.1 Trocar anterior chamber maintainer. https://www.thieme.de/de/q.htm?p=opn/tp/311890101/9781684200979_video_27_01&t=video

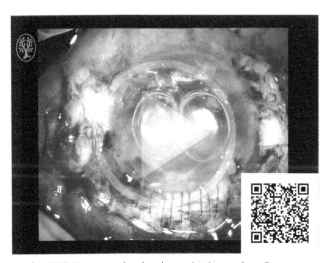

Video 27.2 Trocar anterior chamber maintainer and pre-Descemet endothelial keratoplasty with glued intraocular lens. https://www.thieme.de/de/q.htm?p=opn/tp/311890101/9781684200979_video_27_02&t=video

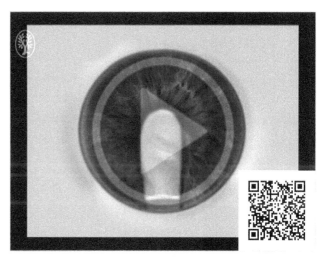

Video 27.3 Vitrectomy assisted phacoemulsification. https://www.thieme.de/de/q.htm?p=opn/tp/311890101/9781684200979_video_27_03&t=video

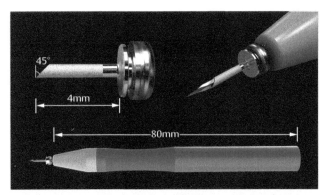

Fig. 27.1 Trocar anterior chamber maintainer—25-G stainless trocar needle and cannula. This is made by Mastel, USA.

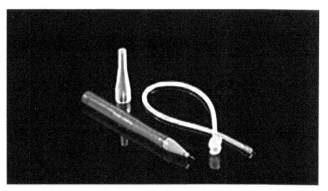

Fig. 27.2 Trocar anterior chamber maintainer surgical package set, which contains the trocar needle with cannula, the protective cover, and the infusion tube line.

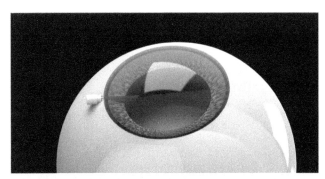

Fig. 27.3 Animation depicting the trocar ACM in place. It is introduced 0.5 mm away from the limbus and enters the anterior chamber above the iris. ACM, anterior chamber maintainer.

possibility of injuring the corneal endothelium with the tip of the trocar blade.

Hence, a special trocar for ACM was designed and it was labeled as trocar ACM (▶ Fig. 27.4a). The newly designed trocar ACM has a shorter blade and has an aluminum dusting on its shaft that prevents its slippage from the scleral wall.

27.3 Device
27.3.1 Trocar Blade

The trocar blade is made up of stainless steel and is 6 mm in length and has an outer diameter of 0.51 mm. It is beveled and the cutting edge of the trocar blade is 2 mm that has a slimmer profile with tapering at both the top and bottom aspects of the blade.

27.3.2 Cannula

The cannula is made of polyamide steel, is beveled with a 45° angulation to the base of the shaft, and has the inner and outer diameter of 0.54 and 0.64 mm, respectively. The angulation allows the cannula to fit properly into the AC with the beveled slope being placed along the corneal endothelial surface. The length of the cannula is 4 mm at one edge of the bevel and is 3.36 mm at the other end of the bevel. The cannula is covered with aluminum dusting to facilitate the cannula to adhere to the scleral wall, thereby negating any chances of spontaneous extrusion.

27.3.3 Infusion Cannula

The length of the infusion cannula is 185 mm. The outer and inner diameter of the tubing is 3.2 and 0.89 mm, respectively, whereas the tubing wall thickness is 1.15 mm.

27.4 Surgical Technique

After conjunctival displacement, at a distance of 0.5 mm from the limbus, the tip of the trocar is inserted in a way that it enters the AC in front of the iris tissue creating an oblique linear incision (▶ Fig. 27.4b, c). The trocar blade is withdrawn and the hub of the cannula is flushed to the surface of the sclera (▶ Fig. 27.4d). An infusion line is then attached to the cannula (▶ Fig. 27.4e, f). After the surgical procedure is over, the infusion is stopped and the cannula is withdrawn from the eye.

27.5 Discussion

The maintenance of a deep AC is a prerequisite for a safe anterior segment surgery. Trocar ACM helps prevent AC collapse apart from serving as an important tool during intraocular lens insertion, post IOL insertion maneuvers, and during vitrectomy or secondary IOL implantation, obviating the need for use of an ophthalmic viscosurgical device. Fluid is the natural milieu of the anterior segment and its use during surgery does not disturb any of the anatomical relationships in the eye. The surgical wound creation for the introduction of ACM necessitates the use of paracentesis wound with a side port incision in the peripheral cornea. The ACM must be exactly the right size and the knife must be withdrawn along the tract of entry as any sideway movement during entry or withdrawal will produce an incision that is too large and the ACM wound will leak. Suturing an incision is often required to prevent postoperative hypotony and also to minimize the continuous leak and the induced postoperative astigmatism. All these shortcomings are outweighed by the use of trocar ACM.

Trocar ACM is placed in position during pre-Descemet's endothelial keratoplasty surgery and an air pump is connected to the trocar ACM (▶ Fig. 27.5). This allows continuous air infusion into the eye during the process of recipient bed preparation that necessitates the performance of descemetorhexis and peeling the diseased Descemet's membrane from

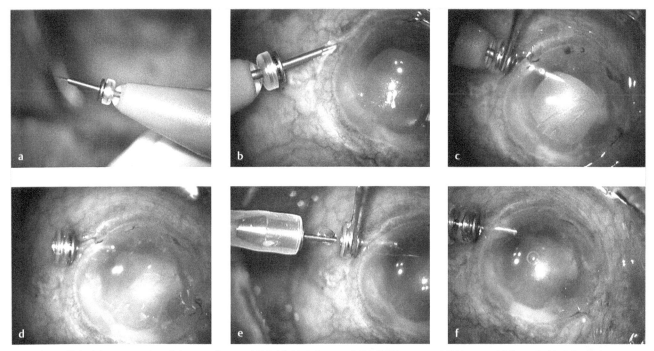

Fig. 27.4 Clinical demonstration of the use of trocar ACM. **(a)** A 25-G trocar ACM. **(b)** The trocar ACM is passed 0.5 mm behind the limbus parallel to the limbus into a half thickness of the sclera. **(c)** The trocar ACM creates an oblique linear incision and enters into the AC above the iris. **(d)** The trocar is removed and only the cannula is left. **(e)** The tubing connects to the cannula. **(f)** The trocar ACM is in place. This can now pass fluid or air into the AC, depending on what the surgeon's requirement. AC, anterior chamber; ACM, anterior chamber maintainer.

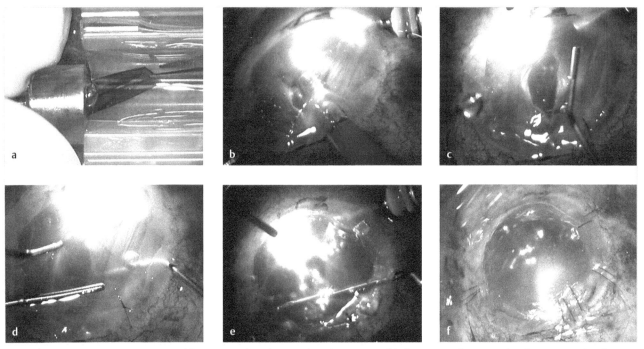

Fig. 27.5 Trocar ACM in PDEK surgery. **(a)** A PDEK graft in the cartridge of an injector. **(b)** The PDEK graft is injected in the AC. Note that the trocar ACM is fixed. **(c)** The PDEK graft is unrolled. At this time, no air is passed through the trocar ACM. **(d)** The graft is unrolled and air will be injected under the graft. **(e)** The air pump is switched ON so that air passes continuously through the trocar ACM into the eye. **(f)** The trocar ACM is removed, and the graft is attached fully. AC, anterior chamber; ACM, anterior chamber maintainer; PDEK, pre-Descemet endothelial keratoplasty.

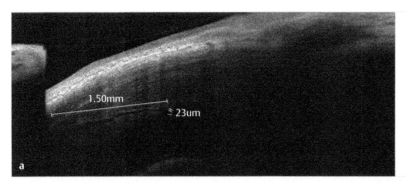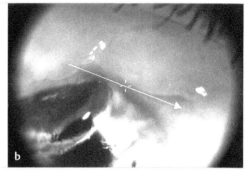

Fig. 27.6 (a, b) Fourier domain optical coherence tomography showing the trocar ACM wound on day 1. Notice that this is a 25-G trocar ACM and the internal ostium on postoperative day 1 is only 23 μm. In 1 week, it is closed totally. ACM, anterior chamber maintainer.

the recipient eye. After the insertion of donor lenticule and partial unscrolling, the air pump is switched ON again. Infusion of air at this stage helps the adherence of donor lenticule to the recipient bed. When the graft is being unscrolled, care should be taken to ensure that the tip of the cannula of trocar ACM does not collide with the donor lenticule as this can damage the endothelial cells and affect the visual outcome of the surgery.

To conclude, trocar ACM helps to maintain the integrity and depth of AC with great precision without compromising on the availability of the working space on the anterior corneal surface for the surgeon (▶Fig. 27.6). It effectively allows the surgeon to switch over between air and fluid infusion as and when required.

References

[1] Pape LG, Balazs EA. The use of sodium hyaluronate (Healon) in human anterior segment surgery. Ophthalmology 1980;87(7):699–705

[2] Pape LG. Intracapsular and extracapsular technique of lens implantation with Healon R. J Am Intraocul Implant Soc 1980;6(4):342–343

[3] Miller D, Stegmann R. Use of sodium hyaluronate in human IOL implantation. Ann Ophthalmol 1981;13(7):811–815

[4] Agarwal A, Narang P, Kumar DA, Agarwal A. Trocar anterior chamber maintainer (T-ACM): improvised technique of infusion. J Cataract Refract Surg 2016;42:185–189

Index

Note: Page numbers set in **bold** or *italic* indicate headings or figures, respectively.